T0206246

Occupational Therapy Assessments for Older Adults

100 Instruments for Measuring Occupational Performance

Occupational Therapy Assessments for Older Adults

100 Instruments for Measuring Occupational Performance

Kevin Bortnick, OTD, OT/L
University of St. Augustine for Health Sciences
Department of Occupational Therapy
St. Augustine, Florida

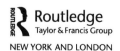

Routledge
Taylor & Francis Group

NEW YORK AND LONDON

Dr. Kevin Bortnick has no financial or proprietary interest in the materials presented herein.

First published in 2017 by SLACK Incorporated

Published 2024 by Routledge
605 Third Avenue, New York, NY 10158

and by Routledge
4 Park Square, Milton Park, Abingdon, Oxon OX14 4RN

Routledge is an imprint of the Taylor & Francis Group, an informa business

© 2017 Taylor & Francis Group

Library of Congress Cataloging-in-Publication Data

Names: Bortnick, Kevin, 1968- author.
Title: Occupational therapy assessments for older adults : 100 instruments
    for measuring occupational performance / Kevin Bortnick.
Description: Thorofare, NJ : SLACK Incorporated, [2017] | Includes
    bibliographical references.
Identifiers: LCCN 2016047799 (print) | ISBN
    9781630913588 (alk. paper) | ISBN
Subjects: | MESH: Occupational Therapy--methods | Needs Assessment | Outcome
    Assessment (Health Care) | Health Status Indicators | Aged
Classification: LCC RM735.3 (print) | NLM WB 555 | DDC
    615.8/5150846--dc23
LC record available at https://lccn.loc.gov/2016047799

ISBN: 9781630913588 (pbk)
ISBN: 9781003525288 (ebk)

DOI: 10.4324/9781003525288

Dedication

This book is in many ways dedicated to all those who in their own way allowed for its creation, such as my parents, family, and professors, since it is from them that I learned the essence of occupational therapy. Here, I must also acknowledge that after completing this manuscript the development of a special appreciation for all of the authors and researchers involved in the advancement of standardized testing, and although I feel a certain affinity with those who spend many hours developing and proving the validity of an assessment, my discourse here is in no way contemporary with their essential work.

Contents

Acknowledgments

Special thanks to Soo Borson, MD, Professor Emerita, University of Washington School of Medicine, Affiliate Professor, University of Washington School of Nursing Dementia Care Tools—Research and Consulting; Suryakumar Shah, PhD, OTD, MEd, OTR, FAOTA, Professor Emerita of Occupational Therapy, AT Still University, Mesa, Arizona; and Roger Watson BSc, PhD, RN, FRSB, FFNMRCSI, FRSA, FHEA, FEANS, FRCP Edin, FRCN, FAAN, Professor of Nursing, Faculty of Health & Social Care, The University of Hull, Hull, UK for their valuable feedback; Brien Cummings, Acquisitions Editor and the SLACK Incorporated team for their help in bringing this project to fruition; and finally, Emily Densten, Project Editor, editor of this work.

About the Author

Kevin Bortnick, OTD, OT/L is an occupational therapist, researcher, and author. He holds a clinical doctorate in occupational therapy from the University of St. Augustine for Health Sciences in St. Augustine, Florida as well as a master's degree from Barry University in Miami Shores, Florida. Raised in Michigan, where he received his undergraduate training in General Studies from the University of Michigan—Ann Arbor, he naturally enjoys the outdoors and conservation. He is currently involved in neurocognitive disorder-related research and is working on his next book. You can follow him on Facebook with the same name.

Introduction

The role of measurement is extremely important and much has been written about the potential benefits of outcome measures, which are typically defined as tools used to document change in one or more constructs over time, help to describe the client's problem, formulate a prognosis, as well as to evaluate the effects of occupational therapy intervention (Jette, Halbert, Iverson, Miceli, & Shah, 2009; Law & Letts, 1989). They are used in research, program evaluation, quality improvement, case management, and utilization review, as well as cost containment therapy practice. Additionally, many such instruments have been developed for use for persons with particular conditions such as traumatic brain injury, stroke, visual perceptual deficits and cognitive impairment, as well as disorders relating to the shoulder, arm, and hand (Jette et al., 2009; Wedge et al., 2013). Outcome measures occupy a unique place in the therapeutic process; in particular, at the beginning or evaluation phase as well as at the end when therapy outcomes are examined and decisions are made about future interventions (American Occupational Therapy Association [AOTA], 2014). The *Occupational Therapy Practice Framework: Domain & Process, 3rd edition* (AOTA, 2014), which is the guiding document of the occupational therapy profession, discusses the use of outcome measures at length and uses the phrase *outcome measure* no less than 4 times, *standardized assessment* once, and the word *assessment* in association with measurement over 10 times. The *Framework* considers them to be essential to practice because they not only identify and measure client contexts and environments but the activity demands and client factors that influence performance skills and performance patterns (AOTA, 2014). The *Framework* also points out that *quantitative* assessment is the preferred method over *qualitative* or non-standardized when available, because they are intrinsically designed to provide objective data about the supports and hindrances to performance. However, it must be noted that each type can purvey unique information and both can aid in the development and refinement of hypotheses about client occupational performance, their strengths and limitations, as well as assist in the creation of goals to address desired outcomes (AOTA, 2014). Many adjectives are used that loosely describe the phenomenon of measurement such as *scale, rating scale*, or *screen*, which is a type of instrument designed to quickly determine if further investigations are warranted and since the occupational therapist will encounter each in research and practice, the following pages can help in that endeavor by providing an in-depth review of 100 instruments, which for the most part are standardized; however, some non-standardized instruments and quick screens are explored as well, testifying to the fact that measurement of client traits is a vibrant and dynamic field encompassing many perspectives. The book is organized by function (i.e., what it is that is being measured, such as upper extremity motor function or driving ability), which is in contrast to other possible arrangements like by *condition*, where major headings might have included cerebral palsy or carpal tunnel syndrome or by *clinical setting*, where sections titled skilled nursing or out-patient rehabilitation would have been created or finally, by *type* of scale such as *self-report questionnaires* and *activity-based rating scales*. Although each taxonomy had its appeal, *function* seemed best able to account for all of the confounding variables relative to the possible arrangement of 100 assessments. However, it must be noted that several (less than 7) did not fit neatly into the function taxonomy such that they were condition specific and pertained to 3 conditions in particular: Parkinson's disease (PD; 2 assessments) and stroke/cerebrovascular accident (CVA; 4 assessments), which were included as a single section titled, "Cerebrovascular Accident and Parkinson's Disease Specific Assessment" as well as one assessment that measures vision related issues and was included in the section titled "Vision and Visual-Perceptual Assessment." This is not to say that other outcome measures within the book should not be used with persons who have those conditions as a number of other scales will still be applicable, such as the 10 or so items that measure activities of daily living or those that quantify motor performance for persons with PD or CVA.

Many assessments were given consideration for inclusion but it was those that had a preponderance of evidence in support of their use including an amount of research, peer-reviewed citations, and general acceptance within the field of occupational therapy that were included. Thus, the choices are narrowed with information presented to the reader in the form of a classification system which may include anywhere from 2 to 10 assessments for each section. A several page discourse per measure then discusses its various properties. The reader is then left to decide which assessment is best and for what situation, which may include such considerations as the time needed to administer and score the measure; the need for specialized equipment or training; the ease of obtaining a copy of the scale, such as its cost and copyright issues; its clinical utility; and its psychometric properties, where aspects of validity and reliability as well as others are discussed (Potter et al., 2014). Considering the amount and type of information purveyed, there are numerous scenarios where this book would have value, such as the fast-paced clinical setting where there is little time to conduct a thorough review of the literature let alone access a database to examine the evidence. At its most basic is the transactional relationship between client and clinician, where according to Unsworth (2000), measuring outcomes involves two parts: demonstrating that client change occurred (the ability to document change through some form of measurement) and attributing the change to therapeutic intervention (therapy effectiveness). Therefore, when the clinician is able to demonstrate through, preferably standardized, measurement that change is due to therapy and not spontaneous recovery or other factors, then therapy effectiveness has been demonstrated. This has numerous ramifications of which the most notable may be for reimbursement.

Elements Included in the Review of Each Outcome Measure

The following are the elements included in the review of each measure:

- Description: A brief record of the measure.

- Psychometrics: A review of the level of research evidence that either supports or does not support the instrument, including such items as inter-rater, intra-rater, and test-retest reliabilities, as well as internal consistencies and construct validities among others.

- Advantages: Synopsis of the benefits of using the measure over others including its unique attributes.

- Disadvantages: A summary of its faults. For example, the amount of research evidence may be limited or the measure may be expensive.

- Administration: Information regarding how to administer, score, and interpret results.

- Permissions: How and where to procure the instrument, such as websites where it may be purchased or journal articles or publications that may contain the scale.

- Summary: A brief summation of important information.

- Contact: Includes authors, organizations, and downloads.

The Role of Outcome Measures in Evidenced-Based Practice

The Centennial Vision (Hopper, 2010) of the occupational therapy profession outlines the need to advance competencies in areas of research, theory, and evidenced-based practice (EBP) to better meet the occupational needs of weakened populations. The utilization of EBP and outcome measures, in particular, are ways for clients to receive the best level of care (Hooper, 2010; Lyon, Brown, & Tseng, 2011). EBP is becoming increasingly important and most would agree that it is the procedure whereby the clinician incorporates the use of current, high quality empirical evidence, clinical expertise, and patient values when making decisions and recommendations resulting in the presentation of the most appropriate and efficient services to his or her clients. It requires the synthesis of information from different theoretical perspectives, the creation and exchange of knowledge from sources such as colleagues and professors, as well as a necessary understanding of the methods used to conduct needs assessments and to make appropriate recommendations based on their results. Grounded in scientific method, it is a process that embraces (1) the development of clinical questions, (2) the assimilation of the best available evidence in order to answer those questions, (3) a systematic and critical appraisal of the evidence, (4) applying evidence to clinical problems, and lastly, (5) the evaluation and revision of the previous steps to identify areas of change for future applications, signifying that knowledge is an uncertain and continuous process that requires participation and continual revision, reflecting its temporary and historical nature (AOTA, 2010; Hooper, 2010; Upton, Stephens, Williams, & Scurlock-Evans, 2014).

The incorporation of EBP into practice allows the clinician to remain up to date with health care trends and efficiencies, stay informed of current perspectives, and understand the methodologies for measuring individual, program, and system outcomes that affect health, well-being, and participation (AOTA, 2010; Thomas & Law, 2013). EBP is also client centered because it takes into account the various competing influences unique to the client and how they affect occupational performance, such as the client's values, beliefs, spirituality, sense of efficacy, and the dynamic interactions between the individual, family, community, and social systems. Working in specialized teams, a supportive environment, having access to research that this book provides as well as holding an advanced degree or having professional autonomy tend to support the use of EBP. Conversely, a lack of understanding about the reasons for involvement in research and poor organization may inhibit its use. A 2013 survey of 473 occupational therapists that examined attitudes, skills, and behaviors toward EBP found that the majority of clinicians perceived EBP to be useful in daily practice and that it improved client-centered care; however, findings also suggested that clinicians predominantly relied on their own clinical expertise to guide clinical decision making, using clinical reasoning based on research evidence less than half of the time (Graham, Robertson, & Anderson, 2013). Other results of that study found that it placed too much demand on workload as well as the perception that there was insufficient relevant evidence available with the most cited perceived barriers to implementing EBP being lack of time, lack of sufficient relevant research, and inadequate access to research literature, all issues addressed by this book (Graham et al., 2013). Those results almost uniformly concurred with an earlier survey by Bennet et al. (2003) that also found that respondents thought that lack of skills in locating research evidence, lack of computing resources, lack of access to research literature as well as the perception that there was not enough evidence in occupational therapy were significant factors that frequently affected its implementation into practice.

Factors Influencing the Incorporation of Evidence-Based Practice

The following factors influence the incorporation of EBP:

- Support
  - Expands knowledge and furthers clinical reasoning
  - Effect on reimbursement
  - Team work (multidisciplinary)
  - Validation of the learned experience
  - Provides a rationale for treatment
  - Discussion of EBP viewpoints
  - Participation in EBP-related activities
  - Organizational support
  - Amount of available research
  - Professional autonomy
  - Access to research
  - Advanced degree
  - Influence of the facility/mandated use
  - Patient suitability
  - Best practice guidelines
- Inhibit
  - Cost of continuing education/workshops
  - Perceptions of low research applicability
  - Poor research skills
  - Inability to interpret findings
  - Inability to translate research into practical use
  - Poor communication
  - Continually changing nature of evidence
  - Competing evidence
  - Complicated testing methodologies
  - Reliance on clinical experience
  - Lack of motivation
  - Could be considered unpaid work
  - Size of case load

Implementation of Evidence-Based Practice

The realization of EBP has become a priority for not only occupational therapy but also for health care professionals in general, as changes in how health care is administered have occurred as a result of increasing costs, reduced staffing, managed care systems, and shorter hospital stays, all of which have served to increase clinician and department accountability (Lin, Murphy, & Robinson, 2010). As clinicians are under more pressure to justify their services, not including EBP in results can affect reimbursement as well. One way for the practitioner to embrace EBP is to have readily available, relevant, and concisely summarized information if it is to become integrated into practice, which, in many ways, is what this book can help to accomplish. Furthermore, greater communication and collaboration among all stakeholders must occur as there is evidence to suggest that knowledge translation requires multiple processes and coordinated efforts and everyone from practitioners to employers have a role in increasing the transfer of knowledge into practice (Lin et al., 2010). du Toit and Wilkinson (2011) propose a unique method for promoting EBP to counter the problems mentioned previously by suggesting that EBP, in and of itself, be viewed as an occupation whereby it encourages the specific roles, values, and habits associated with occupational therapy, which can facilitate its integration at all levels of the profession. By identifying EBP as occupation, its engagement is done in order to fulfill the essential desire to learn something, satisfy curiosities and creativity, develop critical thinking abilities and improve one's understanding of a topic as well as to answer clinical questions. The culmination of EBP, within the academic and professional environment, supports the interpretation, internalization, application, and generation of new research as well as the gathering of factual information from outcome measures (Isaak & Hubert, 1999). EBP as occupation also allows individuals and systems to respond and perform consistently over time, which creates opportunities to recognize the positive experiences while engaging in it and, more importantly, facilitates the development of customs and traditions associated with a research culture and an enhanced occupational identity as a composite sense of who one is and who one wishes to become as an occupational being, which is generated from one's history of occupational participation (Isaak & Hubert, 1999).

As the translation of research into practice can be a complex process, another framework for the reader to consider may be *implementation science* (IS), which is the scientific study of methods to promote the systematic uptake of research findings and other EBPs, like the use of outcome measures, into clinical practice in order to improve the quality and effectiveness of health care (Clark, Park, & Burke, 2013). Understanding the barriers and facilitators that influence the successful implementation of evidence is critical as there is research to suggest that 30% to 45% of patients receive a wide range of professional programs and services that are not based on scientific evidence and 20% to 25% of that care is not needed or may be potentially harmful (Center for Research in Implementation Science and Prevention [CRISP], 2016; Clark et al., 2013). Since increasing the number of evidenced-based interventions that translate into practice can have a direct and positive impact on public health, the steps needed for IS in general to be successful include problem recognition, followed by the acquisition, incorporation, and evaluation of the responding innovation into practice (Craik & Rappolt, 2003). The Model of Research Utilization in Occupational Therapy by Craik and Rappolt (2003), which includes aspects of Occupational Performance Process Model by Fearing et al. (1997) as well as Knott and Wildavsky's (1980) Stages of Knowledge Utilization, further enumerates the IS theory within the occupational therapy context by suggesting that first, interactions between client and practitioner occur, followed by a period of reflection in which the practitioner considers his or her skills and knowledge base to make informed decisions and actions regarding the client's condition. If the answer upon that reflection is no (i.e., unable to make informed decisions and actions), then the research utilization process begins. This is a multi-stage event encompassing an *acquisition stage* where the search for and acquisition of research evidence begins, which may include appropriate outcome measures to use, followed by the *cognition stage*, which entails a critical analysis of that evidence. The next stage is called the *effort stage* where questions such as how the new evidence applies to the client are answered as well as case applications contemplated. The final stage is the *adoption stage* where the clinician hypothesizes occupational outcomes based on the new found evidence, which may also include consultation with peers to gain further insight into how the gathered evidence may be used with this and other clients.

Both models discussed suggest that systemic modifications need to occur, which includes not only practitioners, therapy departments, and organizations but also how research is conducted, because a key concept of the IS model is that for an intervention or an outcome measure to work it must have reach and in order to have reach it must be able to expedite the implementation process (CRISP, 2016). It must also be designed to possess real-world practicality and be readily transferable to a wide range of practice settings. Similarly, outcome measures that are embedded within the World Health Organization's *International Classification of Functioning, Disability, and Health* (WHO-ICF) framework are also desirable as there is an impetus for numerous health professions to adopt a universal view of the disablement process through the continued development and acceptance of the world-wide taxonomy that the WHO-ICF espouses. Conversely, interventions and outcome measures that are viewed as too intensive, demanding too much time or effort, and not adequately packaged or manualized are less likely to be implemented (Clark et al., 2013). Finally, by moving away from traditional models where research findings are generated in a laboratory-like setting and then transmitted to the clinician, an open bi-directional relationship between researcher and practitioner can help to produce research that is relevant to practice (Lencucha, Kothari, & Rouse, 2007). This is achieved through increased involvement in research by practitioners and alludes to the realization of knowledge translation as the end product will take into account their unique practice knowledge. The final concept of the researcher/practitioner model is the belief that as the practitioner once again has clinical practice back at the forefront *communities of knowing* within the profession can develop as they work with others to support the interpersonal, cultural, and environmental factors that influence person-to-person knowledge sharing with the conscious understanding that knowledge is both an empirical and social concept, embedded within community (Lencucha et al., 2007).

TABLE I-1
TYPES OF RESEARCH THAT PRACTITIONERS MAY BE INVOLVED IN AND A HIERARCHY OF THE LEVELS OF THAT EVIDENCE

LEVEL	DESCRIPTION
I	Strong evidence from a systematic review of multiple well-designed randomized controlled trials. Systematic reviews, meta-analyses, randomized controlled trials.
II	Strong evidence from at least one properly designed randomized controlled trial of appropriate size. Two groups, non-randomized studies (such as cohort, case control).
III	Evidence from well-designed trials without randomization, single group pre–post, cohort, time series, or matched case-controlled studies.
IV	Evidence from well-designed non-experimental studies from more than one center or research group. Descriptive studies that include analysis of outcomes such as single-subject design or case series.
V	Evidence from case reports and expert opinion that include narrative literature reviews and consensus statements. Opinions of respected authorities, based on clinical evidence, descriptive studies, or reports of expert committees

Adapted from Arbesman, M., & Lieberman, D. (2011). Methodology for the systematic reviews on occupational therapy for adults with Alzheimer's disease and related dementias. *American Journal of Occupational Therapy, 65,* 491.

Appraising the Evidence

Much of this book delivers fairly basic information where the reader will be able to make interpretations without much consideration; however, the psychometrics section can be technical because the development and validation of an assessment can be a rigorous scientific process, thus many research examples are given. Accounting for all of the possible variables when examining the properties or validating the utility of an assessment can be difficult if not unattainable. Therefore, the reader should consider the evidence presented as a whole and decide how best to internalize the information as several methodologies might be considered. A study by Law and Letts (1989) suggests that the clinician consider six critical review questions when deciding whether or not to use an outcome measure with the first being, what is the purpose of the scale? As outcome measures are typically designed to quantify information for one of three purposes: description, prediction, or evaluation. Second, is the scale clinically useful? This may include such considerations as its cost, time to administer, acceptability, and in what format the measure is delivered. Then, is it a questionnaire completed by proxy or through an interview or is it a performance-based rating scale? Next, is the instrument's construction adequate? This may entail an examination of item selection methodology, the level of measurement purveyed, or what type of scoring paradigm is used. Fifth, is it standardized and if so what is the level of research pertaining to it? Finally, is the scale both reliable and valid? Where reliability would be the estimate of the extent to which the instrument is measuring the true difference between different constructs and may include several subtypes that as a whole will establish its reliability, such as the level of its internal consistency, inter-rater and intra-rater reliability, and test-retest reliability, whereas validity could be considered the degree to which an assessment measures what it is intended to measure.

Types of Reliability

The following are the various types of reliability:

- Inter-rater reliability—the consistent measure of an instrument after several administrations by different individuals such that a highly reliable instrument should produce the same results regardless of who is administering the assessment where perfect agreement between administrations is 1.0. Excellent reliability would be 0.90 or above, between 0.90 and 0.80 good, and between 0.80 and 0.70 typically considered acceptable.

- Intra-rater reliability—a measure of the consistency of an instrument after several administrations by the same individual. If the intra-rater reliability is high the instrument should produce the same results for that person upon repeated administrations, where 1.0 is perfect agreement.

- Internal consistency—a measure of whether the varying items that make up the whole of a scale that propose to measure the same general phenomenon in fact are and produce similar scores, such as questions on a questionnaire where each might address the same yet slightly different aspects of the underlying issue being measured. Often calculated as Cronbach's alpha coefficient, which is an average of all correlations among the different questions in the scale (Peacock & Peacock, 2011).

- Test-retest reliability—the consistent measure of an instrument over time. For example, taking into account confounding variables such as prior test knowledge and health improvement testing at a 1-day interval should produce similar scores that are significantly correlated.

Types of Validity

The following are the various types of validity:

- Discriminant validity—numerical extent to which a test's measurements that are supposed to be unrelated are, in fact, unrelated.

- Divergent validity—extent to which a measure does not strongly correlate with another similar measure of a different construct (i.e., if it correlates too strongly than it is merely the other measure just packaged differently.)

- Construct validity—a measure of how well an instrument measures the characteristics that in its design it has set out to do and is involved whenever a test is to be interpreted as a measure of some attribute or quality that is not operationally defined (Cronbach & Meehl, 1955).

- Content validity—degree to which the elements of an instrument are relevant to and representative of the targeted construct of what it was designed to measure, where elements may be questions, response choices, or instructions (Haynes, Richard, & Kubany, 1995).

- Convergent validity—refers to the degree to which scores of one instrument correlate with the scores of other different instruments that are also designed to measure a similar construct phenomenon.

- External validity—the extent to which a study's results can be generalized to other settings and populations and is an important factor if results are to be achieved beyond merely the laboratory or the population sample of the study.

- Face validity—implies an overall judgment of adequacy of a result without paying close attention to the component parts. In most studies it has a low ranking but may be important in some cases such as items intended to reflect observations and intuitions of clinical experience as well as qualitative studies (de Vet, Terwee, & Bouter, 2003).

- Internal validity—can be considered the extent of a study's results. When considered high, there is confidence to conclude that the observed change in the dependent variable was the product of the manipulation of the independent variable and not other confounding factors.

The inductive approach used to create the psychometric section of each outcome measure reviewed could be considered a collection, reduction, and display of data, with the hope of allowing research findings to emerge from the frequent, dominant, and significant themes gathered from the raw data. As the collection of data is common, another efficient and defendable procedure for its analysis has been proposed by Guba and Lincoln (1981) and is based on the identification of four aspects of trustworthiness considered relevant to both quantitative and qualitative studies and includes examinations of a study's (1) credibility, (2) transferability, (3) dependability, and (4) confirmability (Curtin & Fossey, 2007; Krefting, 1991). What makes the evaluative criteria proposed by Guba and Lincoln unique is that it substitutes reliability and validity with the parallel concept of *trustworthiness* where further criteria outlined by the authors to judge research include its (1) truth value, (2) applicability, (3) consistency, and (4) neutrality (Morse, Barrett, Mayan, Olsen, & Spiers, 2002). With regard to *truth value* the reader would internalize such numerations as to whether the researcher has established confidence in the truth of the findings for the subjects or informants and the context in which the study was undertaken, while *applicability* refers to the degree to which the findings can be applied to other contexts as well as the ability to generalize findings to larger populations (Krefting, 1991), The third criterion of trustworthiness considers the *consistency* of the data, that is to say, whether the findings would be consistent if the inquiry were replicated with the same subjects or in a similar context. Finally, *neutrality* is the degree to which the findings are a function solely of the informants and conditions of the research and not of other biases, motivations, and perspectives (Krefting, 1991).

TABLE I-2
STRATEGIES TO ESTABLISH THE TRUSTWORTHINESS OF RESEARCH THAT ARE PARTICULARLY RELEVANT TO QUALITATIVE STUDIES WHERE STATISTICAL P VALUES ARE TYPICALLY LIMITED
CREDIBILITY
• Field experience of researcher
• Interview technique
• Authority of researcher
• Structural coherence
• Negative case analysis
TRANSFERABILITY
• Comparison of sample to demographic data
• Rich description of details
DEPENDABILITY
• Dense description of methods
• Ability to replicate the study
• Peer review
CONFIRMABILITY
• Confirmability audit
• Audit trail
• Theory development
• Reflexivity
Adapted from Krefting, L. (1991). Rigor in qualitative research: The assessment of trustworthiness. *American Journal of Occupational Therapy, 45*(3), 217.

Conclusion

Encouraging practitioners to expand their thinking about the use of appropriate outcome measures is essential as they have a significant role to play through not only the therapeutic process, but also in the delivery of effective occupational therapy services as a whole, where their utilization can aid in the promotion of health, well-being, and participation for clients with a vast number of conditions and functional performance deficits. The proliferation and use of outcome measures can also help to foster a common language within the occupational therapy community, allowing not only for the comparison of outcomes between clinicians, but those related to diverse intervention approaches as well (American Physical Therapy Association, 2016). Finally, the ability to capture the change that outcome measures characteristically produce can have numerous ramifications. As different instruments may capture different aspects of complex phenomena the selection of an appropriate outcome measure can be a key factor that ultimately affects the value it results in (Coster, 2013).

References

American Occupational Therapy Association. (2010). Specialized knowledge and skills in mental health promotion, prevention, and intervention in occupational therapy practice. *American Journal of Occupational Therapy, 64*(6), S30-S43.

American Occupational Therapy Association. (2014). Occupational therapy practice framework: Domain and process (3rd ed.). *American Journal of Occupational Therapy, 68*(Suppl. 1), S1–S48.

American Physical Therapy Association. (2016). Outcome Measures in Patient Care. Retrieved from www.apta.org/OutcomeMeasures/

Arbesman, M., & Lieberman, D. (2011). Methodology for the systematic reviews on occupational therapy for adults with Alzheimer's disease and related dementias. *American Journal of Occupational Therapy, 65*, 490–496.

Bennett, S., Tooth, L., McKenna, K., Rodger, S., Strong, J., Ziviani, J.,...Gibson, L. (2003). Perceptions of evidence-based practice: A survey of Australian occupational therapists. *Australian Occupational Therapy Journal, 50*(1), 13-22.

Center for Research in Implementation Science and Prevention. (2016). *Dissemination and Implementation Science.* Boulder, CO: University of Colorado. Retrieved from www.ucdenver.edu/academics/colleges/medicalschool/programs/crisp/Pages/default.aspx

Clark, F., Park, D. J., & Burke, J. P. (2013). Dissemination: Bringing translational research to completion. *American Journal of Occupational Therapy, 67*(2), 185-193.

Craik, J., & Rappolt, S. (2003). Theory of research utilization enhancement: A model for occupational therapy. *Canadian Journal of Occupational Therapy, 70*(5), 266-275.

Cronbach, L. J., & Meehl, P. E. (1955). Construct validity in psychological tests. *Psychological Bulletin, 52*, 281-302.

Coster, W. J. (2013). Making the best match: Selecting outcome measures for clinical trials and outcome studies. *American Journal of Occupational Therapy, 67*(2), 162-170.

Curtin, M., & Fossey, E. (2007), Appraising the trustworthiness of qualitative studies: Guidelines for occupational therapists. *Australian Occupational Therapy Journal, 54*(2), 88–94.

de Vet, H., Terwee, C., & Bouter, L. (2003). Current challenges in clinimetrics. *Journal of Clinical Epidemiology, 56*, 1137–1141.

du Toit, S., & Wilkinson, A. (2011). Promoting an appreciation for research-related activities: The role of occupational identity. *British Journal of Occupational Therapy, 74*(10), 489-493.

Graham, F., Robertson, L., & Anderson, J. (2013). New Zealand occupational therapists' views on evidence-based practice: A replicated survey of attitudes, confidence and behaviours. *Australian Occupational Therapy Journal, 60*(2), 120-128.

Hooper, B. (2010). On arriving at the destination of the centennial vision: Navigational landmarks to guide occupational therapy education. *Occupational Therapy in Health Care, 24*(1), 97-106.

Jette, D. U., Halbert, J., Iverson, C., Miceli, E., & Shah, P. (2009). Use of standardized outcome measures in physical therapist practice: Perceptions and applications. *Physical Therapy, 89*(2), 125-135.

Haynes, S. N., Richard, D., & Kubany, E. (1995). Content validity in psychological assessment: A functional approach to concepts and methods. *Psychological Assessment, 7*(3), 238-247.

Isaak, D. J., & Hubert, W. A. (1999). Catalyzing the transition from student to scientist—a module for graduate research training. *BioScience, 49*(4), 321-27. In S. du Toit, & A. Wilkinson. (2011). Promoting an appreciation for research-related activities: The role of occupational identity. *British Journal of Occupational Therapy, 74*(10), 489-493

Krefting, L. (1991). Rigor in qualitative research: The assessment of trustworthiness. *American Journal of Occupational Therapy, 45*(3), 214-222.

Law, M., & Letts, L. (1989). A critical review of scales of activities of daily living. *American Journal Occupational Therapy, 43*(8), 522-528.

Lencucha, R., Kothari, A., & Rouse, M. (2007). The issue is—knowledge translation: A concept for occupational therapy? *American Journal of Occupational Therapy, 61*, 593–596.

Lin, S. H., Murphy, S. L., & Robinson, J. C. (2010). Facilitating evidence-based practice: Process, strategies, and resources. *American Journal of Occupational Therapy, 64*(1), 164–171.

Lyons, C., Brown, T., Tseng, M. H., Casey, J., & McDonald, R. (2011). Evidence-based practice and research utilisation: Perceived research knowledge, attitudes, practices and barriers among Australian paediatric occupational therapists. *Australian Occupational Therapy Journal, 58*(3), 178-186

Morse, J., Barrett, M., Mayan, M., Olsen, K., & Spiers, J. (2002). Verification strategies for establishing reliability and validity in qualitative research. *International Journal of Qualitative Methods, 1*(2), 13-22.

Peacock, J., & Peacock, P. J. (2011). *Oxford handbook of medical statistics.* Oxford, United Kingdom: OUP Oxford.

Potter, K., Cohen, E., Allen, D., Bennett, S., Brandfass, K. G., Widener, G., & Yorke, A. (2014). Outcome measures for individuals with multiple sclerosis: Recommendations from the American Physical Therapy Association neurology section task force. *Physical Therapy, 94*(5), 593-608.

Thomas, A., & Law, M. (2013). Research utilization and evidence-based practice in occupational therapy: A scoping study. *American Journal of Occupational Therapy, 67*(4), e55-65.

Unsworth, C. (2000). Measuring the outcome of occupational therapy: Tools and resources. *Australian Occupational Therapy Journal, 47*(4), 147–158.

Upton, D., Stephens, D., Williams, B., & Scurlock-Evans, L. (2014). Occupational therapists' attitudes, knowledge, and implementation of evidence-based practice: A systematic review of published research. *British Journal of Occupational Therapy, 77*(1), 24-38.

Wedge, F., Braswell-Christy, J., Brown, C., Foley, K., Graham, C., & Shaw, S. (2013). Factors influencing the use of outcome measures in physical therapy practice. *Physiotherapy Theory and Practice, 28*(2), 119–133.

I

Activities of Daily Living (ADLs) and Instrumental Activities of Daily Living (IADLs)

1. Activities of Daily Living (ADL) Profile

2. Activities of Daily Living Questionnaire (ADLQ)

3. Australian Therapy Outcome Measures (AusTOMs)—Third Edition

4. The Frenchay Activities Index (FAI)

5. Instrumental Activities of Daily Living (IADL) Profile

6. Lawton Instrumental Activities of Daily Living (IADL) Scale

7. Melbourne Low-Vision Activities of Daily Living Index (MLVAI)

8. Performance Assessment of Self-Care Skills (PASS)

9. Self-Assessment Parkinson's Disease Disability Scale (SPDDS)

10. Texas Functional Living Scale (TFLS)

Bortnick, K.
Occupational Therapy Assessments for Older Adults: 100 Instruments for Measuring Occupational Performance (pp. 1-26).
© 2017 Taylor & Francis Group.

CHAPTER 1: ACTIVITIES OF DAILY LIVING (ADL) PROFILE

Description

The ADL Profile is both a performance-based assessment and questionnaire that is administered through a semi-structured interview and is designed to measure an individual's occupational performance across three dimensions of everyday activities (personal, home, and community) for individuals with a traumatic brain injury (TBI) (Dutil, Bottari, & Vanier, 2013). The conceptual development of the ADL Profile was based on three theoretical models: (1) the Model of Cerebral Functioning, (2) the Model of Human Occupation, and the (3) Disability Creation Process; and is intended to measure four operational concepts considered necessary for successful activity performance: (1) goal formulation, (2) determination and organization of steps to achieve that goal, (3) planning and execution, and (4) verification of quality controls (Dutil et al., 2013). The ADL Profile has two sections: a performance-based section which includes 21 tasks of which 17 are utilized in the final score and a questionnaire section that measures a person's perception of their life habits pre- and post-injury as well as their satisfaction with their present level of functioning (Dutil et al., 2013). Each task is scored along a 4-level ordinal scale that relates to relative independence in task performance (task score) and the manner in which the task is performed (operation score). A score on any item or activity typically reflects the lowest score as it relates to the four operations of goal attainment (Dutil et al., 2013).

Psychometrics

Original research by the assessment's creators found that test-retest reliability coefficients displayed good stability upon repeated measurements 2 weeks apart with global scores ranging from $r = 0.53$ to 0.93 (Dutil et al., 2013). However, a study by Dell'Aniello-Gauthier (1994) reported only fair inter-rater reliability for the 3 ADL tasks of preparing a hot meal, eating, and obtaining information in which scores had a range of 0.58 to 0.68. Similarly, Rousseau et al. found only poor to fair agreement for inter-rater reliability among 4 occupational therapists with minimal training among a sample of 19 subjects with TBI, $r = 0.23$ to 0.72 (Dutil et al., 2013). Another study by its creators found that 3 factors represented 69% of the variance for the task section of the assessment: one linked to routine activities such as self-care and the other two involving higher physical and complex cognitive skills (Dutil et al., 2013). Alas, a Gervais (1995) study of the assessment's convergent validity found significant correlations between five tasks of the ADL Profile related to personal care and corresponding tasks of the Functional Independence Measure with Kendall's tau $c = 0.40$ to 0.73; $p < .001$ (Poulin & Barfod, 2012).

Advantages

The ADL Profile is a well-designed tool that is both maintained by and can be purchased from the Canadian Association of Occupational Therapy (CAOT) website. Although the assessment is rather extensive, once mastered, the clinician should be able to gain unique insights into the occupational performance of the individual being tested. Lastly, there is a consistent level of evidence in support of its use with the TBI population.

Disadvantages

A 5-day training program is recommended and administration can take up to 7 hours for certain populations across several treatment days. Studies have also noted a substantial amount of variance in its results which may reflect both instability of the assessment itself as well as difficulties associated with measuring performance in TBI populations.

Administration

Administration protocol recommends that the assessment be completed in the person's home or community environment and emphasizes the importance of non-structured observation in a natural setting. This approach allows for the observation of a person's routines and ability to multi-task as opposed to simply the engagement in individual tasks in quick succession. Each item of the ADL Profile is evaluated according to level of performance; thus when a person is able to perform all of the required operations they are considered to be independent and given a score of 2 (Dutil, Forget, Vanier, & Gaudreault, 1990). If the subject is unable to do any of the operations, a score of 0 is given suggesting dependency for the task. When the subject is unable to successfully perform one or more of the operations, they are given a score of 1 which means that assistance is needed to complete the task (Dutil et al., 1990). Under certain conditions a person may receive scores of 7, 8, or 9 if they are unable to perform due to physical or mental state, or if the task is irrelevant (Dutil et al., 1990). The test battery includes three manuals: (1) a description of the instrument, (2) user's guide interviews, and (3) the actual user's guide performance-based assessment. A 5-day training certification is recommended and available at various times through the CAOT website.

Permissions

The ADL Profile can be purchased from the CAOT website for $132. To use in research or publication contact CAOT or its authors at the information below. More information can also be found in the following journal article:

Dutil, E., Forget, A., Vanier, M., & Gaudreault, C. (1990). Development of the ADL profile: An evaluation for adults with severe head injury. *Occupational Therapy in Health Care, 7*(1), 7-22.

Summary

POPULATION	TBI
TYPE OF MEASURE	Performance-based and interview questionnaire component
WHAT IT ASSESSES	Everyday activities related to personal, home, and community
TIME	Up to 7 hours, treatment days
COST	$132

Contact

Carolina Bottari, PhD

University of Montreal

Montreal, Quebec, Canada

Centre de réadaptation Lucie-Bruneau

CAOT-CTTC Bldg

3400-1125 Colonel By Dr

Ottawa, ON K1S 5R1 Canada

Phone: (800) 434-2268

CAOT Store: www.caot.ca/default.asp?pageid =1438

CHAPTER 2: ACTIVITIES OF DAILY LIVING QUESTIONNAIRE (ADLQ)

Description

The Activities of Daily Living Questionnaire (ADLQ) is an informant-based assessment that measures an individual's functional ability and is designed for those with probable neurocognitive disorders (NCD) of the Alzheimer's and related types (Johnson, Barion, Rademaker, Rehkemper, & Weintraub, 2004). The ADLQ specifically measures occupational performance across 6 areas that can provide the clinician with a comprehensive profile of NCD-related deficits in everyday functioning, ranging from basic activities of daily living (ADLs) to more complex activities such as (1) the spectrum of self-care, (2) household maintenance, (3) employment and recreation, (4) shopping and money (5) travel, and lastly, (6) communication (Chu & Chung, 2008; Johnson et al., 2004). The ADLQ comprises 28 items and employs a unique scoring system where individual items are rated along a 4-point Likert scale from 0 (no problem) to 3 (no longer capable of carrying out the task) as well as the possibility of a score of 9 if the item is not applicable and is not factored into results (Chu & Chung, 2008). Scores are calculated according to a specific formula allowing for both *total* and *subscale* scores that can then be expressed as a percentage (0% to 100%) to indicate the level of functional impairment (Chu & Chung, 2008). The assessment can be completed in less than 10 minutes.

Psychometrics

Results derived from a longitudinal study (n = 140) of caregivers of person's with probable NCD of the Alzheimer's or related types showed that the total ADLQ score and each of its subscales were highly reproducible and excluding *employment* and *recreation* at 0.65, all subscales showed high test-retest reliability with coefficients greater than r = 0.86 (Johnson et al., 2004). The same study indicated the ADLQ to be both significantly and negatively correlated with the Mini-Mental State Examination (MMSE), considered the gold standard of cognitive assessment, at −0.38 and positively correlated with the Clinical Dementia Rating Scale at 0.55, where the closer the coefficients are to +1.0 and −1.0 the greater strength of the relationship is between the two assessments (Johnson et al., 2004). When administered to 63 caregivers of persons with NCD internal consistency of the Spanish version (SV-ADLQ) was determined to be high at α = 0.86. The same study found that the technology subscale of the T-ADLQ (which is a revised version of the ADLQ to include 5 technology-specific items relative to the use of a computer, cell phone, ATM, ability to access the

internet, and e-mail use) was significantly correlated with SV-ADLQ total scores at r = 0.76; p < 0.001 (Munoz-Neira et al., 2012). Finally, using a cutoff point of 29.25 SV-ADLQ scores showed a sensitivity and specificity of 0.81 and 0.91, respectively (Munoz-Neira et al., 2012). Research by Chu and Chung (2008) found that factor analysis of the ADLQ-CV (Chinese version) yielded 6 factors that closely resembled the 6 subscales proposed in the original scale and along with the Spanish version suggests cross-cultural relevance of the measure. The ADLQ-CV Cronbach's α coefficients of the subscales ranged from 0.92 to 0.98 and inter-rater reliability for the ADLQ-CV total score was shown to be 0.99. Intra-class correlation coefficients of the 6 subscales ranged from 0.98 to 0.99 (Chu & Chung., 2008).

Advantages

The ADLQ is a fast and relatively easy outcome measure to administer. No special training is required and its scoring grid is well thought out. The ADLQ is also free to use in clinical practice. Originally validated in an outpatient setting, it is considered to be applicable across various client populations where cognitive performance may be of concern. Its scores can also be used to generate a profile description of functional impairment, which can then be used to track the progression of functional decline over time (Munoz-Neira et al., 2012). The ADLQ has also been validated in both the Chinese and Spanish languages and a technology specific version also exists which is designed to gauge a person's ability to use technology (Munoz-Neira et al., 2012).

Disadvantages

Although validity is established, its answers may rely on subjective observational information from the client or caregiver. Another potential limitation is the fact that the ADLQ was developed on the basis of clinical experience; as such, there was no caregiver involvement in the creation of the specific test items (Johnson et al., 2004). Finally, some test items may seem irrelevant or redundant to certain populations being studied such as driving, home maintenance, or home repairs questions that, when factored into scoring, may affect standardization and results.

Administration

The 28-item ADLQ is completed either through client interview or informant based in which answers are based on the person's ability to engage in various ADLs and

IADLs relative to the 6 domains discussed prior. The ADLQ employs a unique formula for scoring as follows:

1. For each section count the total number of questions answered (i.e., questions that are *not* rated as 9) then multiply that number by 3. This equals the total points possible for that section.

2. Add up the total score for the section (i.e., the sum of the responses) and then divide by the total points possible.

3. Multiply that number by 100, which gives the amount of impairment expressed as a percentage where 0% to 33% is suggestive of impairment, 34% to 66% moderate impairment, and 67% or higher is considered severe impairment (Johnson et al., 2004).

Permissions

The ADLQ is free to use in clinical practice and is wholly contained in the following journal article. For research or other purposes contact the author of the assessment at the information that follows.

Johnson, N., Barion, A., Rademaker, A., Rehkemper, G., & Weintraub, S. (2004). The Activities of Daily Living Questionnaire: A validation study in patients with dementia. *Alzheimer Disease and Associated Disorders, 18*(4), 223-230.

Summary

POPULATION	Probable NCD Alzheimer's or other cognitive impairment
TYPE OF MEASURE	Questionnaire, informant based
WHAT IT ASSESSES	ADL performance across 6 domains
TIME	< 10 minutes
COST	Free

Contact

Nancy Johnson, PhD

Cognitive Neurology and Alzheimer's Disease Center

Northwestern University Medical School

Chicago, Illinois

TABLE 2-1
ACTIVITIES OF DAILY LIVING QUESTIONNAIRE EXAMPLE TEST ITEMS
SELF-CARE ACTIVITIES
Dressing
0 = No problems
1 = Independent, but slow or clumsy
2 = Wrong sequence, forgets items
3 = Needs help with dressing
9 = Don't know
TRAVEL
Public Transportation
0 = Uses public transportation as usual
1 = Uses public transportation less frequently
2 = Has gotten lost using public transportation
3 = No longer uses public transportation
9 = Never used public transportation regularly or don't know
SHOPPING AND MONEY
Food shopping
0 = No problem
1 = Forgets items or buys unnecessary items
2 = Needs to be accompanied while shopping
3 = No longer does the shopping
9 = Never had responsibility in this activity or don't know
Adapted from Johnson, N., Barion, A., Rademaker, A., Rehkemper, G., & Weintraub, S. (2004). The Activities of Daily Living Questionnaire: A validation study in patients with dementia. *Alzheimer Disease and Associated Disorders, 18*(4), 228-229.

Chapter 3: Australian Therapy Outcome Measures (AusTOMs)—Third Edition

Description

The Australian Therapy Outcome Measures (AusTOMs), created by Perry et al. (2004), is a performance-based scale designed for therapy departments that measures client outcomes separately as well as combined for occupational therapy, speech pathology, and physical therapy and is based on the United Kingdom Therapy Outcome Measure (TOM). Although the AusTOMs was created specifically for therapists in Australia, several studies have explored its use in other countries and languages as well (Unsworth et al., 2004). AusTOMs was designed according to the three *International Classification of Functioning, Disability, and Health* (ICF) construct domains of impairment, activity and its limitations, and participation and its restriction, and a fourth domain taken from the original TOM which was thought to be particularly useful for occupational therapists—distress/well-being (Unsworth, 2008). The occupational therapy section consists of 12 scales that explore the association of 4 domains of activities of daily living (ADL) performance: (1) impairment, (2) activity, (3) limitation, participation/restriction, and (4) wellbeing (Chen & Yen-Eng, 2015). Administration requires that particular scales be selected based on client assessment and therapy goals; thus not all 12 scales need to be completed (Unsworth, 2015). Client performance is then rated across the 4 domains of each scale using an 11-point ordinal scale from 0 (complete problem) to 5 (no problem) in which half points can also be used (Unsworth, 2008). Assessment time can be as little as 10 minutes but may vary depending on the number of scales selected.

Table 3-1
The 12 Scales of the Australian Therapy Outcome Measures
1. Learning and applying knowledge
2. Functional walking and mobility
3. Upper limb use
4. Carrying out daily life tasks and routines
5. Transfers
6. Using transport
7. Self-care
8. Domestic life—home
9. Domestic life and managing resources
10. Interpersonal interactions and relationships
11. Work, employment, and education
12. Community life, recreation, leisure, and play

Adapted from Unsworth, C., & Duncombe, D. (2014). *AusTOMs for Occupational Therapy* (3rd ed.). Melbourne, Victoria, Australia: La Trobe University.

Table 3-2
Australian Therapy Outcome Measures Administration Protocol
1. Assess the client using usual standardized or non-standardized methods.
2. Establish occupational therapy goals with the client using usual methods.
3. Select occupational therapy scales that reflect current goals.
4. Make a rating for each of the 4 domains of selected scales.
5. Implement occupational therapy program.
6. Re-evaluate goals and/or reassess the client using assessment methods.

Adapted from Unsworth, C., & Duncombe, D. (2014). *AusTOMs for Occupational Therapy* (3rd ed.). Melbourne, Victoria, Australia: La Trobe University.

Psychometrics

Using 7 therapists who rated 11 written case studies, Scott, Unsworth, Fricke, and Taylor (2006) calculated intra-rater reliability coefficients for each domain and found that reliability coefficients were $r = 0.74$ for the Impairment domain, 0.88 for the Activity Limitation domain, 0.81 for the Participation Restriction domain, and 0.94 for the Distress/Well-being domain. A subsequent study of 15 occupational therapists who rated 11 case studies found that inter-rater reliability of the Self-care and Transfers scales using the Swedish translation ranged from $r = 0.76$ to 0.85 and 0.80 to 0.90, respectively (Fristedt, Elgmark Andersson, & Unsworth, 2013). The same study found that intra-rater reliability across all 12 AusTOMs-OT scales was $r = 0.84$ (Fristedt et al., 2013). Examining the correlations of the AusTOMs and the EQ-5D, Unsworth et al. (2004) found that the self-care activity limitation subscale had moderate to strong correlations with the EQ-5D Self Care subscale at $r = -0.65$ upon admission, whereas the upper limb use subscale correlation was $r = 0.71$ with the EQ-5D Health Status subscale. Using data from 506 participants, Abu-Awad, Unsworth, Coulson, and Sarigiannis (2014) found that most clients made statistically significant improvements over time in relation to their participation between admission and discharge suggesting that assessment has sensitivity to change in the rehabilitation setting. Finally, a study by Unsworth (2005) indicated that the most frequently used scales were self-care, upper limb use, transfers, and functional walking and mobility.

Advantages

There is a fair amount of literature in support of the AusTOMs for use in clinical practice and no special training or certifications are needed. Developed to be a collective outcome measure for occupational therapy, physical therapy, and speech pathology departments, its adoption in rehabilitation settings can foster interpersonal communications among the therapy professions (Unsworth et al., 2004). The AusTOMs can be used separately by respective departments as well. Also, the fact that the AusTOMs draws on the Classification of Impairment, Disabilities, and Handicaps domains suggests that it is a culturally relevant assessment. The University of La Trobe—Australia maintains a website devoted to the measure where it can be downloaded free of charge.

Disadvantages

One possible limitation of the assessment is the fact that it is contextualized to Australian allied health practice and reflects the ways in which speech pathology, occupational therapy, and physical therapy are provided there (Perry et

al., 2004). More research may be needed as well with regard to its validity, reliability, sensitivity to change, and clinical usefulness across a number of diagnoses (Perry et al., 2004).

Administration

During assessment the clinician chooses one or more scale and then begins to gather information on occupational performance through interview, observation, clinical judgment, or the results of non-standardized or standardized testing. The compilation of those results are then considered relative to the 11-point scoring system of the chosen scale, which varies depending on the activity. AusTOMs scoring delivers a global rating for each of the 4 domains of (1) impairment, (2) activity, (3) limitation, participation/restriction, and (4) well-being for each scale affording the clinician unique insights into client occupational strengths and weaknesses. Table 3-3 provides scoring examples of the measure.

TABLE 3-3	
ACTIVITY LIMITATION SCALE SCORING	
0	Does not walk or move self around at all
1	Severe limitation in walking or moving self, maximum assistance required.
2	Moderate/severe limitation, needs a person to give moderate hands on assistance such as steadying or guidance, or constant verbal cueing
3	Moderate limitation, needs verbal prompts or supervision, set-up.
4	Mild limitation, able to walk/move but lacks quality or needs extra time.
5	No limitation, independent, with or without the use of adaptive equipment including wheelchair in a reasonable time.
0.5 points possible	

Adapted from Unsworth, C. (2005). Measuring outcomes using the Australian Therapy Outcome Measures for Occupational Therapy (AusTOMs-OT): Data description and tool sensitivity. *British Journal of Occupational Therapy, 68*(8), 354.

Permissions

The AusTOMs is available free of charge and can be obtained from the La Trobe University website where it, as well as other resources, can be downloaded. Use of the

AusTOMs in research or publication can be obtained by contacting the lead researcher of the measure at the information following. More information can be found in the following original publication:

Unsworth, C., & Duncombe, D. (2014). *AusTOMs for Occupational Therapy.* (3rd ed). Melbourne, Victoria, Australia: La Trobe University.

Summary

POPULATION	General
TYPE OF MEASURE	Performance-based rating scale
WHAT IT ASSESSES	ADLs/IADLs, cognitive, social
TIME	≥ 10 minutes
COST	Free

Contact

Carolyn Unsworth, BSc, OT, PhD

School of Allied Health

La Trobe University

Melbourne, Victoria, Australia

Web: http://austoms.com/about/

Chapter 4: The Frenchay Activities Index (FAI)

Description

Developed by Holbrook and Skilbeck, (1983), the Frenchay Activities Index (FAI) is a questionnaire that is used to measure instrumental activities of daily living (IADLs) in patients following stroke. The FAI is designed to measure more complex levels of independence and social survival, beyond only basic-ADLs or IADLs and consists of 15 items that address both the frequency and successful performance of those activities over a 3- to 6-month time frame (Tooth, McKenna, Smith, & O'Rourke, 2003). Ten items of the measure refer to everyday activities that the person has engaged in during the past 3 months, while 5 items relate to seasonal activities accomplished during the last 6 months. The FAI is further delineated into 3 subscales that relate to *domestic activities* (items 1 to 5) *leisure/work* (items 7, 9, 11, 13, and 15), and the *outdoors* (items 6, 8, 10, 12, and 14). Each of the activities is then scored along a variable 4-point scale (range: 0 to 3 points) based on frequency of engagement with higher scores representing more participation. The FAI can be completed in less than 10 minutes.

Psychometrics

A study by Post and de Witte (2003) of 45 outpatient subjects post cerebrovascular accident (CVA) showed good inter-rater reliability for FAI total scores (r=0.90 at the 95% confidence interval) where 11 out of the 15 items displayed good agreement. Items showing poor agreement were local shopping, social occasions, actively pursuing a hobby, and paid work. Similarly, a client/informant based study by Piercy, Carter, Mant, and Wade (2000) of 59 persons who were either post-CVA or their caregiver found that the kappa statistic for 9 of the 15 items had a good level of agreement between 2 research interviews (0.64 to 0.80) while the other 6 items only showed fair or moderate strength of agreement (0.26 to 0.52). Sarker, Rudd, Douiri, and Wolfe (2012) found a significant correlation between the FAI and the Barthel Index (r=0.80) among 238 subjects 3 months post-stroke. Another study found that the FAI ability to detect change was moderate (0.59) for chronic stroke patients between 6 and 12 months post-stroke when compared with the Stroke Adapted Sickness Impact Profile (r=0.63) (Schepers, Visser-Meily, Ketelaar, & Lindeman, 2006). Early research of individuals 65 years of age and older found that mean scores of the FAI were 40.86 for the control group, 35.90 (pre-stroke), and 30.19 (post-stroke) demonstrating its ability to detect change (Schuling, de Haan, Limburg, & Groenier, 1993).

Advantages

The FAI is a relatively quick assessment that can be completed in <10 minutes and requires no special training or certifications to administer. A strength of the FAI may be in the quickness in which it can be completed, which can help determine if a more thorough evaluation is needed. Also, there is a fair amount of research in support of its use in clinical practice. The FAI is located in the public domain and is free to use in clinical practice.

Disadvantages

Research by Appelros, (2007), among pre- and post-stroke individuals, found the existence of a floor effect post-stroke, where as many as 43 patients (17%) of the study received the lowest possible score (15 points). Furthermore, scoring of

Table 4-1
The 15 Items of the Frenchay Activities Index

1. Preparing main meals	8. Walking outside > 15 minutes
2. Washing up	9. Pursuing a hobby
3. Washing clothes	10. Driving a car/bus ride
4. Light house work	11. Travel outings/car rides
5. Heavy house work	12. Gardening
6. Local shopping	13. House/car maintenance
7. Social occasions	14. Reading books
	15. Gainful work

Adapted from Wendel, K., Stahl, A., & Iwarsson, S. (2013). Inter-rater agreement of a modified and extended Swedish version of the Frenchay Activities Index (FAI). *European Journal of Ageing, 10*(3), 249.

individual items tended to conglomerate at the minimum and maximum point range for individual items. Also, the FAI requires the ability to accurately recall activities over a 3- to 6-month time frame, which may be confusing for some and lead to bias. Additionally, Wu, Chuang, Lin, and Horng (2011) suggest that some items on the FAI are redundant. For example, the items of light and heavy housework may not be clearly distinguishable, as are assessing social occasions and travel outings and car rides.

Administration

The FAI is a questionnaire that is completed as either a self-report or by proxy through an interview format. During assessment the person must recall his or her amount of occupational engagement in various ADL and IADL activities over a 6-month time frame that, for the most part, relate to social participation and civic life. The FAI uses several 4-point scales (0 to 3) depending on the particular domain of questions being asked. For example, the question regarding the amount of time in the last 6 months one has undertaken reading books would be scored as (0) never, (1) 1 to 2 times in 6 months, (2) 3 to 12 times in 6 months, (3) at least weekly. The question "In the last 6 months how often have you undertaken gainful work?" would be scored as (0) none, (1) up to 10 hours a week, (2) 10 to 30 hours/week, (3) over 30 hours/week. Specific inclusion/exclusion criteria are outlined for each question to accurately score an individual as well. The question relating to books requires that the book be a full length book and not a periodical or magazine; however, it could be an audio book. For the question pertaining to work, it must be paid work and not volunteer work and the amount should be averaged out over a 6-month time frame.

Permissions

The FAI is free to use in clinical practice. To use in research or publication contact the developers of the assessment or the Oxford journals where it was originally published. Reprint requests can also be made through the Copyright Clearance Center website. More information about the FAI can be found in the following article:

Holbrook, M., & Skilbeck, C. (1983). An activities index for use with stroke patients. *Age and Ageing, 12*(2), 166-70.

Summary

POPULATION	General
TYPE OF MEASURE	Self-report, interview or proxy questionnaire
WHAT IT ASSESSES	More complex ADLs/IADLs
TIME	≤10 minutes
COST	Free

Contact

Clive E. Skilbeck, Associate Professor

School of Psychology

University of Tasmania—Australia

Hobart, Australia

Web: http://media-experts.utas.edu.au/Details. aspx?expertId=321

Chapter 5: Instrumental Activities of Daily Living (IADL) Profile

Description

The Instrumental Activities of Daily Living (IADL) Profile is a performance-based measure designed for those with traumatic brain injury (TBI) that is typically administered in the subject's home and/or community. The assessment quantifies a person's ability to engage in IADLs as well as their level of independence in those IADLS (Bottari, Dassa, Rainville, & Dutil, 2009a). The test is composed of 29 items revolving around 8 tasks of which 6 are designed to accomplish the goal of the client being able to receive guests for a meal and include such things as putting on outdoor clothing, going to the grocery store, shopping for groceries, preparing a hot meal for guests, having a meal with guests, and cleaning up after the meal (Bottari et al., 2009a). The two remaining tasks are single complex IADLs considered necessary for continued independence: obtaining information and making a budget (Bottari et al., 2009a). During the assessment subjects receive minimal instructions and are left to formulate goals in order to plan, engage, and carry out the meal preparation and independence tasks (Bottari et al., 2009a). Each operation is scored using a 5-level ordinal scale relative to performance (dependence, verbal and physical assistance, verbal or physical assistance, independence with difficulty, and independence) that specifically address whether the subject's main difficulties pertain to goal formulation, planning, carrying out the task, and/or attaining the initial task goal, all important components of executive function (Bottari, Dassa, Rainville, & Dutil, et al., 2009b). The IADL Profile is unique in that it attempts to assess the real world functional performance of individuals; thus some components can take a considerable amount of time and energy such as grocery shopping, preparing a hot meal, or having a meal with guests.

Psychometrics

A study of 30 subjects with severe TBI found excellent intra-rater agreement 4 four raters at 0.94 (Bottari, Dassa, Rainville, & Dutil, 2010). Its creators have also noted a good level of inter-rater agreement (r = 0.80) as well as excellent internal consistency for all scales (α = 0.95) with a range of 0.81 to 0.98 (Bottari et al., 2009b). A factor analysis of the assessment supported the following six correlated factors that explained 74% of the variance which suggests good uni-dimensionality of the assessment: (1) going to grocery store/shopping for groceries, (2) having a meal with guests/cleaning up, (3) putting on outdoor clothing, (4) obtaining information, (5) making a budget, and (6) preparing a hot

meal for guests (Bottari et al., 2009a). Further research suggested that the indices of injury severity, measures of executive function, education, age, and environmental factors may account for up to 12% to 28% of the variance in IADL Profile scores (Bottari et al., 2009a). Two outcome measures have shown to be modestly correlated with the IADL Profile, the Tower of London test (r = 0.37) and the Working Memory Index of the Wechsler Memory Scale–III (r = 0.38) (Bottari et al., 2009a). Alas, where a score of 4 equates independence and a score of 0 dependence, Bottari et al. (2010) found that mean scores on the IADL Profile of 30 subjects with TBI were 2.94 going to grocery store/shopping for groceries; 3.57 having a meal with guests/cleaning; 3.61 putting on outdoor clothing; 2.22 obtaining information; 1.30 making a budget; and 3.23 preparing a hot meal for guests.

Advantages

There is a fair amount of research in support of the assessment for use in clinical practice for the TBI population. The IADL Profile also has the ability to document the effects of executive function on IADL engagement and expands on the previous work of the ADL Profile also included in this manual. The assessment also may contribute to a better understanding of executive function deficits through its analysis of everyday IADLs. Due to incomplete literature relative to diverse patient populations there is an opportunity for research oriented individuals to expand the knowledge base of the assessment.

Disadvantages

There is a limited amount of a research outside of what has been established by its creators and most is confined to the TBI population. The assessment requires administration in the home and community environment which may impede testability for many clients. The IADL Profile also requires a significant amount of set up and time to administer and can be fatiguing for some populations (Bottari et al., 2010).

Administration

The authors stress that it is important to be forthcoming during initial discussions with the client in order to develop an understanding that the IADL Profile is a real world-type of assessment with the ultimate goal of evaluating a person's ability to function alone in the community environment following his or her injury, as most occupational therapy assessments do not necessarily ask clients to perform real world activities such as grocery shopping. Once testing begins the clinician uses a non-structured approach and employs naturalistic observations and a minimal amount of cueing, if possible, as the subject plans, formulates, initiates, and engages in tasks. Occupational performance is then rated relative to the amount and type of assistance needed such as: requiring only verbal or physical assistance or whether the subject was independent with difficulties.

Permissions

Use of the assessment in clinical practice, research and/or publication can be obtained by contacting its creators or the publishers of the original work at the information below. Further information can be found in the following journal articles.

Bottari, C., Dassa, C., Rainville, C., & Dutil, E. (2010). A generalizability study of the Instrumental Activities of Daily Living Profile. *Archives of Physical Medicine & Rehabilitation, 91*(5), 734-742.

Bottari, C., Dassa, C., Rainville, C., & Dutil, E. (2010). The IADL Profile: Development, content validity, intra- and interrater agreement. *Canadian Journal of Occupational Therapy, 77*(2), 90-100.

Summary

POPULATION	TBI
TYPE OF MEASURE	Functional performance
WHAT IT ASSESSES	IADLs; level of independence
TIME	≥1 hour for some components
COST	n/a

Contact

Caroline Bottari, PhD

University of Montreal

Montreal, Quebec, Canada

Web: www.readap.umontreal.ca/la-recherche/professeurs-chercheurs/carolina-bottari-ph-d/

CHAPTER 6: LAWTON INSTRUMENTAL ACTIVITIES OF DAILY LIVING (IADL) SCALE

Description

The Lawton Instrumental Activities of Daily Living (IADL) Scale is an 8-item questionnaire administered either by proxy, through interview, or as a self-report that is designed to evaluate a person's ability to engage in more complex activities thought necessary for functioning in community settings by assessing the following 8 areas of occupational performance: (1) the ability to use a telephone, (2) shopping, (3) food preparation, (4) housekeeping, (5) laundry, (6) mode of transportation, (7) responsibility for own medications, and (8) ability to handle finances (Graf, 2008). The Lawton IADL Scale takes approximately 10 minutes to complete and is scored using a 2-point rating scale (0 or 1). During assessment the informant picks the most correct answer from several choices, of up to 5 for each item. Total scores can range from 0 to 8 with higher scores indicating better functioning.

TABLE 6-1

EXAMPLE ITEMS OF THE INSTRUMENTAL ACTIVITIES OF DAILY LIVING SCALE

RESPONSIBILITY FOR OWN MEDICATIONS

1	Is responsible for taking medication in correct dosages at correct time
0	Takes responsibly if medication is prepared in advance in separate dosages
0	Is not capable of dispensing own medication

SHOPPING

1	Takes care of all shopping needs independently
0	Shops independently for small purchases
0	Needs to be accompanied on any shopping trip
0	Completely unable to shop

Adapted from Graf, C. (2008). The Lawton Instrumental Activities of Daily Living Scale. *American Journal of Nursing, 108*(4), 60.

Psychometrics

Original research by Lawton and Brody (1969) found that the measure was highly reproducible with test-retest reliability coefficients of 0.96 (n=97) and 0.93 (n=168), respectively. Work of two independent raters included in the original study also found inter-rater agreement to be good at 0.85 between total scores. The IADL scale was found to correlate well with several outcome measures such as the Physical Self-Maintenance Scale at 0.61, Mental Status Questionnaire at 0.48, Behavior and Adjustment Rating Scales at 0.44, and the Physical Classification at 0.40 (Lawton & Brody, 1969). Burton et al. (2009) found that the correlation between the self- and informant-based versions of the scale was 0.69. Between age and education for the self-report it was 0.24 and –0.10 and for the informant-report it was 0.22 and –0.10. The IADL scale also showed a significant negative correlation with the Scales of Independent Behavior-Revised; and since each test is both a self- and informant-based measure, concurrent validity was compared between each separately. For the self-report it was –0.58 and for the informant versions it was –0.69. A study of falls by Chu, Chiu, and Chi (2006) found that when comparing the IADL Scale with the Barthel Index, Tinetti Balance Scale and gait speed, after gait speed the IADL Scale was able to predict the occurrence of falls among community dwelling residents over 65 years old. A study by Cromwell, Eagar, and Poulos (2003) found that three IADL items (telephone use, self-medication, and handling finances) were statistically associated with cognitive impairment. A similar study found four IADL items were associated with cognitive impairment regardless of age, sex, or education: telephone use, use of transportation, self-medication, and handling finances (Barberger-Gateau et al., 1992). A study by McGrory, Shenkin, Austin, and Starr (2014) found shopping and food preparation to be the most difficult items and considered to be lost first in the disablement process while telephone use was the least difficult, suggesting that a person reporting challenges with telephone use is unlikely to be able to perform any other task on the scale. Conversely, if a person reports no problems with shopping or food preparation they will likely have no limitations with other tasks.

Advantages

There is a good amount of evidence in support of the Lawton IADL Scale for use in clinical practice and it is widely accepted as a valid and reliable measure for use in elderly populations (Barberger-Gateau et al., 1992). Administration is easy and can be completed in less than 10 minutes. Several scoring paradigms have been developed to address the perceived lack of sensitivity to small changes inherent in the original. Also, results can provide useful information about the capacity of an individual to live in the community-based setting.

Disadvantages

Developed in 1969, the Lawton IADL Scale has remained relatively unchanged and because of the simple scoring system (0 or 1 with a high score of 8) some researchers have noted a lack of sensitivity to detect small changes in functional status. Others have noted that although statistical differences fall within acceptable limits, gender bias may exist for items relating to food preparation, laundry, and housekeeping.

Administration

The Lawton IADL Scale is a questionnaire that is completed by proxy, as a self-report, or through interview where the subject is asked to consider items relative to his or her ability to engage in activities considered important for independence. Several researchers have suggested and tested different scoring models to improve the sensitivity of the measure and its ability to document change beyond the original dichotomous scale of (0 = less able, 1 = more able) to include a 3-point scale (1 = unable, 2 = needs assistance, 3 = independent) as well as a 4-point scale. A study examining all 3 scoring systems found reliability estimates to be high respectively for each scoring system at r = 0.80, 0.88, and 0.87, suggesting near equal validity when using the original or more complex scoring systems (Graf, 2008).

Permissions

The assessment is located in the public domain and is free to use in clinical practice. It can also be found in its entirety in several publications as well as online. Permission to use in research and/or publication can be obtained by contacting the publishers of the original work or the Copyright Clearance Center at the information following. Further information can be found in the following journal article:

Lawton, M. P., & Brody, E. M. (1969). Assessment of older people: Self-maintaining and instrumental activities of daily living. *The Gerontologist, 9,* 179-186.

Summary

POPULATION	General
TYPE OF MEASURE	Self-report, interview, or proxy questionnaire
WHAT IT ASSESSES	ADL/IADLs; level of independence
TIME	< 10 minutes
COST	Free

Contact

Copyright Clearance Center

222 Rosewood Drive

Danvers, MA 01923

Phone: (855) 239-3415

E-mail: info@copyright.com

Web Address: www.copyright.com

Chapter 7: Melbourne Low-Vision Activities of Daily Living Index (MLVAI)

Description

The Melbourne Low-Vision Activities of Daily Living Index (MLVAI), developed by Haymes, Johnston, and Heyes (2001b), is an assessment designed to measure the impact vision-related issues have on functional performance and is composed of 25 standardized items that are divided into two sections. In part A, the clinician observes and grades a person's performance as they engage in 16 instrumental activities of daily living (ADLs), such as writing a check, reading an account, or using the telephone. In part B, the person completes a 9-item questionnaire pertaining to their perceived ability to engage in ADLs such as preparing meals, shopping, doing housework, and grooming (Haymes, Johnston, & Heyes, 2002). Scoring for part A involves the clinician observing and rating the subject's performance based on ability, independence, efficiency, and speed of performance. In part B the subject is asked to report and rate their own performance of more basic ADLs (Haymes et al., 2002). Each item of the MLVAI is rated on a 5-level descriptive scale from 0 to 4 and the total score is derived by summing each item with a maximum possible score of 100 with higher scores suggesting more impairment (Haymes et al., 2002). The MLVAI takes approximately 20 minutes to complete.

Table 7-1

Example Items of the Melbourne Low-Vision Activities of Daily Living Index

OBSERVED ITEMS

- Identifying coins
- Naming colors
- Buttoning a shirt
- Threading a sewing needle
- Telling the time: wrist watch
- Telling the time: wall clock
- Reading a digital display

Adapted from Haymes, A., Johnston, A., & Heyes, A. (2001b). The development of the Melbourne Low-Vision ADL Index: A measure of vision disability. *Investigative Ophthalmology and Visual Science, 42*(6), 1216.

Psychometrics

Research by its developers showed that the MLVAI demonstrated good internal reliability with a Cronbach's alpha of 0.96, and an intra-class correlation coefficient of 0.95 for overall reliability (Haymes et al., 2001b). The Spearman's correlation coefficient for test–retest reliability was 0.94 and the inter-rater reliability was 0.90 or higher for 10 practitioners (Haymes et al., 2001b). Overall, there was a moderately high correlation with vision impairment (r = −0.68); however, when each section of the test was examined individually it was determined to be r = −0.80 for part A visual acuity and r = -0.49 for part B basic self-care ADLs, suggesting that the MLVAI is a valid instrument for detecting the effects of low-vision on occupational performance (Haymes et al., 2001b). A second study also by its creators found that age, near word acuity, results of an administered Melbourne Edge Test, contrast sensitivity, and visual field accounted for 82.2% of the variance of MLVAI total scores, thus validating the content of the exam (Haymes et al., 2002). A subsequent study of a modified version was evaluated, which entails weighting each item (ADL) by importance to the person being tested along a 5-level scale from 0 to 4 where the study of 97 subjects indicated an internal reliability of 0.94 (Haymes et al., 2001b). Further results determined a strong correlation with near-word acuity at 0.78, followed by Melbourne Edge Test contrast sensitivity at −0.72, and visual field at −0.52 (Haymes et al., 2001a).

Advantages

The MLVAI is unique in that it is an ADL/vision-specific assessment, thus making it relevant to the occupational therapy profession. Also, there is potential for the interested researcher to use the MLVAI in future validation studies due to the limited amount of research in support of its clinical use.

Disadvantages

There is an insufficient amount of research pertaining to the MLVAI outside of that involving its creators, as well as a lack of comparison with other gold standard assessments to adequately establish its content validity as an effective measure of the low-vision panacea. Thus, its author suggests that items on the assessment should be used and adapted as necessary during the development of the client's occupational profile.

Administration

In part A (16 items) the clinician observes and rates client functional performance along a 5-point scale (0 to 4) where examples include telling time with a wrist watch, using a telephone book, reading newspaper print, reading a medicine label, reading a digital display, and recognizing faces, which are scored as (0) very unsatisfactory, (1) unsatisfactory, (2) borderline, (3) satisfactory, or (4) very satisfactory. In part B the client subjectively rates their performance across 9 tasks/items. The maximum possible score of the MLVAI is 100.

TABLE 7-2
PART B SELF-REPORT ITEM SCORING
0. Very unsatisfactory: Complete inability to perform task
1. Unsatisfactory: Ability to perform task, but only with a great deal of help
2. Unsatisfactory: Ability to perform task, but only with a great deal of help
3. Satisfactory: Ability to perform task without help, but slowly or with some difficulty
4. Very satisfactory: Ability to perform task independently, quickly, and efficiently
Adapted from Haymes, A., Johnston, A., & Heyes, A. (2001b). The development of the Melbourne Low-Vision ADL Index: A measure of vision disability. *Investigative Ophthalmology and Visual Science,* 42(6), 1216.

Permissions

Use of the MLVAI assessment can be obtained by contacting the copyright holders or its creators at the following information. Its description is contained in its entirety in the following journal article:

Haymes, A., Johnston, A., & Heyes, A. (2001b). The development of the Melbourne Low-Vision ADL Index: A measure of vision disability. *Investigative Ophthalmology and Visual Science, 42*(6), 1215-1225.

Summary

POPULATION	Suspected visual impairment
TYPE OF MEASURE	Functional performance and self-report questionnaire
WHAT IT ASSESSES	ADL/IADL performance and self-perceived abilities
TIME	20 minutes
COST	Free

Contact

Dr. Sharon Bentley

Optometry and Vision Sciences

University of Melbourne—Australia

Melbourne, Victoria, Australia

Chapter 8: Performance Assessment of Self-Care Skills (PASS)

Description

The Performance Assessment of Self-Care Skills (PASS) is an outcome measure designed to document change in functional status through the observation and rating of an individual's occupational performance of selected activity of daily living (ADL)/instrumental activity of daily living (IADL) tasks (Holm & Rogers, 2008). PASS is composed of 26 items that are categorized into 1 of 4 functional domains: 5 that relate to *functional mobility*; 3 to *personal self-care*; 14 involving IADLs that emphasize *cognitive performance*; and 4 that emphasize *physical performance* (Holm & Rogers, 2008). Designed to assist practitioners in both treatment and discharge planning, it can help to identify the type and amount of assistance required for successful task performance, as well as risks to safety and the specific point of task breakdown (Holm & Rogers, 2008). There are two versions of PASS available, the PASS-Clinic and the PASS-Home, where both versions are generally the same with the exception of some materials, which differ for each setting. For example, task materials are provided in the clinic, whereas the home version the client uses task materials typically found in the home (Holm & Rogers, 2008). During the assessment the clinician rates client performance based on their ability to safely, independently, and adequately complete tasks using a progressive system of least to most assistive prompts. Each of the 3 scoring domains uses a 4-point scale (0 to 3) that relate to the type and amount of prompts given as well as level of safety. Time to complete PASS can be as long as 60 minutes.

Table 8-1

Example Domains and Activities on the Performance Assessment of Self-Care Scale

FUNCTIONAL MOBILITY
- Bed transfer
- Stair use
- Toilet/bathtub/shower transfer
- Indoor walking

BASIC ADLS
- Oral hygiene
- Trimming toe nails
- Getting dressed

COGNITIVE IADLS
- Shopping
- Bill paying by check
- Checkbook balancing
- Mailing bills
- Telephone use
- Medication management

Adapted from Holm, M. (2010). Online Assessment of Self-Care Skills: ACIE Award 2009. University of Pittsburgh. Retrieved from: www.pitt.edu/~facaffs/acie/holm.html, slides 12, 18 and 22.

Psychometrics

Developers of the measure confirmed good inter-rater reliability for the scoring domains of independence relative to both the clinic and home versions at $r = 0.92$ and $r = 0.96$ as well as for safety at $r = 0.93$ and 0.97, and adequacy at $r = 0.90$ and 0.88 (Holm, 2010). Using data from multiple clinical studies ($n = 941$) other research has shown the PASS to have good to excellent test–retest reliabilities for independence at $r = 0.092$ to 0.96 and for the safety domain of $r = 0.89$ to 0.90 as well as an inter-rater agreement of 0.96 for independence and 0.97 for safety (Chisholm, Toto, Rainia, Holm, & Rogers, 2014). Inter-rater reliability established by Foster (2014) found similar results using 6 raters among 25 subjects (12 with Parkinson's disease, 13 without) where the percentage of agreement for the 3 scoring domains was 0.95 for independence (range: 0.92 to 0.98), 0.92 for adequacy (range 0.85 to 0.96), and 0.90 for safety (range 0.85 to 0.95). A study discussed by Neistadt (2000) found that the percent agreement between two observers, whether done in the clinic or the home, ranged between 0.96 and 0.99. A study by Ciro, Anderson, Hershey, Prodan, and Holm (2015) of community dwelling individuals ($n = 12$) with mild cognitive impairment found that PASS scores were significantly lower in participants with mild cognitive impairment (median score 40.6) with an average Mini-Mental State Exam (MMSE) score of ≥ 24 than in the control group (44.2) with an MMSE of ≥ 27, suggesting that PASS has the ability to detect small changes in IADL ability. Finally, a case study of a person with acute stroke during a 14-day inpatient rehabilitation found that the mean PASS score improved from 1.1 to 2.9 at discharge, suggesting that changes were clinically meaningful (Skidmore et al. 2011).

Advantages

There is a fair amount of literature in support of the PASS assessment for use in clinical practice among a variety of client populations. It has also been translated into several languages. PASS could be considered a unique tool in that it rates task safety and independence separately contrary to most instruments that propose that to be independent one must be safe during the complex person–task–environment transaction (Chisholm et al., 2014). Also, the clinician can administer only those tasks deemed applicable and if none of the 26 available are, the clinician can develop his or her own using a template contained in the test kit (Chisholm et al., 2014). The test manual as well as support material can be obtained by contacting its creators for a nominal fee.

Disadvantages

Scoring for the assessment can be complex where amount and type of prompts must be considered. Administration time can also be significant (1 to 3 hours) depending on the number and type of tasks chosen from the 26 core tasks available.

Administration

PASS is composed of 26 items as well as a template to create additional items if needed where each activity is presented to the client along with verbal instructions and placement of task objects. Some items may require set-up and, initially, the clinician observes that all environmental conditions are met before commencing the assessment. PASS encompasses 5 domains and includes such items as stair use, which requires the subject to ascend a set of stairs turn around on the landing and descend stairs; whereas the shower transfer activity necessitates the person to enter the shower turn around 180 degrees and exit the shower. Similarly, items pertaining to teeth require the person to manipulate toothpaste, brush teeth, and rinse mouth, while for dentures the person would need to prepare a denture solution then remove, clean, and reinsert dentures (Holm, 2010). As the client attempts a task the practitioner provides and scores the level of assistance needed using least to most assistive prompts which are then folded into varying 4-point ordinal scales from 0 to 3, where 3 suggests complete independence and 0 dependence or where 3 suggests safe practices and 0 when there is a risk to safety of such severity that task was stopped or taken over to prevent harm (Chisholm et al., 2014).

TABLE 8-2
TYPES OF PROMPTS USED BY THE PERFORMANCE ASSESSMENT OF SELF-CARE SKILLS
• Verbal encouragement
• Verbal non-directive
• Verbal directive
• Gestures
• Task/environment rearrangement
• Demonstration
• Physical guidance
• Physical support
• Total assistance
Adapted from Foster, E. R. (2014). Instrumental activities of daily living performance among people with Parkinson's disease without dementia. *American Journal of Occupational Therapy, 68*(3), 355.

Permissions

Use of the PASS in practice, research, or publication can be obtained by contacting its creators at the contact information that follows. The test kit itself can be obtained by contacting the developers of the assessment. More information can be found in the following textbook chapter:

Holm, M., & Rogers, J. (2008). The performance assessment of self-care skills (PASS). In B. J. Hemphill-Pearson (Ed.), *Assessments in occupational therapy mental health.* (2nd ed., pp. 102-110). Thorofare, NJ: SLACK Incorporated.

Summary

POPULATION	General
TYPE OF MEASURE	Functional performance
WHAT IT ASSESSES	ADLs/IADLs, level of assistance, types of prompts
TIME	1 to 3 hours
COST	Nominal

Contact

Margo Holm PhD, OTR/L

Professor Emerita

University of Pittsburgh

School of Health and Rehabilitation Sciences

Pittsburgh, Pennsylvania

Joan C. Rogers, PhD., OTR/L, FAOTA

Department Chair-Occupational Therapy

University of Pittsburgh

School of Health and Rehabilitation Sciences

Pittsburgh, Pennsylvania

Chapter 9: Self-Assessment Parkinson's Disease Disability Scale (SPDDS)

Description

The Self-Assessment Parkinson's Disease Disability Scale (SPDDS) by Brown, MacCarthy, Jahanashi, and Marsden (1989) is a Parkinson's disease (PD) specific questionnaire that consists of 24 items that address individual performance of activities of daily living (ADLs) and is administered either by proxy or as a self-assessment. During administration the individual is asked to quantify to what extent he or she is able to perform outlined ADLs without help and includes such items as inserting and removing an electric plug, pouring milk from a bottle or carton, getting up out of an armchair, getting out of bed, getting dressed, and picking up an object from the floor (Biemans, Dekker, & van der Woude, 2001). The assessment contains 24 items and uses a 5-point Likert scale (1 to 5) for each item outlined as follows: (1) able to do alone and without difficulty, (2) able to alone with a little effort, (3) able to do alone with a lot of effort or a little help, (4) able to do but only with a lot of help, or (5) unable to do at all (Stallibrass, Sissons, & Chalmers, 2002). Scores range from 24 to 120 with higher scores indicative of more severe impairment. The assessment can be completed in less than 10 minutes.

Psychometrics

To establish the validity of the SPDDS, 330 subjects with PD living at home were first asked to complete a self-assessment followed by one that was rater-administered among a subgroup of 30 subjects. Overall, results showed that the SPDDS had high internal consistency with a Cronbach's alpha coefficient of $\alpha = 0.97$ as well as excellent reliability ($r = 0.97$) suggesting good uni-dimensional hierarchy (Biemans et al., 2001). An examination of individual scores found that people had the least problems with washing and brushing their teeth while turning in bed, traveling by public transport, and writing letters were the most difficult (Biemans et al., 2001). Subgroup scores showed the relationship between self-report and skilled observation across 11 selected items was only moderately correlated at $r = 0.66$ with a range of 0.52 (using a telephone) to 0.82 (making cup of tea of coffee) implying only moderate to high associations (Biemans et al., 2001). A study by Stallibrass et al. (2002) of 93 persons with clinically confirmed idiopathic PD showed that pre- and post-intervention scores were statistically different at 33.3 (SD = 8.7) and 31.0 (SD = 7.9), respectively, thus indicating the assessments discriminant validity.

Advantages

The SPDDS is a relatively quick and simple outcome measure to administer and can be completed in less than 10 minutes either by proxy or as a self-report. No special training is needed and it can be a good tool to measure the effects of rehabilitative interventions over time. The assessment is also unique in that it is a PD ADLs specific.

Disadvantages

There is a limited amount of research in support of the SPDDS for use in clinical practice and access to the full standardized assessment may not be readily available.

Administration

During assessment the rater is asked to consider their own or the subject's ability to engage in 24 common ADL and IADL tasks and then to rate that performance using the provided scale relative to the amount of independence or level of difficulty for successful performance.

Table 9-1
Example Items of the Self-Assessment Parkinson's Disease Disability Scale
• Brushing teeth
• Using a telephone
• Making tea or coffee
• Holding and reading a newspaper
• Walking up or down the stairs
• Cutting food with a knife and fork
• Opening a can with a can opener
• Turning over in bed
• Travelling by public transport
• Writing a letter
Adapted from Biemans, M., Dekker, J., & van der Woude, L. H. V. (2001). The internal consistency and validity of the Self-Assessment Parkinson's Disease Disability Scale. *Clinical Rehabilitation, 15*(2), 224.

Permissions

The SPDDS is free to use in practice. To use in research contact the journal in which it was originally published or those associated with its development. More information can be found in the following publications.

Brown, R. G., MacCarthy, B., Jahanashi, M., & Marsden, C. D. (1989). Accuracy of self-reported disability in patients with Parkinsonism. *Archives of Neurology, 46,* 955–959.

Wade, T. (1992). *Measurement in neurological rehabilitation.* New York, New York: Oxford University Press.

Summary

POPULATION	PD
TYPE OF MEASURE	Self-report/proxy questionnaire
WHAT IT ASSESSES	ADL/IADL performance
TIME	< 10 minutes
COST	Free

Contact

Richard Brown, Professor

Kings College

Department of Psychology

London, United Kingdom

Marjan Jahanashi, PhD

Institute of Neurology

Chapter 10: Texas Functional Living Scale (TFLS)

Description

The Texas Functional Living Scale (TFLS) by Cullum et al. (2001) is a performance-based assessment that measures instrumental activities of daily living (IADLs) across 4 subscales: time, money and calculation, communication, and memory. Initially designed for those with neurocognitive disorders (NCDs), subsequent studies suggest that it may be useful across a number of diagnoses where IADL engagement is of primary concern (Binegar, 2007). The TFLS contains 24 activities that assess various aspects of IADLs such as using an analog clock, calendar, check book, phone, and setting a microwave. Other tasks include calculations involving time and money as well as recall of information within a 15-minute span (Drozdick & Cullum, 2011). Scores range from 0 to 5 for each activity with a maximum possible score of 52. Total scores and cumulative percentages are recorded for each of the 4 subscales and an overall T-score is calculated for the entire test. The TFLS takes approximately 15 to 20 minutes to administer and higher scores are suggestive of better IADL functioning.

Psychometrics

Original research by the authors of 21 subjects with NCD of the Alzheimer's type and 21 controls demonstrated a strong correlation between the TFLS and the Mental State Examination at r=0.92, whereas the TFLS was only moderately correlated with the Blessed Dementia Rating Scale (Cullum et al., 2001). The same study showed 1-month test-retest reliability to be high as well as a strong correlation between the subscale scores and the total score at r=>0.90 for most items was noted (Cullum et al., 2001). Another study by Binegar, Hynan, Lacritz, Weiner, and Cullum (2009), in their examination of individuals with mild cognitive impairment, found no significant relationship between TFLS and Mini Mental State scores for either intervention or control group at r=0.26 for the intervention group while the normal control group the relationship was r=0.25; however, a moderate correlation was noted when both groups scores were combined at r=0.34. Further analyses determined the sensitivity and specificity scores for the observed cohort ranged from 40 to 52 where a cutoff score of 48 represented the highest combination of sensitivity (0.57) and specificity (0.63), yielding a percent accurate group classification of 0.60. Lyon (2012) found that correlations between TFLS T-Score and Wechsler Memory Scale (WMS–IV) subtest scores ranged from 0.46 (Logical Memory II) to 0.60 (Logical Memory I, Verbal Paired Associates II, and Visual Reproduction

I) suggesting that memory is moderately related to IADLs performance. Drozdick and Cullum (2011) found that the correlations between the TFLS T-score and the Wechsler Adult Intelligence Scale (WAIS-IV) were higher in the overall clinical sample (i.e., traumatic brain injury, NCD, autism, or major depression) than in the normative group where the subtest scores of the WAIS were moderate to highly correlated (range=0.63 to 0.80).

Advantages

The TFLS is a brief and easily administered performance-based measure of daily functional capabilities that is sensitive to level of cognitive impairment and has shown to be applicable in patients with varying degrees of NCD (Cullum et al., 2001). Initial research has also demonstrated good reliability, internal consistency, and convergent and discriminant validity with several measures of global cognitive status and behavioral functioning (Cullum et al., 2001). No special training or certifications are required for its administration. The TFLS is managed by and can be purchased from Pearson Psych Corp.

Disadvantages

The TFLS is a relatively new outcome measure and more supportive data is needed to ascertain its utility in a variety of clinical populations (Drozdick & Cullum, 2011). Another potential downside may be found in the design of the cue card system used where Lindsey-Glenn and Strang (2010) note that the black-and-white line drawings may be difficult for some people to use or interpret. For example, the microwave oven may be suggestive of a poor representation where using real objects or models of real objects might be more effective. A similar argument can be made concerning those cue cards provided for the water bill, writing a check, and addressing an envelope in which their appearance may make it difficult for persons with developmental disabilities to make accurate inferences.

Administration

During administration the client may be asked to respond to items containing oral and visual cues depending on the nature of the particular item being assessed, such as writing a check or looking up information in a phone book (Lindsey-Glenn & Strang, 2010). For example, a client may be asked to point to the date on a calendar. A correct response given would earn 3 points, whereas 2 points would be given if they point to only the correct week but not the correct day, and 1 point if they point to the correct month only, etc. (Binegar, 2007). Other activities include telling time on a traditional clock, making change, paying a bill, using a phone and phonebook, managing medications, and making a snack. The test kit contains stimulus cards for some of the items as well as a list of other items needed, which includes a calendar, stop watch, and various coin and bill denominations. Explicit instructions and scoring interpretation guidelines are included in the manual.

Permissions

The TFLS is an assessment battery that can be purchased from Pearson at the information that follows for a cost of $163. Use in research or publication can also be obtained by contacting Pearson or its creators at the addresses below. Further information can be found in the following original journal article.

Cullum, C., Saine, K., Chan, L., Martin-Cook, K., Gray, K., & Weiner, M. (2001). Performance-based instrument to assess functional capacity in dementia: The Texas Functional Living Scale. *Neuropsychiatry, Neuropsychology, and Behavioral Neurology, 14*(2), 103-108.

Summary

POPULATION	NCD, suspected cognitive impairment
TYPE OF MEASURE	Performance-based
WHAT IT ASSESSES	Abilities relative to time, money and calculation, communication, and memory
TIME	15 to 20 minutes
COST	$163

Contact

Munro Cullum, PhD.

University of Texas Southwestern Medical Center

Dallas, Texas

Web: http://profiles.utsouthwestern.edu/profile/11587/c-munro-cullum.html

Pearson Customer Support

P.O. Box 599700

San Antonio, TX 78259

Phone: (800) 627-7271

Email: clinicalcustomersupport@pearson.com

Web: www.pearsonclinical.com/therapy/products/100000222/texas-functional-living-scale-tfls.html

References

Abu-Awad, Y., Unsworth, C., Coulson, M., & Sarigiannis, M. (2014). Using the Australian Therapy Outcome Measures for Occupational Therapy (AusTOMs-OT) to measure client participation outcomes. *British Journal of Occupational Therapy, 77*(2), 44–49.

Appelros, P. (2007). Characteristics of the Frenchay Activities Index one year after a stroke: A population-based study. *Disability and Rehabilitation, 29*(10), 785-790

Barberger-Gateau, P., Commenges, D., Gaagnon, M., Letenneur, L., Sauvel, C., & Dartigues, J. F. (1992). Instrumental activities of daily living as a screening tool for cognitive impairment and dementia in elderly community dwellers. *Journal of the American Geriatric Society, 40*, 1129–1134.

Biemans, M., Dekker, J., & van der Woude. L. (2001). The internal consistency and validity of the Self-Assessment Parkinson's Disease Disability Scale. *Clinical Rehabilitation, 15*(2), 221-228.

Binegar, D. (2007). *Performance on the Texas Functional Living Scale (TFLS) in mild cognitive impairment.* Unpublished doctoral dissertation, The University of Texas Southwestern Medical Center at Dallas, Texas.

Binegar, D., Hynan, L., Lacritz, L., Weiner, M., & Cullum, C. M. (2009). Can a direct IADL measure detect deficits in persons with MCI? *Current Alzheimer Research, 6*(1), 48–51.

Bottari, C., Dassa, C., Rainville, C., & Dutil, E. (2009a). The criterion-related validity of the IADL Profile with measures of executive functions, indices of trauma severity and sociodemographic characteristics. *Brain Injury, 23*(4), 322-335.

Bottari, C., Dassa, C., Rainville, C., & Dutil, E. (2009b). The factorial validity and internal consistency of the Instrumental Activities of Daily Living Profile in individuals with a traumatic brain injury. *Neuropsychological Rehabilitation, 19*(2), 177-207.

Bottari, C., Dassa, C., Rainville, C., & Dutil, E. (2010). A generalizability study of the Instrumental Activities of Daily Living Profile. *Archives of Physical Medicine and Rehabilitation, 91*(5), 734-742.

Brown, R. G., MacCarthy, B., Jahanashi, M., & Marsden, C. D. (1989). Accuracy of self-reported disability in patients with Parkinsonism. *Archives of Neurology, 46*, 955–959.

Burton, C., Strauss, E., Bunce, D., Hunter, M., & Hultsch, D. (2009). Functional abilities in older adults with mild cognitive impairment. *Gerontology, 55*(5), 570-581.

Chen, Z., & Yen-Eng, J. (2015). Use of the Australian Therapy Outcome Measures for Occupational Therapy (AusTOMs-OT) in an early supported discharge programme for stroke patients in Singapore. *British Journal of Occupational Therapy.* 1–6 (Published online before print), doi:10.1177/0308022614562582

Chisholm, D., Toto, P., Raina, K., Holm, M., & Rogers, J. (2014). Evaluating capacity to live independently and safely in the community: Performance Assessment of Self-Care Skills. *British Journal of Occupational Therapy, 77*(2), 59–63.

Chu, L., Chiu, A., & Chi, I. (2006). Impact of falls on the balance, gait, and activities of daily living functioning in community-dwelling Chinese older adults. *The Journals of Gerontology. Series A, Biological Sciences and Medical Sciences, 61*(4), 399-404.

Chu, T., & Chung, J. (2008). Psychometric evaluation of the Chinese version of the activities of daily living questionnaire (ADLQ-CV). *International Psychogeriatrics, 20*(6), 1251-1261.

Ciro, C., Anderson, M., Hershey, L., Prodan, C. I., & Holm, M. (2015). Instrumental activities of daily living performance and role satisfaction in people with and without mild cognitive impairment: A pilot project. *American Journal of Occupational Therapy, 69*(3), 1-10.

Cromwell, D., Eagar, K., & Poulos, R. (2003). The performance of Instrumental Activities of Daily Living Scale in screening for cognitive impairment in elderly community residents. *Journal of Clinical Epidemiology, 56*(2), 131-137.

Cullum, C., Saine, K., Chan, L., Martin-Cook, K., Gray, K., & Weiner, M. (2001). Performance-based instrument to assess functional capacity in dementia: The Texas Functional Living Scale. *Cognitive and Behavioral Neurology, 14*(2), 103-108.

Dell'Aniello-Gauthier, M. (1994). *Metrological study of a mini-profile measuring instrument of functional status of elderly victims of cerebrovascular accident.* Quebec, Canada: Université de Sherbrooke.

Drozdick, L., & Cullum, C. M. (2011). Expanding the ecological validity of WAIS-IV and WMS-IV with the Texas Functional Living Scale. *Assessment, 18*(2), 141-155.

Dutil, E., Bottari, C., & Vanier, M. (2013). ADL Profile. Canadian Association of Occupational Therapists: COAT-ACE. Retrieved from www.caot.ca/default.asp?pageid=1438

Dutil, E., Forget, A., Vanier, M., & Gaudreault, C. (1990). Development of the ADL profile: An evaluation for adults with severe head injury. *Occupational Therapy in Health Care, 7*(1), 7-22.

Foster, E. R. (2014). Instrumental activities of daily living performance among people with Parkinson's disease without dementia. *American Journal of Occupational Therapy, 68*(3), 353-362.

Fristedt, S., Elgmark Andersson, E., & Unsworth, C. A. (2013). The inter-rater and test-retest reliability of the self-care and transfer scales, and intra-rater reliability of all scales of the Swedish Translation of the Australian Therapy Outcome Measures for Occupational Therapy (AusTOMs-OT-S). *Scandinavian Journal of Occupational Therapy, 20*(3), 182-189.

Gervais N. (1995). *Comparison of ADL profile and the Functional Independence Measure: Trait validity.* Quebec, Canada: University of Montreal.

Goverover, Y., Kalmar, J., Gaudino-Goering, E., Shawaryn, M., Moore, N., & DeLuca, J. (2005). The relation between subjective and objective measures of everyday life activities in persons with multiple sclerosis. *Archives of Physical Medicine and Rehabilitation, 86*(12), 2303–2308.

Graf, C. (2008). The Lawton Instrumental Activities of Daily Living Scale. *American Journal of Nursing, 108*(4), 53-62.

Haymes. S., Johnston, A., & Heyes, A. (2001a). A weighted version of the Melbourne Low-Vision ADL Index: A measure of disability impact. *Optometry and Vision Science, 78*(8), 565-79.

Haymes, A., Johnston, A., & Heyes, A. (2001b). The development of the Melbourne Low-Vision ADL Index: A measure of vision disability. *Investigative Ophthalmology and Visual Science, 42*(6), 1215-1225.

Haymes, A., Johnston, A., & Heyes, A. (2002). Relationship between vision impairment and ability to perform activities of daily living. *Ophthalmic and Physiological Optics, 22*, 79-91,

Holbrook, M., & Skilbeck, C. E. (1983). An activities index for use with stroke patients. *Age and Ageing, 12*(2), 166-170.

Holm, M. (2010). Online Assessment of Self-Care Skills: ACIE Award 2009. University of Pittsburgh. Retrieved from www.pitt.edu/~facaffs/acie/holm.html

Holm, M., & Rogers, J. (2008). The Performance Assessment of Self-Care Skills (PASS). In B. J. Hemphill-Pearson (Ed.), *Assessments in occupational therapy mental health* (2nd ed., pp. 102-110). Thorofare, NJ: SLACK Incorporated.

Johnson, N., Barion, A., Rademaker, A., Rehkemper, G., & Weintraub, S. (2004). The Activities of Daily Living Questionnaire: A validation study in patients with dementia. *Alzheimer Disease and Associated Disorders, 18*(4), 223-230.

Lawton, M. P., & Brody, E. M. (1969). Assessment of older people: Self-maintaining and instrumental activities of daily living. *The Gerontologist, 9*, 179-186.

Lindsey-Glenn, P., & Strang, J. (2010). Review of the Texas Functional Living Scale. In R. A. Spies, J. F. Carlson, & K. F. Geisinger. (Eds.), *The eighteenth mental measurements yearbook.* Ipswich, MA: Buros Institute of Mental Measurements.

Lyon, J. L. (2012). TFLS/WMS-IV: Comparison of the Texas Functional Living Scale and Wechsler Memory Scale—Fourth Edition in a mild Alzheimer disease sample. Retrieved from http://images.pearsonclinical.com/images/assets/tfls/ComparisonoftheTFLSandWMSIV.pdf

McGrory, S., Shenkin, S., Austin, E., & Starr, J. (2014). Lawton IADL scale in dementia: Can item response theory make it more informative? *Age and Ageing, 43*(4), 491.

Munoz-Neira C., Lopez, O., Riveros, R., Nunez-Huasaf, J., Flores, P., & Slachevsky, A. (2012). The Technology–Activities of Daily Living Questionnaire: A version with a technology-related subscale. *Dementia and Geriatric Cognitive Disorders, 33*, 361-371.

Neistadt, M. (2000). *Occupational therapy evaluations for adults: pocket guide.* Baltimore, MD: Lippincott, Williams, & Wilkins.

Piercy, M., Carter, J., Mant, J., & Wade, D. (2000). Inter-rater reliability of the Frenchay Activities Index in patients with stroke and their careers. *Clinical Rehabilitation, 14*(4), 433-440.

Perry, A., Morris, M., Unsworth, C., Duckett, S., Skeat, J., & Reilly, K. (2004). Therapy outcome measures for allied health practitioners in Australia: The AusTOMs. *International Journal for Quality in Health Care, 16*(4), 285-291.

Post, M., & de Witte, L. (2003). Good inter-rater reliability of the Frenchay Activities Index in stroke patients. *Clinical Rehabilitation, 17*, 548-552

Poulin, V., & Barfod, V. (2012). ADL Profile. Health and Stroke Foundation: Canadian partnership for Stroke Recovery. Retrieved from www.strokengine.ca/psycho/adl_psycho/.

Sarker, S., Rudd, A., Douiri, A., & Wolfe, C. (2012). Comparison of 2 extended activities of daily living scales with the Barthel Index and predictors of their outcomes: Cohort study within the South London Stroke Register (SLSR). *Stroke, 43*(5), 1362-1369.

Schepers, V., Visser-Meily, A., Ketelaar, M. & Lindeman, E. (2006). Poststroke fatigue: Course and its relation to personal and stroke-related factors. *Archives of Physical Medicine and Rehabilitation, 87*(2), 184-188.

Schuling, J., de Haan, R., Limburg, M., & Groenier, K. (1993). The Frenchay Activities Index assessment of functional status in stroke patients. *Stroke, 24*(8), 1173-1177.

Scott, F., Unsworth, C. A., Fricke, J., & Taylor, N. (2006). Reliability of the Australian Therapy Outcome Measures for occupational therapy self-care scale. *Australian Occupational Therapy Journal, 53*(4), 265-276.

Skidmore, E., Holm, M., Whyte, E., Dew, M., Dawson, D., & Becker, J. (2011). The feasibility of meta-cognitive strategy training in acute inpatient stroke rehabilitation: Case report. *Neuropsychological Rehabilitation, 21*(2), 208-223.

Stallibrass, C., Sissons, P., & Chalmers, C. (2002). Randomized controlled trial of the Alexander technique for idiopathic Parkinson's disease. *Clinical Rehabilitation, 16*(7), 695-708.

Tooth, L., Mckenna, K., Smith, M., & O'Rourke, P. (2003). Further evidence for the agreement between patients with stroke and their proxies on the Frenchay Activities Index. *Clinical Rehabilitation, 17*(6), 656.

Unsworth, C. (2005). Measuring outcomes using the Australian Therapy Outcome Measures for Occupational Therapy (AusTOMs-OT): Data description and tool sensitivity. *British Journal of Occupational Therapy, 68*(8), 354- 366.

Unsworth, C. (2008). Using the Australian Therapy Outcome Measures for Occupational Therapy (AusTOMs-OT) to measure outcomes for clients following stroke. *Topics in Stroke Rehabilitation, 15*(4), 351-364.

Unsworth, C. (2015). AusTOMs Australian Therapy Outcome Measures. La Trobe University. Retrieved from www.latrobe.edu.au/school-allied-health/clinicians/australian-therapy-outcome-measures-austoms

Unsworth, C., Duckett, S., Duncombe, D., Perry, A., Skeat, J., & Taylor, N. (2004). Validity of the AusTOM scales: A comparison of the AusTOMs and EuroQol-5D. *Health and Quality of Life Outcomes, 2*(64), 1-12.

Unsworth, C., & Duncombe, D. (2014). *AusTOMs for Occupational Therapy* (3rd ed.). Melbourne, Victoria, Australia: La Trobe University.

Wendel, K., Stahl, A., & Iwarsson, S. (2013). Inter-rater agreement of a modified and extended Swedish version of the Frenchay Activities Index (FAI). *European Journal of Ageing, 10*(3), 247-255.

Wu, C., Chuang, L., Lin, K., & Horng, Y. (2011). Responsiveness and validity of two outcome measures of instrumental activities of daily living in stroke survivors receiving rehabilitative therapies. *Clinical Rehabilitation, 25*(2), 175-183.

II

Basic Activities of
Daily Living (B-ADLs)

Bortnick, K.
*Occupational Therapy Assessments for Older Adults: 100 Instruments for
Measuring Occupational Performance* (pp. 27-38).
© 2017 Taylor & Francis Group.

Chapter 11: The Barthel Index (BI)

Description

The Barthel Index (BI) is a standardized activities of daily living (ADLs) assessment designed to quantify level of occupational performance by observing how well a person performs basic ADLs. The BI is composed of 10 items related to a client's ability to feed him- or herself, bathe, groom, dress, bowel and bladder management, toilet use, ability to transfer, mobility, and ability to use stairs. The BI uses a unique scoring algorithm where 2 items are evaluated with a 2-point scale (0 and 5 points), 6 items are evaluated with a 3-point scale (0, 5, or 10 points), and 2 items are evaluated with a 4-point scale (0, 5, 10, or 15 points). Scores can range from 0 to 100 with higher scores indicating better ADL performance. The assessment can be completed in 10 to 15 minutes where a score of 0 to 20 suggests total dependence, 21 to 60 severe dependence, 61 to 90 moderate dependence and 91 to 95 slight dependence (Shah, Vanclay, & Cooper, 1989).

Psychometrics

Original research by Mahoney and Barthel (1965) has shown an inter-rater reliability median of 0.96 with a range from 69% to 100% suggesting excellent agreement. The same study reported good instrument sensitivity evidenced by its ability to detect changes in ADLs in response to rehabilitation. A study of 5 physical therapist raters with 7 subjects found that inter-rater agreement was 0.80 and had a range of 0.70 to 0.88 (Loewen & Anderson, 1988). A systematic review and meta-analysis by Duffy, Gajree, Langhorne, Stott, and Quinn (2013) found two high quality studies displaying excellent inter-rater reliability of r = 0.93 at a 95% confidence interval. Another study of 22 subjects with 1 physiotherapist rater found that test-retest agreement ranged from r = 0.77 to perfect agreement for the 10 items of the BI (Green, Forster, & Young, 2001). A study by Hartigan and O'Mahony (2011) found a strong correlation between BI scores when rated by doctors and nurses (Spearman's ρ = 0.70), whereas the correlation among only doctors was 0.74 and between only nurses it was 0.83. Finally, a study by Sarker, Rudd, Douiri, and Wolfe (2012) demonstrated good concurrent validity between the Frenchay Activities Index and Barthel Index at r = 0.80 among 238 subjects 3 months post-cerebrovascular accident.

Advantages

The BI is easy to administer, can be completed in 10 to 15 minutes, no special training is required, and it is simple to score. There is a good amount of research in support of its use in clinical practice and at one time was considered a gold standard of ADL assessment.

Disadvantages

The BI has been limited by inherent ceiling and floor effects in its scoring system. When ceiling/floor effects occur in data-gathering, there is a pooling of scores at either the upper or lower levels reported by the instrument. The modified version of the BI by Shah et al. (1989) was designed, in many respects, to address this problem.

Administration

The BI is an observational tool where the clinician observes the client performing specific basic ADLs thought critical for independence in which they are scored according to level of performance. Activities outlined on the assessment include feeding; moving from wheelchair to bed and returning, as well as sitting up in bed; the ability to wash face; comb hair; shave; clean teeth; getting on and off of a toilet including handling clothes, wiping, and flushing; bathing self; walking or propelling a wheelchair on a level surface; managing stairs; dressing, which includes tying shoes and fastening fasteners; and the ability to control bowels and bladder (Mahoney & Barthel, 1965). The cumulative score is calculated by summing each item scored. BI scores are multiples of 5 with a range of 0 to 15 and may vary for each item. Total scores have a range from 0 meaning the person is completely dependent, to 100 which suggests complete independence in basic ADLs, thus higher scores represent a higher degree of independence (Kwon, Hartzema, Duncan, & Lai, 2004).

Permissions

The BI can be accessed through the Mapi Research Trust education information dissemination website and can be used in clinical practice or publication if requested first. A user agreement for the measure is necessary if it is to be used for commercial or research purposes. Distribution fees may be requested according to the study design and context of use of the questionnaire. Furthermore, the Maryland State Medical Society holds the original copyright for the BI where it can be accessed through the Copyright Clearance Center at www.copyright.com. Search under "Maryland State Medical Journal," the journal in which the index was initially published. If requested, it may be used (certain royalties may apply). More information can be found in the following original journal article:

Mahoney, F. I., & Barthel, D. (1965). Functional evaluation: The Barthel Index. *Maryland State Medical Journal, 14,* 56-61.

Summary

POPULATION	General
TYPE OF MEASURE	Performance based
WHAT IT ASSESSES	Basic ADLs
TIME	10 to 15 minutes
COST	Free

Contact

Mapi Research Trust

27, rue de la Villette

69003 Lyon, France

Phone: +33 (0) 472-13-65-75

Email: PROinformation@mapi-trust.org.

Website: www.mapi-trust.org

MedChi, The Maryland State Medical Society

1211 Cathedral Street

Baltimore, MD 21201

Phone: (800) 492-1056

Web address: www.copyright.com or www.medchi.org

CHAPTER 12: FUNCTIONAL INDEPENDENCE MEASURE (FIM)

Description

The Functional Independence Measure (FIM) scale, introduced by Granger et al. (1984), is an interactive observational tool that the clinician can use to grade an individual's level of performance while engaging in activities of daily living (ADLs). It is a quantitative hierarchical measure that includes 7 levels that differentiate major gradations in activity performance from independence (7) to dependence (1) and is considered a classification system the clinician can use to judge a client's ability to carry out an activity independently vs his or her need for assistance from another person or a device. If help is needed the scale quantifies that need where the need for assistance (burden of care) translates to the time/energy that another person must expend to serve the dependent needs of the impaired individual to achieve and maintain a certain quality of life. Higher scores on the FIM thus denote persons that have a higher level of independence and require a smaller amount of assistance. The FIM scale contains a total of 18 items and the sum of all 18 items gives the client's total score, which can range from 18 to 126. Developed by the Uniform Data System for Medical Rehabilitation (UDSMR), its unique software database provides the clinician as well as therapy teams with a way of collecting rehabilitation data in a consistent manner where participating units can report FIM scores, along with client demographics which can then be included within comparative reports generated by the National Rehabilitation Reporting System (Fioravanti, Bordignon, Pettit, Woodhouse, & Ansley, 2012). Facilities can then use these reports to compare programs and client populations with other similar facilities as well as for internal program evaluation.

TABLE 12-1
ACTIVITIES OF THE FUNCTIONAL INDEPENDENCE MEASURE
SELF-CARE
• Eating
• Grooming
• Dressing (upper body)
• Dressing (lower body)
• Toileting
MOBILITY
• Transfers (bed, chair, and wheelchair)
• Transfers (toilet)
• Transfers (shower)
LOCOMOTION
• Walk, wheelchair
• Stairs
COMMUNICATION
• Comprehension
• Expression
• Social cognition
• Interaction
• Problem solving
• Memory
Adapted from Kushner, D., Peters, K. M., & Johnson-Greene, D. (2014). Evaluating use of the Siebens domain management model during inpatient rehabilitation to increase functional independence and discharge rate to home in stroke patients. *PM&R, 7*(4), 359.

Psychometrics

A literature review by Glenny and Stolee (2009) found that the internal consistency of the FIM ranged from $\alpha = 0.88$ to 0.97, while intra-rater reliability had a range of r= 0.94 to 0.98 and inter-rater reliability was r=0.80 to 0.99 among older adults. Fioravanti et al. (2012) found that at admission, there was a moderate correlation between the FIM motor scores and Assessment of Motor and Process Skills (AMPS) motor measures (r=0.54) and between the FIM cognitive scores and AMPS process measures (r=0.56). However, at discharge, FIM motor and AMPS motor measures were only weakly correlated (r=0.29), whereas FIM cognitive and AMPS process measures continued to be moderately correlated (r=0.48). An early study of the FIM also investigated concurrent validity of the same measures in a community-dwelling population of older adults with memory impairment where results demonstrated a moderate relationship between FIM cognitive scores and AMPS process measures, and FIM motor scores and AMPS motor measures with r=0.62 for both relationships (Robinson & Fisher, 1996). An examination of FIM scores by Timbeck and Spaulding (2004) found that persons who scored less than 37 upon admission to a rehabilitation unit rarely got discharged home, whereas an FIM score of less than 50 typically meant dependent with self-care activities upon discharge. Those that scored 90 or greater tended to be independent with most ADLs and were usually discharged home; however, it was found that at a score of 80 a person might be discharged home depending on the availability of caregiver support suggesting good predictive value.

Advantages

A good amount of literature exists in support of the FIM for use in clinical practice and it is a comprehensive way for the clinician to measure a client's level of ADL participation across a wide range of activities. The UDSMR maintains a helpful interactive website for the FIM measure and use of their proprietary software allows for the uniform reporting and examination of data sets across many people and populations through their unique interactive database. Terminology associated with FIM has wide spread acceptance as well (i.e., minimum, moderate, or maximum assistance).

Disadvantages

Although many clinicians may employ simplified versions of FIM in their practice, the scale is a type of data entry system that must be purchased and used accordingly to achieve true standardization. Grading ADL performance can also be difficult because it relies on the skilled observation abilities of the clinician who must, for example, be able to delineate a person's ability to do a percentage of a task

such as: The client was only able to do 40% of a transfer vs 55%. FIM requires certification prior to its administration and although training in all aspects of the assessment is available through UDSMR, the FIM system and associated software can be difficult and time consuming to implement in therapy departments.

Administration

FIM is an interactive observational tool in which the clinician grades a person's ability to complete 18 ADL tasks along a continuum from 0% to 100% as well as quantifies the amount of assistance needed to complete those task items. An example *Locomotion: Walk/Wheelchair* item would include walking one time from a standing position, or if using a wheelchair, once from the seated position across a level surface (Cloud, Johnson, & Lauinger, 1995). A score of 5 (supervision) would be attained if while walking the subject required only standby supervision, cuing, or coaxing to go a minimum of 150 feet, whereas if in a wheelchair, the person also only required standby supervision, cuing, or coaxing to go the minimum distance of 150 feet. (Cloud et al., 1995).

TABLE 12-2	
ACTIVITIES OF THE FUNCTIONAL INDEPENDENCE MEASURE	
7	Person is completely independent
6	Modified independence (patient requires use of a device, but no physical assistance).
5	Person requires only supervision or setup to complete task.
4	Minimal contact assistance (patient can perform 75% or more of the task)
3	Moderate assistance (patient can perform 50% to 74% of the task)
2	Maximal assistance (patient can perform 25% to 49% of the task)
1	Total assistance (patient can perform less than 25% of the task or requires more than one person to assist)
0	Activity does not occur

Permission

The FIM Instrument is a trademark of the UDSMR, a division of UB Foundation Activities, Inc. and several software versions are available that are created for particular populations such as sub-acute, skilled nursing, outpatient, and adult day. Permission to use in research, clinical practice, or publishing can be obtained by contacting the copyright holder at the address that follows. More information can be found in the following article.

Keith, R., Granger, C., Hamilton, B., & Sherwin, F. (1987). The functional independence measure. *Advances in Clinical Rehabilitation, 1,* 6-18.

Summary

POPULATION	General
TYPE OF MEASURE	Performance based
WHAT IT ASSESSES	Basic ADLs
TIME	< 10 minutes/task (18 tasks)
COST	Subscription price varies

Contact

Uniform Data System for Medical Rehabilitation

270 Northpointe Parkway, Suite 300

Amherst, New York 14228

Phone: (716) 817-7800

Email: info@udsmr.org

Web: www.udsmr.org/WebModules/FIM/Fim_About. aspx

Chapter 13: Katz Index of Independence in Activities of Daily Living

Description

The Katz Index of Independence in Activities of Daily Living, by Katz, Ford, Moskowitz, Jackson, and Jaffe (1963), is an outcome measure designed to quantify an individual's capacity to engage in basic activities of daily living (B-ADLs). Through assessment, functional status is determined by the clinician as he or she observes the person perform 6 activities related to (1) feeding, (2) continence, (3) transferring, (4) going to the toilet, (5) dressing, and (6) bathing. The Katz Index employs a unique Guttman-like hierarchy that follows the pediatric development model which argues that as a child matures, the simplest activity which is eating, is mastered first, followed by continence, then transferring, toileting, dressing, and bathing, in order of increasing complexity; thus as a person ages or experiences illness and performance is lost, it is lost in the reverse order from bathing to eating (LaPlante, 2010). The assessment uses a distinctive scoring system as well that delivers an item score as well as a total score expressed as levels of dependence from A, which is considered independent to G, representing the most of possible dependent grades (i.e., requiring assistance in all 6 activities). Although, there are only 6 items, there are several scoring possibilities in relation to the amount of assistance needed per task and the number of tasks where that assistance is needed (Strauss, Aguero-Torres, Kareholt, Winblad, & Fratiglioni, 2003). The quantitative notation of some type of assistance needed per task suggests more dependence. The Katz Index can be completed in less than 30 minutes; however, any single item can be completed in less than 5 minutes.

Psychometrics

Original research by its authors determined that the Katz Index had and inter-rater reliability of r = 0.95 and correlated with a mobility scale at 0.50 and a house confinement scale at 0.39. A later Guttmann analysis of 100 subjects found that the coefficients of scalability had a range of r = 0.74 to 0.88, suggesting that the index formed a successful cumulative scale (Brorsson, & Asberg, 1984; Katz, Downs, & Grotz, 1970; Katz et al., 1963). A Turkish translation also found high inter-rater reliability at r = 0.99 as well as high test–retest reliability (0.99), and moderate levels of internal consistency at α = 0.84 among an outpatient clinic population of n = 211 (Arik et al., 2015). A cross-sectional study by Gerrard (2013) of 13,507 skilled nursing facility subjects (average age: 81 years, majority White female) determined *eating* to be the easiest item and *bathing* the most difficult item confirming the developmental model discussed earlier. A study of 460 acutely admitted older patients (mean age 78 years) and their proxies exhibited moderate to good levels of overall agreement relative to Katz Index scores at 0.70 to 0.90, which increased as their Mini-Mental State Exam (MMSE) scores increased. For example, when subjects scored ≤ 15 agreement was 0.70, whereas for those with MMSE scores between 16 to 23 there was 0.79 agreement, and for persons with scores ≥ 24 there was 0.90 agreement (Pol, Buurman, de Vos, & Rooij, 2011). Two studies of the predictive validity of Katz Index (n = 124 and n = 106) for cerebrovascular accident (CVA) subjects, who were assessed by an occupational therapist, determined that 96 and 94% of those graded A to C on days 5 to 7 after stroke were discharged within 1 month, whereas 96% and 92% of those graded D to G stayed in the hospital longer than 1 month or had died, while 62% and 68% of subjects graded as G died within 1 month, suggesting that the Katz Index is a valid tool for early prognosis and rehabilitation planning of CVA outcomes (Asberg & Nydevik, 1991).

Advantages

There is a significant amount of research in support of the Katz Index and it requires no training or certifications for use in clinical practice. Several modifications also exist, such as the trichotomous scoring version (i.e., three levels of independence/dependence), as well one that uses as a simplified scoring system where each item is scored as either (1) independent or (0) with totals expressed along a numerical scale from (0 to 6). The Katz Index has been around since 1963 and can facilitate a common language because it is used by many health professions. The measure has been adapted and translated into numerous languages highlighting its cross-cultural relevancy as well.

Disadvantages

The presence of floor/ceiling effects can occur in scoring; thus, the appropriateness of its use should be considered relative to patient populations.

Administration

During assessment the clinician first observes and grades client performance relative to task items along a continuum of independent or dependent using standardized instructions and although independence typically suggests without supervision, direction, or active personal assistance, each item has specific inclusion/exclusion criteria. For example, in the bathing task independence is considered assistance only in bathing a single part (as back or disabled extremity) or bathes self completely, whereas dependence is assistance in bathing more than one part of the body, assistance in getting in or out of tub, or does not bathe self. Independence for the transfer item is the ability to move in and out of bed independently or move in and out of chair independently (with or without the use of mechanical supports), while dependence is assistance in moving in or out of bed and/or chair or does not perform one or more transfers (MacDowell, 2006). Item tasks are them summed along a hierarchical grading scale form (A) independent in all task to (G) dependent in all tasks as follows:

TABLE 13-1
GRADING HIERARCHY OF THE KATZ INDEX

A	Independent in feeding, continence, transferring, going to toilet, dressing, and bathing
B	Independent in all but one task
C	Independent in all but bathing and one additional task
D	Independent in all but bathing, dressing, and one additional task
E	Independent in all but bathing, dressing, going to toilet, and one additional task
F	Independent in all but bathing, dressing, going to toilet, transferring, and one additional task
G	Dependent in all six functions
Other	Dependent in at least two functions, but not classifiable as C, D, E, or F

Adapted from MacDowell, M. (2006). *Measuring health: A guide to rating scales and questionnaires* (p. 76). New York, New York: Oxford University Press.

Permissions

The Katz Index is located in the public domain and is readily available from many websites on the Internet; however, to use in research or publication contact the original journal where it has been published or the Copyright Clearance Center. More information can be found in the following article:

Katz, S., Ford, A.B., Moskowitz, R. W., Jackson, B. A., & Jaffe M. W. (1963). Studies of illness in the aged. The index of ADL: A standardized measure of biological and psychosocial function. *JAMA, 185*, 914-919.

Summary

POPULATION	General
TYPE OF MEASURE	Performance based
WHAT IT ASSESSES	B-ADLs
TIME	<30 minutes total; 5 minutes/item (6 items)
COST	Free

Contact

Copyright Clearance Center
222 Rosewood Drive
Danvers, MA 01923
Phone: (855) 239-3415
E-mail: info@copyright.com
Web Address: www.copyright.com

Chapter 14: Modified Barthel Index (MBI)

Description

Based on the original Barthel Index, the Modified version by Shah, Vanclay, and Cooper (1989) is also designed to assess an individual's ability to engage in basic activities of daily living (ADLs) by measuring level of performance and the degree of independence a person is from needing assistance to complete task items. The Modified Barthel Index (MBI) covers the same 10 domains as the original: (1) bowel control, and (2) bladder control, as well as help with (3) grooming, (4) toilet use, (5) feeding, (6) transfers, (7) walking, (8) getting dressed, (9) climbing stairs, and (10) bathing. While the BI uses only a 3-point scale the MBI uses a 5-point scale. This was done in part to address inherent floor/ceiling effects found in the original and an inability to correctly classify persons who only needed some form of assistance. The graduated scale uses the same parameters and is more sensitive to small improvements in functional independence while still maintaining the qualities of the original (Shah et al., 1989). The MBI is also scored along the same compendium as the original with 0 to 15 for each item and a total score range of 0 to 100; thus it can be said that the MBI does not cause any additional difficulty nor increase the implementation time (10 to 15 minutes) while improving the internal consistency and providing better discrimination of functional ability (Shah et al., 1989).

Table 14-1

Five Item Scale of the Modified Barthel Index

RANGE: 0 TO 15
1. Unable to perform task
2. Attempts task, but unsafe
3. Moderate help required
4. Minimal help required
5. Fully independent

Table 14-2

Three Item Scale of the Original Barthel Index

RANGE: 0 TO 15
1. Unable to perform task
2. Needs assistance
3. Fully independent

Psychometrics

The MBI has been shown to have high content reliability with a Cronbach's coefficient alpha of internal consistency of $\alpha = 0.90$ recorded at the commencement of rehabilitation (Shah, et al. 1989). Kucukdeveci et al. (2000) found that the internal consistency of the MBI in spinal cord injury patients was good ($\alpha = 0.88$ to 0.90) and inter-rater reliability sufficient at the item level (kappa 0.50 to 0.78) as well as good for the overall inter-rater agreement as the intra-class correlation coefficient was 0.77. The same study found correlations between the MBI and American Spinal Injury Association motor scores ranged from $r = 0.58$ to 0.82 excluding personal hygiene at 0.25 and feeding at 0.27, respectively. Results of the Chinese version MBI-C suggests cross-cultural stability according to data from two sets of inter-rater reliability indices that were obtained by conducting the MBI-C and the MBI concurrently on a total of 15 people with stroke. This was evidenced by the mean total scores on the MBI-C and the MBI which were similar at 57.2 (SD = 20.4) and 60.5 (SD = 22.3) (Leung, Chan, & Shah, 2007). That study also found the most inter-rater consistent item for the MBI was personal hygiene (k = 0.85) while the least consistent item was toileting (k = 0.63), whereas the most inter-rater consistent item among the MBI-C items was transfer (k = 1.00), and the least consistent item was stair climbing (k = 0.81) (Leung et al., 2007).

Advantages

There is a significant amount of research in support of the MBI's use in clinical practice. The development of the MBI was based on the work of the original Barthel Index, once a gold standard of ADL assessment. It is easy and quick to administer, 10 to 15 minutes, and there is no special training required. Scoring parameters are well thought out which has resulted in improved discriminate ability.

Disadvantages

Possible limitations of the measure point to the fact that although the MBI builds on a significant amount of previous work relative to the original, there is limited direct evidenced-based research for a number of conditions such as neurocognitive disorders of the Alzheimer's and related types suggesting more research is needed to definitively apply the MBI to other populations in a similar fashion as the original.

Administration

The MBI is an activity-based observational tool in which the clinician observes and grades client performance across 10 specific ADLs using a 5-item scale (range 0 to 15) where 6 items are scored as (0) unable to perform task, (2) substantial help required, (5) moderate help provided, (8) minimal help required, or (10) fully independent; 2 items scored as (0) unable to perform task, (1) substantial help required, (3) moderate help provided, (4) minimal help required, or (5) fully independent; and 2 items scored as (0) unable to perform task, (3) substantial help required, (8) moderate help provided, (12) minimal help required, or (15) fully independent (Shah, 1998; Shah et al., 1989). The cumulative score is calculated by summing each item score with higher scores suggesting a greater degree of independence in ADL functioning. The following scoring norms, as outlined by its developers, quantifies an individual's level of dependency one might find for particular scoring ranges.

Permissions

Consent to use the MBI in practice, research, or publication can be obtained by contacting its creator or copyright holders at the following information. The MBI was published by Wiley & Sons in *Compendium of Quality of Life Measures* by Sam Salek (1998). More information about the tool can be found in the following original research article:

Shah, S., Vanclay, F., & Cooper, B. (1989). Improving the sensitivity of the Barthel Index for stroke rehabilitation. *Journal of Clinical Epidemiology, 42*, 703-709.

Summary

POPULATION	General
TYPE OF MEASURE	Performance based
WHAT IT ASSESSES	Basic ADLs
TIME	10 to 15 minutes
COST	Free

Contact

Dr. Suryakumar Shah

A.T. Still University

Department of Occupational Therapy

Kirksville, Missouri

TABLE 14-3
MODIFIED BARTHEL INDEX SCORING AND PREDICTED LEVELS OF ASSISTANCE

LEVEL	MBI SCORES	DEPENDENCY LEVELS	HOURS OF HELP NEEDED/WEEK TO ATTEND TO ADL AND IADL NEEDS
1	0 to 24	Total	27.0
2	25 to 49	Severe	23.5
3	50 to 74	Moderate	20.0
4	75 to 90	Mild	13.0
5	91 to 99	Minimal	< 10.0

Adapted from Shah, S. (1998) Modified Barthel Index or Barthel Index (Expanded) In S. Salek. (Ed). *Compendium of quality of life instruments Part II.* Chichester, PA: Wiley & Sons; Shah, S., Vanclay, F., & Cooper, B. (1989). Improving the sensitivity of the Barthel Index for stroke rehabilitation. *Journal of Clinical Epidemiology, 42*(8), 703-709.

REFERENCES

Arik, G., Varan, H. D., Yavuz, B. B., Karabulut, E., Kara, O., Kilic, M. K.,... Cankurtaran, M. (2015). Validation of Katz Index of Independence in Activities of Daily Living in Turkish older adults. *Archives of Gerontology and Geriatrics, 61*(3), 344-350.

Asberg, K. H., & Nydevik, I. (1991). Early prognosis of stroke outcome by means of Katz Index of Activities of Daily Living. *Scandinavian Journal of Rehabilitation Medicine, 23*(4), 187-191.

Brorsson, B. & Asberg, K. (1984). Katz index of independence in ADL: Reliability and validity in short-term care. *Scandinavian Journal of Rehabilitation Medicine, 16*(3), 125-132. In I. MacDowell. (2006). *Measuring health: A guide to rating scales and questionnaires.* New York, New York: Oxford University Press.

Cloud, J. A., Johnson, D. C., & Lauinger, T. A. (1995). *Functional Independence Measurement Scale: Analysis of variables to determine predictability to stroke patient's discharge site.* Masters Thesis. Paper 248. Grand Valley State University. Grand Valley, MI.

Duffy, L., Gajree, S., Langhorne, P., Stott, D., & Quinn, T. (2013). Reliability (inter-rater agreement) of the Barthel Index for Assessment of stroke survivors systematic review and meta-analysis. *Stroke, 44*, 462-468.

Fioravanti, A., Bordignon, C., Pettit, S., Woodhouse, L., & Ansley, B. (2012). Comparing the responsiveness of the Assessment of Motor and Process Skills and the Functional Independence Measure. *Canadian Journal of Occupational Therapy, 79*, 167-174.

Gerrard, P. (2013). The hierarchy of the activities of daily living in the Katz Index in residents of skilled nursing facilities. *Journal of Geriatric Physical Therapy, 36*(2), 87-91.

Glenny, C., & Stolee, P. (2009). Comparing the Functional Independence Measure and the interRAI/MDS for use in the functional assessment of older adults: A review of the literature. *BMC Geriatrics, 9*(52), 1-12.

Green, J., Forster, A., & Young, J. (2001). A test-retest reliability study of the Barthel Index, the Rivermead Mobility Index, the Nottingham extended Activities of Daily Living Scale and the Frenchay Activities Index in stroke patients. *Disability and Rehabilitation, 23*(15), 670-676.

Hartigan, I., & O'Mahony, D. (2011). The Barthel Index: Comparing inter-rater reliability between nurses and doctors in an older adult rehabilitation unit. *Applied Nursing Research, 24*, e1-e7.

Katz, S., Downs, T. H., & Grotz, R. (1970). Progress in development of the index of ADL. *The Gerontologist, 10*, 20-30. In I. MacDowell. (2006). *Measuring health: A guide to rating scales and questionnaires.* New York, New York: Oxford University Press.

Katz, S., Ford, A. B., Moskowitz, R. W., Jackson, B. A., & Jaffe M. W. (1963). Studies of illness in the aged. The index of ADL: A standardized measure of biological and psychosocial function. *JAMA, 185,* 914-919. In I. MacDowell. (2006). *Measuring health: A guide to rating scales and questionnaires.* New York, New York: Oxford University Press.

Kucukdeveci, A., Yavuzer, G., Tennant, A., Suldur, N., Sonel, B., & Arasil, T. (2000). Adaptation of the Modified Barthel Index for use in physical medicine and rehabilitation in Turkey. *Scandinavian Journal of Rehabilitation Medicine, 32*(2), 87-92.

Kushner, D., Peters, K. M., & Johnson-Greene, D. (2014). Evaluating use of the Siebens domain management model during inpatient rehabilitation to increase functional independence and discharge rate to home in stroke patients. *PM&R, 7*(4), 354–364.

Kwon, S., Hartzema, A., Duncan, P., & Lai, S. (2004). Disability measures in stroke relationship among the Barthel Index, the Functional Independence Measure, and the Modified Rankin Scale. *Stroke, 35,* 918-923.

LaPlante, M. P. (2010). The classic measure of disability in activities of daily living is biased by age but an expanded IADL/ADL measure is not. *Journal of Gerontology: Social Sciences, 65B*(6), 720–732,

Leung, S., Chan, C., & Shah, S. (2007). Development of a Chinese version of the Modified Barthel Index validity and reliability. *Clinical Rehabilitation, 21*(10), 912-922.

Loewen, S., & Anderson, B. (1988). Reliability of the Modified Motor Assessment Scale and the Barthel Index. *Physical Therapy, 68,* 1077-1081.

MacDowell, I. (2006). *Measuring health: A guide to rating scales and questionnaires.* New York, New York: Oxford University Press. New York.

Mahoney, F. I., & Barthel, D. (1965). Functional evaluation: The Barthel Index. *Maryland State Medical Journal, 14,* 56-61.

Pol, M., Buurman, B., de Vos, R., & Rooij, S. (2011). Patient and proxy rating agreements on activities of daily living and the instrumental activities of daily living of acutely hospitalized older adults. *Journal of the American Geriatrics Society, 59*(8), 1554-1556.

Robinson, S., & Fisher, A. (1996). A study to examine the relationship of the Assessment of Motor and Process Skills (AMPS) to other tests of cognition and function. *British Journal of Occupational Therapy, 59,* 260-263. In A.M. Fioravanti, C. M. Bordignon, S. M. Pettit, L. J. Woodhouse, & B. J. Ansley. (2012). Comparing the responsiveness of the Assessment of Motor and Process Skills and the Functional Independence Measure. *Canadian Journal of Occupational Therapy, 79*(3), 167-174.

Sarker, S. Rudd, A., Douiri, A., & Wolfe, C. (2012). Comparison of 2 extended activities of daily living scales with the Barthel Index and predictors of their outcomes: Cohort study within the South London Stroke Register (SLSR). *Stroke, 43*(5), 1362-1369.

Shah, S. (1998) Modified Barthel Index. In Salek, S. (Ed.). *Compendium of quality of life instruments* (pp. 1-6). Boston, MA: Wiley and Sons.

Shah, S., Vanclay, F., & Cooper, B. (1989). Improving the sensitivity of the Barthel Index for stroke rehabilitation. *Journal of Clinical Epidemiology, 42*(8), 703-709.

Strauss, E., Aguero-Torres, H., Kareholt, I., Winblad, B., & Fratiglioni, L. (2003). Women are more disabled in basic activities of daily living than men only in very advanced ages: A study on disability, morbidity, and mortality from the Kungsholmen project. *Journal of Clinical Epidemiology, 56*(7), 669-677.

Timbeck, R., & Spaulding, S. (2004). Ability of the Functional Independence Measure to predict rehabilitation outcomes after stroke: A review of the literature. *Physical and Occupational Therapy in Geriatrics, 22*(1), 63-76.

III

Balance and Mobility

Bortnick, K.
*Occupational Therapy Assessments for Older Adults: 100 Instruments for
Measuring Occupational Performance* (pp. 39-59).
© 2017 Taylor & Francis Group.

CHAPTER 15: BERG BALANCE SCALE (BBS)

Description

The Berg Balance Scale (BBS) by Berg et al. (1989) is a performance-based measure designed to quantitatively assess a person's balance and fall risk. Originally designed for older community-dwelling adults through direct observation of their performance, the BBS has shown to be valid across multiple patient populations where balance is of primary concern (Berg, Wood-Dauphinee, Williams, & Maki, 1992). The assessment consists of 15 items that measure the person's ability to maintain balance, either statically or while performing various functional movements, for a specified duration of time (Blum & Korner-Bitensky, 2008). Each item is scored along a 5-point scale of 0 to 4 where 0 indicates the lowest level of function and 4 the highest. The maximum possible score is 56 and is indicative of less fall risk. The BBS takes less than 30 minutes to complete.

TABLE 15-1
EXAMPLE ACTIVITIES ON THE BERG BALANCE SCALE
• Standing with eyes closed
• Standing with feet together
• Reaching forward with outstretched arm
• Retrieving object from floor
• Turning to look behind
• Turning 360 degrees
• Placing alternate foot on stool
• Standing with one foot in front
• Standing on one foot
Adapted from Stevenson, T. (2001). Detecting change in patients with stroke using the Berg Balance Scale). *Australian Journal of Physiotherapy, 47*(1), 30.

Psychometrics

Early research by its author involving 32 individual raters across a number of therapy disciplines using 35 stroke patients and 28 elderly rehabilitation residents found that initial results showed excellent agreement for both inter- and intra-rater reliability with intra-class correlation coefficients of r=0.98 and 0.97, respectively. In addition, standardized Cronbach's alpha estimates were high in both elderly residents ($\alpha=0.87$) and stroke patients ($\alpha=0.98$), indicating strong internal consistency (Berg, 1992). A longitudinal study, also involving its author, of elderly and stroke subjects examined at baseline, and at 3, 6, and 9 months, and at 2, 4, 6, and 12 weeks (stroke) found that Cronbach's alphas at each evaluation were greater than 0.83 and 0.97 showing strong internal consistency for the measure (Berg, Wood-Dauphine, & Williams, 1995). A study by Conradsson et al. (2007) (n=45; mean age, 82 years; mean Mini-Mental State Examination, 17.5) found test-retest reliability to be excellent at r=0.97 where the mean score was 30.3 points. Subsequent research, also involving stroke patients, found that correlations between the BBS and the Barthel Index were excellent with a range of 0.80 to 0.94 (Blum & Korner-Bitensky, 2008). The same study found that correlations between the BBS and Fugl-Meyer balance subscale were considered adequate to excellent with a range of 0.62 to 0.94. Results of a study by Chou et al. (2006) generally concur with results mentioned previously where they too found excellent correlations between the BBS and the Barthel Index at 0.88 and between the BBS and the motor functioning subscale of the Fugl-Meyer Assessment (0.71) 2 weeks post-stroke. (Blum & Korner-Bitensky, 2008). A study by Muir, Berg, Chesworth, and Speechley (2008) argued that dichotomizing the BBS at a score of 45 (those above and those below) resulted in the following probabilities for falling: 58% (20/34) of people with BBS scores at or below 45 fell, whereas only 39% of people (60/153) with scores above 45 fell. Further analysis suggested that the optimal single cutoff value for any fall was 54 and that for multiple falls it was 53 and for injurious falls it was also 54. The high cutoff values required to optimize sensitivity in each fall outcome category suggest that balance impairment alone may not define increased fall risk and that falls are frequent among people with scores above 45 (Muir, Berg, Chesworth, & Speechley, 2008). Finally, an examination to identify elderly people (age range: 65 to 94 years old) who are at risk for falling found that at a cutoff score of 35 the BBS had a sensitivity of 30% and specificity of 96%, at 40 the sensitivity was 45% and specificity was 96%, and at the suggested cutoff score of 45 sensitivity was 64% and specificity was 90% (Riddle & Stratford, 1999).

Advantages

Riddle and Stratford (1999) argue that the BBS is an easy-to-administer, safe, simple, and reasonably brief measure of balance for elderly people that has a good amount of research in support of its use in clinical practice. The assessment can also be used to monitor several aspects of the therapeutic process such as a person's response to treatment. The BBS could also be considered a naturalistic type of assessment since elements resemble common everyday activities. No special training or certifications are needed and it has also displayed high inter- and intra-rater agreement as well as strong correlations with other accepted outcome measures.

Disadvantages

Falls and the risk of falling in general can be complex, and several mechanisms may complicate the issue (i.e., disease process, medication, cognitive decline, or the aging process) increasing a person's chances of falling, thus quantifying that risk may be difficult. The problem is highlighted by the fact that validation efforts that have argued that a cutoff score of 45/56 is necessary for independent ambulation and that failure to reach this score indicate a need to consider a gait aid, provision of assistance or supervision have not generally been accepted. As Stevenson, Connelly, Murray, Hugget, and Overend (2010) suggest, currently there is not enough evidence for using BBS scores to prescribe gait aids as limitations of the identified threshold values resulted in the misclassification of >25% of subjects involving clients who were 65 years of age or older who were able to complete the 2-Minute Walk Test with or without a gait aid, suggesting further research is needed to identify threshold values along with specific subject populations. Other studies have also noted the presence of floor/ceiling effects.

Administration

The BBS is an activity-based observational tool whereby the rater scores client performance as he or she engages in 14 balance activities. Of the maximum possible score of 56 its author suggests the following interpretation of results: 0 to 20, wheelchair bound; 21 to 40, walking with assistance; 41 to 56, independent ambulation; and scores ≤45 as indicative of a high risk of falling. There is also some research to suggest that a change of 8 points is necessary to document a change in function between 2 administrations. Tools needed are a stop watch; 2 chairs, 1 with arm rests; measuring tape/ruler; an object to pick up off the floor; 15 feet of walkway; and a step stool.

Permissions

The BBS is free to use in clinical practice. Use of the measure in research and/or publication can be obtained by contacting the creator of the original work at the address following or contacting the Copyright Clearance Center pertaining to the authors' various publications. Further information can be found in the following journal article:

Berg, K., Wood-Dauphinee, S., Williams, J., & Maki, B. (1992). Measuring balance in the elderly: Validation of an instrument. *Canadian Journal of Public Health*, *83*(2), S7-11.

Summary

POPULATION	General
TYPE OF MEASURE	Performance based
WHAT IT ASSESSES	Fall risk
TIME	<30 minutes
COST	Free

Contact

Katherine Berg, PhD, PT

Executive Chair, Rehabilitation Sciences

Chair and Associate Professor

Department of Physical Therapy

University of Toronto

Toronto, Ontario, Canada

CHAPTER 16: BRUNEL BALANCE ASSESSMENT (BBA)

Description

The Brunel Balance Assessment (BBA) is an activity-based outcome measure developed to quantify the reacquisition of balance post-stroke by using a hierarchical design that incorporates the progression of functional performance as a person recovers, which is thought to occur in a sequence across the 4 domains of (1) assisted balance, (2) independent balance, (3) static balance, and finally (4) dynamic balance. The BBA comprises 12 levels from sitting to standing, to altered base of support and eventual movement where the first and easiest skill to attain is *static sitting balance with upper limb support* and the hardest is *advanced changes of the base of support*. Thus, as a person's perceived change in balance ability progresses or regresses to different levels of the hierarchy the BBA can document that change (Tyson, & DeSouza, 2004). The BBA has 3 sections: a sitting section (3 subtests), standing (3 subtests), and stepping (6 subtests). Each section can be used individually or in conjunction with each other for a complete assessment of the individual (Tyson, 2004). Each section is further divided into several levels, which are achieved by increasing the demand on balance ability (Tyson, 2004). Example items include sitting forward and reaching, standing with arms raised, and a 5-meter walk test with an aid. The BBA uses a 12-point ordinal scale (0 to 12) as well as some pass/fail items with lower scores indicative of decreased abilities. Time to complete the BBA is less than 30 minutes.

TABLE 16-1
REACQUISITION OF BALANCE ACCORDING TO THE BRUNEL BALANCE ASSESSMENT
• Supported sitting
• Static sitting balance
• Dynamic sitting balance
• Supported standing balance
• Static standing balance
• Dynamic standing balance
• Static double stance balance
• Supported single stance
• Dynamic double stance
• Initial change of base of support
• Dynamic single stance
• Advanced change of the base of support
Adapted from Tyson, S. (2004). *Brunel Balance Assessment* (BBA) (1st ed., p. 5). Manchester, United Kingdom: Centre for Research and Human Performance Research, University of Salford.

Psychometrics

During development, criterion validity was assessed by comparing the BBA with other accepted outcome measures and results showed that correlation coefficients were 0.83 when compared to the sitting section of the Motor Assessment Scale, 0.97 with the Berg Balance Test, and 0.95 with the Rivermead Mobility Index, indicating good validity relative to other established measures. The internal consistency Cronbach's alpha coefficient for the measure was $\alpha = 0.93$ (Tyson & DeSouza, 2004). The coefficients of reproducibility and scalability were 0.99 and 0.69 respectively. Lastly, test-retest and inter-rater reliability were both high with 100% agreement (Tyson & DeSouza, 2004). The BBA has also shown to have fair predictive value. Using balance disability as a predictor of future function Tyson, Hanley, Chillala, Selley, and Tallis (2007) found that at 3 months those with limited sitting balance (0% to 22%) and standing balance (25% to 50%) recovered independent functional mobility, whereas those people who could initially walk recovered independent functional mobility at a rate of 66% to 84%.

Advantages

The BBA scale is easy to use and the clinical value of the test is increased by the ability to use all or part of the assessment by employing a hierarchical design where difficulty increases with each item; thus when a subject fails an item he or she can be assumed to fail all higher items and conversely, if the subject passes an item, it can be assumed that he or she would pass all of the lower items. This means that not all items need to be tested and testing can stop once the subject has failed an item reducing the time and effort required by both clinician and subject (Tyson & DeSouza, 2004). Another advantage to this type of assessment is that it gives information about what a patient can or cannot do, rather than how many activities they may able to do (Tyson & DeSouza, 2004).

Disadvantages

The amount of peer-reviewed literature in support of its use outside of that authored or co-authored by its creator is limited. The BBA can also be a relatively complex if the clinician must test all levels, which could take up to 1 hour to complete. Its reliability is also thought to decrease with less-experienced health care professionals (Tyson, 2004). Finally, the assessment requires some set up and the use of various tools as well as an amount of space to perform all activities.

TABLE 16-2
ACTIVITIES OF THE BRUNEL BALANCE ASSESSMENT
1. Supported sitting—30 seconds
2. Sitting arm raise test—3 or more arm lifts in 15 seconds
3. Sitting forward reach test—more than 7 cm
4. Supported standing test—30 seconds
5. Standing arm raise test—3 or more arm lifts in 15 seconds
6. Standing forward reach test—more than 5 cm
7. Timed step standing test—static step standing 30 seconds
8. Walk with aid—5 meters in 60 seconds
9. Weight shift test—3 or more shifts in 15 seconds
10. Walk without an aid—5-meters in 60 seconds
11. Tap test—2 or more taps in 60 seconds
12. Step-up test—1 or more in 15 seconds
Adapted from Tyson, S. (2004). *Brunel Balance Assessment (BBA)* (1st ed., p. 6). Salford, United Kingdom: Centre for Research and Human Performance Research, University of Salford.

Administration

During assessment the client is asked to perform each subsection item in hierarchical fashion until he or she gets to the level that is the limit of their functional ability. Subjects are allowed 3 chances to pass each item. When the client is unable to pass after 3 tries, the test is completed and the score within that level is used as a measure of performance and noted along the 12-point hierarchical ordinal scale. For example, if an individual were to achieve a level 4 (supported standing balance) they would be able to stand supported for 30 seconds. If he or she failed the level relating to dynamic standing balance they would be unable to stand supported and do 3 arm lifts in 15 seconds. Required items include a base or suitable seating, a 1-meter ruler, a step up block that is 7.5 to 10 cm high, a stopwatch, tape to mark a 5-meter walkway, and 2 stools or chairs.

Permissions

The Centre for Research and Human Performance Research at the University of Salford, United Kingdom has published an examination manual developed by its creators that can be found at the information following. Use of the BBA in research or publication can be obtained by contacting the developer of the battery also at the information following or contacting the journal where it was published. More information can be found in the following article:

Tyson, S., & DeSouza, L. (2004). Development of the Brunel Balance Assessment: A new measure of balance disability post stroke. *Clinical Rehabilitation, 18*(7), 801-810.

Summary

POPULATION	Cerebrovascular accident; general
TYPE OF MEASURE	Performance based; hierarchy
WHAT IT ASSESSES	Reacquisition of balance following injury
TIME	< 30 minutes
COST	Free

Contact

Sarah Tyson, FCSP, MSc, PhD

Professor of Rehabilitation

University of Manchester

Manchester, United Kingdom

Stroke & Vascular Research Centre School of Nursing, Midwifery & Social Work

Web: www.nursing.manchester.ac.uk/staff/sarahtyson

Examiner's manual: http://usir.salford.ac.uk/4886/1/new_BBA_manual.pdf

CHAPTER 17: COMMUNITY BALANCE AND MOBILITY SCALE (CB&M)

Description

The Community Balance and Mobility Scale (CB&M) is an activity-based outcome measure designed to evaluate the balance and mobility of individuals who are functioning at a high level yet have persistent balance problems (Knorr, Brouwer, & Garland, 2010). Initially validated among ambulatory patients after traumatic brain injury (TBI), it has also been able to capture the decline in balance that occurs with aging in healthy individuals, thus supporting its validity and sensitivity for use with a number of possible populations (Howe, Inness, & Wright, 2011). The CB&M can assess a wide range of advanced mobility and balance abilities in order to identify postural instability and evaluate change following intervention with respect to independence and considers such things as capacity for velocity and distance (Inness et al., 2011). As a 13-item scale, it measures performance of more challenging balance and mobility tasks that require speed, precision, accuracy, and sequencing of movement components thought to represent the underlying motor skills necessary for successful occupational performance which also includes bending, turning, or looking while walking and equilibrium reactions (Howe, Inness, Venturini, Williams, & Verrier, 2006; Takacs, Garland, Carpenter, & Hunt, 2014). Individual scores range from 0 to 5 and each item uses various unique scoring criteria relevant for that particular activity. The CB&M has a maximum total score of 96 (some items have left and right tested separately and 1 item carries a bonus point) where higher scores are indicative of better mobility and less fall risk. The assessment requires an amount of space, roughly 30 feet by 6 feet, for a track as well as some set up. The CB&M can take up to 1 hour to complete.

TABLE 17-1
PERFORMANCE-BASED ACTIVITIES OF THE COMMUNITY BALANCE AND MOBILITY SCALE
• Unilateral stance—right and left
• Tandem walk
• 180 tandem pivot
• Lateral foot scooting—right and left
• Hopping forward—right and left
• Crouch and walk
• Lateral dodging
• Walking and looking—right and left
• Running with controlled stop
• Forward to backward walking
• Walk, look, and carry—right and left
• Descending stairs
• Step-ups—right and left
Adapted from Howe, J., & Inness, E. (2006). *Community Balance and Mobility Scale* (pp. 3-4). Toronto, Canada: University Health Network: Toronto Rehabilitation Institute.

Psychometrics

A study of 25 knee osteoarthritis patients determined test-retest reliability to be high at r = 0.95 at the mean 8-day range (Takacs et al., 2014). Developmental research by Howe et al. (2006) using 2 convenience samples (n = 36; 32) of ambulatory patients with traumatic brain injury demonstrated strong inter- and intra-rater reliability at r = 0.98, an internal consistency of α = 0.96, as well as good initial test-retest reliabilities of r = 0.98, and 0.89 5 days later; however, only a moderate content and construct validity was determined at 0.62 and 0.64 using physical therapist global ratings and maximal walking velocity as determinants. The same study found that individuals who were able to successfully reintegrate back into the community had scores that were significantly different than those that could not and suggested that a cutoff score of 50 be considered as an indicator of future occupational performance (Howe et al., 2006). Testing of a stroke-specific population demonstrated moderate to high correlation coefficients (range = 0.70 to 0.83) between the Berg Balance Scale, and Timed Up and Go test (Knorr, et al. 2010). It was also moderately correlated with Chedoke-McMaster Stroke Assessment leg and foot scores at 0.61 and 0.63, respectively (Knorr et al., 2010). Whereas, the study by Takacs et al. (2014), discussed earlier, had somewhat different results when they found it correlated with the Timed Up and Go test at r = −0.74 and 0.52 with the Berg Balance scale. While Liu-Ambrose, et al. (2006) found that the CB&M showed only a moderate correlation with the Physical Activity Scale for the Elderly at r = 0.37; however, its correlation with the Activities-Specific Balance Confidence Scale was slightly better at 0.48 among a sample of 98 women aged 75 to 86 years.

Advantages

The CB&M occupies a specific position in balance assessment evidenced by its ability to investigate the performance of high functioning individuals. Initially designed for use with ambulatory patients after a TBI, it has been validated in other populations as well. In a study of healthy individuals ages 30 to 59 years old, the CB&M proved sufficiently difficult as to prevent the occurrence of a ceiling effect, where only 3 of the 90 individuals were able to obtain a perfect score of 96 (Rocque, Bartlett, Brown, & Garland, 2005). The same study observed significant declines in total scores in the 50 to 59 year age category for women but not for men, highlighting its sensitivity in detecting possible gender-specific physical decline at that age cohort (Rocque, Bartlett, Brown, & Garland, 2005).

Disadvantages

There is a limited amount of research in support of its use in clinical practice, which may be a result of the fact that it is a relatively new assessment. The CB&M can also take up to 1 hour to complete in certain client populations and requires a fair amount of set up as well as access to various items that may not be readily available such as a stairway (8 steps minimum).

Administration

While testing, the client is asked to complete specific activities and is graded according to the amount of time it takes to complete the task, their ability to perform, as well as level of assistance required. Subjects are scored on the first trial; however, in cases where it is clear that the individual did not understand the task a second trial is allowed. A scoring example for the single-leg stance activity would be 0 if the person was unable to sustain a unilateral stance independently, 1 if he or she only sustained it for 2 to 4 seconds, 2 for 5 to 9 seconds, 3 for 10 to 19 seconds, 4 for 20 seconds, and 5 if he or she was able to maintain the stance for 45 seconds (Liu-Ambrose et al., 2006). The CB&M requires specific items that include access to a full flight of stairs (8 steps); stop watch (digital preferred); an average size laundry basket or large rigid box of same dimensions; 1 2-pound and 1 7.5-pound weight; a visual target used in item 8 (a paper circle 20 cm in diameter with a 5-cm diameter black circle in the middle); and a bean bag. All tasks are to be performed without ambulation aides (with one exception, item 12—descending stairs). Instructions for testing and scoring are clearly outlined in the examiner's manual.

TABLE 17-2		
COMMUNITY BALANCE AND MOBILITY SCALE SCORING NORMS: HEALTHY INDIVIDUALS		
AGE	N	MEAN
20 to 29 years old	24	88.71
30 to 39 years old	27	86.33
40 to 49 years old	23	84.35
50 to 59 years old	26	77.43
60 to 69 years old	17	64.94
70 to 79 years old	4	49.75
n = 121		

Adapted from Howe, J., Inness, E., & Wright, V. (2011). *The Community Balance and Mobility Scale.* The Center for Outcome Measurement in Brain Injury. Retrieved from www.tbims.org/combi/cbm/cbmprop.html

Permissions

Use of the CB&M in research or publication can be obtained by contacting the developer of the measure at the information following or by contacting the journal in which the original work was published. Further information can be found in the following publications:

Howe, J., Inness, E., Venturini, A., Williams, J. I, &, Verrier, M. (2006) The Community Balance and Mobility Scale: A balance measure for individuals with traumatic brain injury. *Clinical Rehabilitation, 20,* 885-95.

Summary

POPULATION	TBI; general
TYPE OF MEASURE	Performance based
WHAT IT ASSESSES	Higher level balance and mobility
TIME	≤1 hour
COST	Free

Contact

Jo-Anne Howe, DipP&OT, BScPT

University of Toronto

Toronto Rehabilitation Institute

Toronto, Ontario, Canada

Web: www.physicaltherapy.utoronto.ca/faculty/jo-anne-howe

Examiner's manual: www.uhn.ca/TorontoRehab/ Health_Professionals/Documents/TR_HCP_ SUPP_CBMScale.pdf

Liz Inness, BScPT, MSc

University of Toronto

Toronto Rehabilitation Institute

Toronto, Ontario, Canada

CHAPTER 18: DYNAMIC GAIT INDEX (DGI)

Description

The Dynamic Gait Index (DGI), by Shumway-Cook et al. (1995), is designed to assess dynamic postural control in older adults and is used to quantify walking ability and fall risk as well as determine changes in gait and balance throughout the therapeutic process. Validated among several conditions such as multiple sclerosis, stroke, Parkinson's disease, older adults with dizziness or balance problems, and relatively healthy independent older adults, the DGI has 8 tasks and includes such items as stepping over an obstacle where the subject is asked to walk at their normal speed up to and over a shoebox, as well as gait with horizontal head turn where the person must look both left and right while walking for a time (Herman, Inbar-Borovsky, Brozgol, Giladi, & Hausdorff, 2009). A newly modified version also exists with slight changes to the original 8 items as well as an expanded scoring system for better sensitivity. Both measures are based on a person-environment model of mobility which argues that particular environmental demands must be met in order to achieve functional performance, which can be categorized into one of several dimensions representing those external demands that have to be met for an individual to be mobile within their environment, such as the ability to navigate successfully through existing ambient conditions. Performance of both the original and modified versions are based on a combination of gait performance (GP), level of assistance (LOA), and time to complete the activity (T). Scoring of the original DGI uses a single 4-point ordinal scale for each item (range 0 to 3); however, for the mDGI, separate scores are applied to performance relative to (1) the time it takes to complete each task, (2) LOA needed, which uses a 3-point scale, and (3) GP, which uses a 4-point scale that differs slightly for each task. Lower scores are indicative of decreased performance. Although, the DGI requires some set up, once done it can be completed in less than 15 minutes.

TABLE 18-1
TASK ITEMS OF THE DYNAMIC GAIT INDEX
• Walking
• Walking while changing speed
• Walking while turning the head horizontally
• Walking while turning the head vertically
• Walking with pivot turn
• Walking over obstacles
• Walking around obstacles
• Stair climbing

Adapted from Jonsdottir, J., & Cattaneo, D. (2007). Reliability and validity of the Dynamic Gait Index in persons with chronic stroke. *Archives of Physical Medicine & Rehabilitation, 88*(11), 1411.

TABLE 18-2
DIMENSIONS OF FUNCTIONAL PERFORMANCE
• Distance
• Temporal conditions
• Ambient conditions
• Terrain
• Physical load
• Attention
• Postural transitions
• Density (i.e., obstacles)

Adapted from Shumway-Cook, A., Taylor, C., Matsuda, P., Studer, M. T. & Whetten, B. (2013). Expanding the scoring system for the Dynamic Gait Index. *Physical Therapy, 93*(11), 1494.

Psychometrics

A study of 25 subjects post-stroke determined that intra-class correlation coefficients for test-retest and inter-rater reliability were both good at r=0.96 and 0.96. The reliability of single item scores was also moderate to good with a range of r=0.55 to 0.93 (Jonsdottir & Cattaneo, 2007). The same study found a moderate positive correlation with the Berg Balance Scale and the Activities-Specific Balance Confidence Scale at 0.83 and 0.68, whereas the Timed Walking Test and the Timed Up and Go tests were negatively correlated at −0.73 and −0.77 (Jonsdottir & Cattaneo, 2007). Vestibular research by Whitney, Wrisley, & Furman (2003) showed that the DGI and Berg Balance Scale were moderately but significantly correlated as well at r=0.71. In the same study of subjects 14 to 90 years of age, it was determined that at a score of ≤18 persons were 2.7 times more likely to have reported a fall in the previous 6 months. The sensitivity of the DGI at a score ≤18 was also reported to be 0.70 with a specificity of 0.51, whereas at a score ≤19 the positive predictive value was 0.50 and the negative predictive value was 0.87 (Forsberg, Andreasson, & Nilsagard, 2013; Whitney, Marchetti. Schadee, & Wrisley, 2004). Exploratory research of the mDGI found good inter-rater agreement with coefficients ranging from r=0.90 to 0.98 for T scores, 0.59 to 0.88 for GP scores, and 0.84 to 1.0 for LOA scores. Test-retest results for T were r=0.91 while for the GP and LOA subtests it was 0.91 and 0.87, respectively (Shumway-Cook, Taylor, Matsuda, Studer, & Whetten, 2013). Factor analysis of the mDGI showed that a 4-factor solution explained 95% of the variance in task scores. Factor 1, posture, which includes horizontal head turns, vertical head turns, and pivot turn; factor 2, temporal, composed of usual pace, change of pace, pivot turn, and around obstacles; factor 3, terrain, which includes stairs; and lastly, factor 4, density, consisting of avoidance of static and dynamic obstacles (Shumway-Cook, Matsuda, & Taylor, 2015).

Advantages

There is a good amount of DGI research among various patient populations in support of its use in clinical practice and once set up it is a relatively quick measure that requires no certifications. Established research also suggests that the DGI can be good indicator of those at risk for falls. For example, a study by Whitney et al. (2003) found that there was agreement between the Berg Balance Scale and DGI in 44 of 70 patients (63%); and of the 26 patients where there was no agreement, 25 were identified as having an increased risk of falls by the DGI but not by the Berg Balance Scale. Preliminary research of the modified version, with its expanded scoring system, has shown it to be both a valid and reliable assessment that can give the

clinician increased insight into client mobility by providing a greater range of measurement as well as enabling the ability to monitor improvement or deterioration in any one of the three expanded scoring categories not seen in the original (i.e., LOA, GP, and T; Shumway-Cook et al., 2013).

Disadvantages

Dye, Eakman, and Bolton (2013) highlighted results showing a ceiling effect in community-dwelling populations and in people with primary complaints of dizziness. Other studies have noted that two of the items of the DGI, *gait with pivot turn* and *step around obstacles*, have displayed ceiling effects as well, which was further evidenced by a Finnish study of subjects with neurological disorders that found similar problems for the same items. Head-turns have also been difficult in some populations as reports of dizziness have been noted, while the item involving stepping over obstacles may also present difficulties (Forsberg, Andreasson, & Nilsagard, 2013). The original DGI scoring system may have some limitations as it uses a rating system that incorporates the concepts of LOA, GP, and T into one score without a clear explanation of the relative contribution of each found in the newly modified scoring system (Shumway-Cook et al., 2013).

Administration

Both the original and modified versions test 8 aspects of gait where item 1 is considered a baseline that examines the ability of the subject to walk under low-challenging conditions (i.e., self-paced, level surface, level gait), while the remaining 7 items explore the subject's ability to adapt gait to increasing task demands and changing environmental dimensions. The assessment requires some set up as well as enough space to create a small obstacle course and items needed include a shoebox (original DGI), cones, access to stairs, and access to a walkway. The DGI maximum score is 24 and research suggests that scores less than 19 are predictive of falls in the elderly. The mDGI has a score range of 0 to 64 with the subtests of T (range 0 to 24), GP (range 0 to 24), and LOA (range 0 to 16) (Shumway-Cook et al., 2013). An example item of the DGI includes *steps* where the person is asked to walk up a flight of stairs (using the rail if necessary) then turn around at the top and walk down, which would be scored as (3) normal—alternating steps with no rail; (2) mild impairment—alternates feet and must use rail; (1) moderate impairment—uses 2 feet per stair and must use rail; and (0) severe impairment—cannot do activity safely.

Permissions

Both versions of the DGI are free to use in clinical practice. Their use in research or publication can be obtained by contacting their creators at the information that follows or contacting the original publications which contain the assessments. More information can be found in the following journal article:

Shumway-Cook, A., Taylor, C., Matsuda, P., Studer, M., & Whetten, B. (2013). Expanding the scoring system for the Dynamic Gait Index. *Physical Therapy, 93*(11), 1493-1506.

Summary

POPULATION	General
TYPE OF MEASURE	Performance based
WHAT IT ASSESSES	Dynamic postural control and fall risk
TIME	< 15 minutes after set up
COST	Free

Contact

Marjorie Woollacott, PhD

Institute of Neuroscience

University of Oregon

Eugene, Oregon

Web: http://uoneuro.uoregon.edu/ionmain/htdocs/index.html

Anne Shumway-Cook, PT, PhD

Professor Emeritus, Rehabilitation Medicine

University of Washington

Seattle, Washington

CHAPTER 19: RIVERMEAD MOBILITY INDEX (RMI)

Description

The Rivermead Mobility Index (RMI) is a standardized assessment of mobility originally designed for persons with either head injury or stroke but has subsequently been validated in other populations as well. Currently there are 2 versions available. The first is the original 15-item RMI, derived from the Rivermead Motor Assessment, which comprises 14 self-reported items and 1 direct observation item. The assessment includes such items as observing and grading the patient's ability to stand for 10 seconds or their self-reported ability of picking up an article off the floor. Each item is scored as either 0, unable to perform or 1, able to perform. A maximum score of 15 points is possible with higher scores indicative of better mobility. The modified version, which includes an expanded scoring system, was developed in response to the original's inability to detect small changes because of its two item scoring system (Lennon & Johnson, 2000). The m-RMI is now only a direct observational tool as well and is more stroke detailed with increased sensitivity to the effects of therapy (Lennon & Johnson, 2000). This is done by using an extended 6-point scoring system as well as a reduction on the number of items from 15 to only 8 that are stroke specific and include (1) turning over, (2) lying to sitting, (3) sitting balance, (4) sitting to standing, (5) standing, (6) transfers, (7) walking indoors, and (8) stairs. The m-RMI is scored as follows: (0) unable to perform, (1) assistance of 2 people, (2) assistance of 1 person, (3) requires supervision or verbal instruction, (4) requires an aid or an appliance, and (5) independent. A maximum score of 40 is possible with higher scores indicative of increased mobility. Both assessments take less than 15 minutes to complete.

Psychometrics

Early studies of the original RMI by Collen, Wade, Robb, and Bradshaw (1991) concluded that the RMI correlated significantly with the Barthel Index (0.91) and aspects of the Functional Ambulation Category Scale at 0.89 and with its mobility category at 0.85, gait speed (0.82), balance (0.67), and 6-minute distance (0.63), but not with the actual number of falls (0.30). A study by Hsieh, Hsueh, and Mao (2000) of stroke patients (n=38) showed that the RMI scores were moderately to significantly correlated with the Barthel Index and Berg Balance Scale scores at > 0.60 and > 0.80, and that subjects improved by more than 3 points during their stay indicating that the RMI is sensitive to change over time. Lennon and Johnson (2000) established content validity and inter-rater and test-retest reliability by assessing subjects (n = 30) with two independent raters in two different settings, an elderly care unit and a stroke rehabilitation unit using the modified version of the RMI. Results showed that it was responsive to change as well as highly reliable between raters with intra-class correlation coefficients of r = 0.98 and high internal consistency with a Cronbach's alpha of $\alpha = 0.93$. The highest level of agreement was for standing and the lowest level was for walking indoors.

Advantages

The two versions of the RMI are simple and quick assessments that target mobility items that are relevant to the clinician. The noted floor/ceiling effect in the original RMI have arguably been reduced in the modified version as it is considered more sensitive to change. Tentative research results support the use of both versions in practice as reliable and valid assessment tools. The Rivermead batteries only require a minimum of training to administer.

Disadvantages

There is a limited amount of peer reviewed evidence pertaining to the m-RMI. Also, the suppression of 7 items in comparison to the original 15-item tool could potentially have an impact on its content validity (i.e., it now may be assessing a totally different phenomenon) suggesting that further studies are needed and among different client populations as well (Hsieh et al., 2000). A study by Hsueh et al. (2003) found the RMI to have a limited score range and a notable floor effect at ≤ 14 days post-stroke. Indicating that it may not be able to adequately characterize patient mobility in the early stages following a CVA, a problem not found in the m-RMI during the same study.

Administration

The m-RMI is an 8-item observational tool of functional performance in which the therapist grades the client's ability to perform certain movements relative to balance that uses a 6-point Likert scale as follows: (1) unable to perform, (2) assistance of 2 people, (3) assistance of 1 person, (4) requires supervision or verbal instruction, (5) requires an aid or an appliance, and (6) independent. The maximum score for the m-RMI is 40. The original 15-item scale is composed of both observation and activities, employs only a 2-response scoring system (0 or 1), and has a maximum score of 15. Higher scores are indicative of better mobility for both scales.

TABLE 19-1
EXAMPLE ACTIVITIES OF THE ORIGINAL 15-ITEM RIVERMEAD MOBILITY INDEX
1. Turning over
2. Lying to sitting
3. Sitting balance
4. Sitting to standing
5. Standing
6. Transfers
7. Walking indoors
8. Stairs
9. Walking outside (even ground)
10. Walking inside without an aid
11. Picking up an article from the floor
12. Walking outside (uneven ground)
13. Bathing
14. Stairs
15. Running
Adapted from Franchignoni, F., Tesio, L., Benevolo, E., & Ottonello, M. (2003). Psychometric properties of the Rivermead Mobility Index in Italian stroke rehabilitation inpatients. *Clinical Rehabilitation*, *17*(3), 277.

Collen, F., Wade, D., Robb, G., & Bradshaw, C. (1991). The Rivermead Mobility Index: A further development of the Rivermead Motor Assessment. *International Disability Studies, 13*, 50–54

Lennon, S., & Johnson, L. (2000). The modified Rivermead Mobility Index: Validity and reliability *Disability & Rehabilitation, 22*(18), 833-839.

Summary

POPULATION	Cerebrovascular accident; traumatic brain injury; general
TYPE OF MEASURE	Performance based
WHAT IT ASSESSES	Balance and mobility
TIME	< 15 minutes after set up
COST	Free

Permissions

The RMI batteries are free to use in practice and are located in their entirety in several journals as well as on the Internet. Their use in publication or research can be obtained by contacting the authors of the respective measure or where published. Further information can be found in the following journal articles:

Contact

Professor Sheila Lennon

Head of Physiotherapy

Flinders University School of Medicine

Bedford Park, Australia

Web: www.flinders.edu.au/people/sheila.lennon#publications

Louise Johnson, PhD, BSc(Hon), MCSP

School of Health Studies

University of Bradford—School of Life Sciences

Bradford, West Yorkshire, United Kingdom

Web: www.southampton.ac.uk/healthsciences/about/staff/lj1b06.page?p

Chapter 20: Timed Up and Go Test (TUG)

Description

The Timed Up and Go Test (TUG) is a relatively quick outcome measure developed to test a person's balance and fall risk. During assessment the subject is asked to rise from a seated position, walk 3 meters, turn around and sit back down while the clinician records the amount of time taken to complete the activity. The TUG is a widely used and simple measure of basic mobility and has shown to compare well with other measures of balance and function (Large, Gan, Basic, & Jennings, 2006). Based on the original Get up and Go Test by Mathias, et al. (1986) which was originally scored along an ordinal scale of 1 to 5 as well as the observer's perception of fall risk, Podsiadlo and Richardson (1991) modified the test by timing the task rather than only scoring it qualitatively (Chaya & Vidhu, 2011). Scoring norms have been established for a number of age groups and the assessment can be completed in less than 5 minutes.

Psychometrics

A study of 51 people with neurocognitive disorders of the Alzheimer's type by Ries, Ecternach, Nof, Gagnon, and Blodgett (2009) found test-retest reliability to very high at r = 0.99. Noren, Borgen, Bolin, and Stenstrim (2001) established similar results for inter-rater reliability using 3 raters at r = 0.99. TUG scores have also shown to correlate well with the Berg Balance Scale scores at 0.81 and Barthel Index at 0.78 (Podsiadlo & Richardson, 1991). An investigation of fall risk among elderly persons found that those unable to do the TUG due to nonphysical disability had the highest fall rate (11%), followed by those with physical disability (9%), while those able to do the Timed Up and Go had the lowest fall rate (6%) suggesting that physical impairment alone is not a good predictor for falls among the elderly (Large et al., 2006). Expanding on that research, Mirelman et al. (2014) found that persons with mild cognitive impairment had less walking consistency, smaller pitch range during transitions, lower angular velocity during turning and required more time to complete the turn-to-walk activities of the TUG. Meanwhile, several studies have established confidence intervals that can be used to note performance that is worse than average specifically if they exceed 9.0 seconds for 60 to 69 year olds, 10.2 seconds for 70- to 79-year-olds, and 12.7 seconds for individuals 80 to 99 year olds (Bohannon, 2006). While cutoff levels for the TUG at a score of 13.5 seconds or longer produced an overall correct prediction rate of 90% (Shumway-Cook, Brauer, & Woollacott, 2000).

Advantages

There is a significant amount of research to support its use in clinical practice. TUG is a relatively quick and simple outcome measure that requires a minimum amount of tools and set up (a tape measure, stop watch, tape for the floor mark, and a chair) and can be completed in less than 5 minutes. No special training is required and scoring is based on the amount of time needed to complete the activity.

Disadvantages

Although the TUG has been shown to be useful for evaluating functional mobility, the literature suggests that its predictive value and diagnostic accuracy for identifying future falls is not as straight forward, further validating results of research pertaining to other fall assessments that suggest that fall-risk falls are a complex issue that have many variables that are difficult to predict (Beauchet et al., 2011).

Administration

During assessment the subject is asked to (1) rise from a seated position, (2) walk 3 meters, and (3) return and sit back down. Timing begins just as the person attempts to rise from the chair and is stopped when the person is seated again after walking 3 meters. Regular footwear and customary walking aids should be used during the assessment.

TABLE 20-1				
SELECTED NORMS FROM A META-ANALYSIS OF 21 STUDIES COMPRISING HEALTHY OLDER ADULTS				
AGE	**N**	**TIME**	**95% CONFIDENCE INTERVAL**
60 to 69 years old	176	8.1	7.1 to 9.0
70 to 79 years old	798	9.2	8.2 to 10.2
80 to 89 years old	1102	11.3	10.2 to 12.7
60 to 99 years old	4394	9.4	8.9 to 9.9
n = 4395				

Adapted from Bohannon, R. (2006). Reference values for the Timed Up and Go Test: A descriptive meta-analysis. *Journal of Geriatric Physical Therapy 29*(2), 68.

Permissions

The TUG is located in the public domain and is free to use in clinical practice. To use in research or publication contact the author at the information following or the journal in which it was published. Further information can be found in the following original journal article:

Podsiadlo, D., & Richardson, S. (1991). The timed 'Up and Go' Test: A test of basic functional mobility for frail elderly persons. *JAGS: Journal of American Geriatric Society, 39,* 142-148.

Summary

POPULATION	General
TYPE OF MEASURE	Performance based
WHAT IT ASSESSES	Fall risk, balance
TIME	< 5 minutes
COST	Free

Contact

Diane Podsiadlo, BSc, PT

CLSC de Notre-Dame-de-Grace

Chapter 21: Tinetti Falls Efficacy Scale (FES)

Description

The Falls Efficacy Scale (FES) by Tinetti, Richman, and Powell (1990) is a standardized questionnaire designed to quantify a person's fear of falling. Operationalized by two related but separate constructs, falls self-efficacy and balance confidence, the assessment is loosely based on Bandura's Self-Efficacy theory, which proposes that an individual's perceived ability has an effect on functional performance regardless of actual ability. Also, several investigators have argued that fear of falling may be more extensive of a problem in the elderly than actual falling; thus, the ability to quantify that fear is important for occupational therapy practitioners (McAuley, Mihalko, and Rosengren, 1997; Schepens, Sen, Painter, & Murphy, 2012). Through analysis, the FES examines the person's degree of confidence at avoiding a fall during 10 relatively non-hazardous activities of daily living (ADLs), such as cleaning the house, taking a bath or shower, or reaching into cabinets or closets (Tinetti et al., 1990). The assessment can be completed as an interview or as a self-report measure where each item is rated from 1, very confident to 10, not confident at all. FES scores range from 0 to 100, with higher scores suggestive of a greater fear of falling. A modified international version (FES-I) of the measure also exists that has an expanded 16 items scored along a 4-point scale from 1, not at all concerned to 4, very concerned. The FES-I is designed to include more demanding and challenging activities, which may be of interest for higher functioning individuals, such as walking on a slippery surface, walking in a place with crowds, going out to a social event (i.e., family gathering or club meeting), walking up or down a slope, reaching for something above your head or on the ground, and visiting a friend or relative (Delbaere et al., 2010). Both the FES and FES-I can be completed in less than 10 minutes.

Table 21-1
Example Items of the Falls Efficacy Scale
• Cleaning the house
• Getting dressed and undressed
• Preparing a simple meal
• Taking a bath or shower
• Simple shopping
• Getting in and out of a chair
• Going up and down stairs
• Walking around the neighborhood
• Reaching into cabinets or closets
• Answering the door or phone
Adapted from Tinetti, M., Richman, D., & Powell, L. (1990). Falls efficacy as a measure of fear of falling. *Journal of Gerontology, 45*(6), P241.

Psychometrics

Hauer et al. (2010) found test-retest reliability to be good with a range of $r = 0.81$ to 0.88, whereas internal reliability was 0.89 to 0.92. They also found that scores differed between administration methods in cognitively impaired individuals (i.e., self-report or interview) but not in the cognitively intact group, indicating that impaired persons may express less concern about falling in self-reports. Original research in 2 samples of community-living elderly persons showed good test-retest reliability at r = 0.71, and that subjects who reported avoiding activities because of fear of falling had higher FES scores, representing lower self-efficacy or confidence than subjects not reporting fear of falling (Tinetti et al., 1990). A later study, also by its creators, found that the FES was able to stratify scores among a group cohort where 57% denied a fear of falling, 24% acknowledged fear but denied effect on activity, and 19% acknowledged avoiding activities because of a fear of falling. Furthermore, 24% of recent fallers vs 15% of non-fallers acknowledged activity restriction due to fear of falling (Tinetti, Mendes de Leon, Doucette, & Baker, 1994).

Advantages

The FES is a relatively quick and simple questionnaire that can be used across a number of patient populations as a self-report or interview-based measure. There is a considerable amount of research in support of its use in clinical practice and no special training is required. There are several modified versions available and the more complex 16-item (FES-I) international version has been well validated. The FES-I maintains a website devoted to the measure where translations and research information can be found.

Disadvantages

The FES scale has been critiqued for its poor discriminant validity and some argue that it may be difficult for respondents to distinguish between their self-confidence in performing a task and their actual ability to perform the task (Edwards & Lockett, 2008). The scale has also yielded results that may be erroneous for subjects with good mobility where data from a sample of 1103 subjects ≥ 72 years old, who were ambulatory within the household, showed that 39% had scores with highest perceived efficacy, 38% moderate, and only 23% low self-efficacy (Edwards & Lockett, 2008).

Administration

Assessment requires the individual to rate his or her perceived fear of falling while performing various ADLs along a numerical rating scale from 1 (very confident) to 10 (not confident at all). The FES has maximum score of 100 points where a score greater than 70 indicates that the person has a fear of falling.

Permissions

The FES and FES-I are free to use in clinical practice. Use of either, in research or publication, can be obtained by contacting their creators at the information following or contacting the publisher that contain the assessments. More information can be found in the following journal articles:

Tinetti, M., Richman, D., & Powell, L. (1990). Falls efficacy as a measure of fear of falling. *Journal of Gerontology, 45*(6), P239-P243

Yardley, L., Beyer, N., Hauer, K., Kempen, G., Piot-Ziegler, C., & Todd C. (2005). Development and initial validation of the Falls Efficacy Scale-International (FES-I). *Age Ageing, 34*(6), 614-619.

Summary

POPULATION	General
TYPE OF MEASURE	Self-report or interview questionnaire
WHAT IT ASSESSES	Fall risk, balance, self-efficacy
TIME	< 10 minutes
COST	Free

Contact

Mary Elizabeth Tinetti, MD

Yale University School of Public Health

New Haven, Connecticut

Web: http://publichealth.yale.edu/people/mary_tinetti. profile

Chris Todd, PhD

The University of Manchester, United Kingdom

The School of Nursing, Midwifery and Social Work

Web: www.nursing.manchester.ac.uk/staff/Chris Todd/

Web: www.profane.eu.org/fesi.html

REFERENCES

Beauchet, O., Fantino, B., Allali, G., Muir, S., Montero-Odasso, M., & Annweiler, C. (2011). Timed Up and Go Test and risk of falls in older adults: A systematic review. *Journal of Nutrition, Health & Aging, 15*(10), 933-938.

Berg, K. (1992). Measuring balance in the elderly: Development and validation of an instrument. McGill University. Graduate thesis. Retrieved from http://digitool.Library.McGill.CA:80/R/-?func=dbin-jump-full&object_id=39553&silo_library=GEN01

Berg, K., Wood-Dauphine, S., & Williams, J. (1995). The Berg Balance Scale: Reliability assessment with elderly residents and patients with an acute stroke. *Scandinavian Journal of Rehabilitation Medicine, 27,* 27–36.

Berg, K., Wood-Dauphinee, S., Williams, J., & Maki, B. (1992). Measuring balance in the elderly: Validation of an instrument. *Canadian Journal of Public Health, 83,* S7-S11.

Blum, L., & Korner-Bitensky, N. (2008). Usefulness of the Berg Balance Scale in stroke rehabilitation: A systematic review. *Physical Therapy, 88*(5), 559-566.

Bohannon, R. (2006). Reference values for the Timed Up and Go Test: A descriptive meta-analysis. *Journal of Geriatric Physical Therapy 29*(2), 64-68.

Chaya, G., & Vidhu, S. (2011). Functional performance in community-dwelling elderly people: Six-Minute Walk Test, Berg Balance Scale, Timed Up and Go Test and Gait Speeds. *Indian Journal of Physiotherapy and Occupational Therapy, 5*(4), 29-33.

Chou, C., Chien, C., Hsueh, I., Sheu, C., Wang, C., & Hsieh, C. (2006). Developing a short form of the Berg Balance Scale for people with stroke. *Physical Therapy, 86*(2), 195-204.

Collen, F., Wade, D., Robb, G., & Bradshaw, C. (1991). The Rivermead Mobility Index: A further development of the Rivermead Motor Assessment. *International Disability Studies, 13,* 50–54

Conradsson, M., Lundin-Olsson, L., Lindelöf, N., Littbrand, H., Malmqvist, L., Gustafson, Y., & Rosendahl, E. (2007). Berg Balance Scale: Intrarater test-retest reliability among older people dependent in activities of daily living and living in residential care facilities. *Physical Therapy, 87*(9), 1155-1163.

Delbaere, K., Close, J., Mikolaizak, A., Sachdev, P., Brodaty, H., & Lord, S. (2010). The Falls Efficacy Scale International (FES-I). A comprehensive longitudinal validation study. *Age and Ageing, 39,* 210–216.

Dye, D., Eakman, A., & Bolton, K. (2013). Assessing the validity of the Dynamic Gait Index in a balance disorders clinic: An application of Rasch analysis. *Physical Therapy, 93*(6), 809-818.

Edwards, N., & Lockett, D. (2008). Development and validation of a modified Falls-Efficacy Scale. *Disability and Rehabilitation: Assistive Technology, 3*(4), 193-200.

Franchignoni, F., Tesio, L., Benevolo, E., & Ottonello, M. (2003). Psychometric properties of the Rivermead Mobility Index in Italian stroke rehabilitation inpatients. *Clinical Rehabilitation, 17*(3), 273–282.

Forsberg, A., Andreasson, M., & Nilsagard, Y. (2013). Validity of the Dynamic Gait Index in people with multiple sclerosis. *Physical Therapy, 93*(10), 1369-1376.

Hauer, K., Yardley, L., Beyer, N., Kempen, G., Dias, N., Campbell, M.,... Todd, C. (2010). Validation of the falls efficacy scale and falls efficacy scale international in geriatric patients with and without cognitive impairment: Results of self-report and interview-based questionnaires. *Gerontology, 56*(2), 190-199.

Herman, T., Inbar-Borovsky, N., Brozgol, M., Giladi, N., & Hausdorff, J. (2009). The Dynamic Gait index in healthy older adults: The role of stair climbing, fear of falling and gender. *Gait Posture, 29*(2), 237–241.

Howe, J., & Inness, E. (2006). *Community Balance and Mobility Scale.* Toronto, Ontario, Canada: University Health Network: Toronto Rehabilitation Institute.

Howe, J., Inness, E., Venturini, A., Williams, J., & Verrier, M. (2006). The Community Balance and Mobility Scale: A balance measure for individuals with traumatic brain injury. *Clinical Rehabilitation, 20,* 885-895.

Howe, J., Inness, E., & Wright, V. (2011). *The Community Balance and Mobility Scale.* The Center for Outcome Measurement in Brain Injury. Retrieved from www.tbims.org/combi/cbm/cbmprop.html

Hsieh, C. L., Hsueh, I. P., & Mao, H. F. (2000). Validity and responsiveness of the Rivermead Mobility Index in stroke patients. *Scandinavian Journal of Rehabilitation Medicine, 32*(3), 140-142.

Hsueh, I., Wang, C., Sheu, C., & Hsieh, C. (2003). Comparison of psychometric properties of three mobility measures for patients with stroke. *Stroke, 34*(7), 1741-1745.

Inness, E., Howe, J., Niechwiej-Szwedo, E., Jaglal, S., McIlroy, W. E., & Verrier, M. C. (2011) Measuring balance and mobility after traumatic brain injury: Validation of the Community Balance & Mobility Scale (CB&M). *Physiotherapy Canada, 63*(2), 199- 208.

Jonsdottir, J., & Cattaneo, D. (2007). Reliability and validity of the Dynamic Gait Index in persons with chronic stroke. *Archives of Physical Medicine & Rehabilitation, 88*(11), 1410-1415.

Knorr, S., Brouwer, B., & Garland, S. (2010). Validity of the Community Balance and Mobility Scale in community-dwelling persons after stroke. *Archives of Physical Medicine & Rehabilitation, 91*(6), 890-896.

Large, J., Gan, N., Basic, D., & Jennings, N. (2006). Using the Timed Up and Go Test to stratify elderly inpatients at risk of falls. *Clinical Rehabilitation, 20*(5), 421-428.

Lennon, S., & Johnson, L. (2000). The modified Rivermead Mobility Index: Validity and reliability. *Disability and Rehabilitation, 22*(18), 833-839.

Liu-Ambrose, T., Khan, K., Donaldson, M., Eng, J., Lord, S., & McKay, H. (2006). Falls-related self-efficacy is independently associated with balance and mobility in older women with low bone mass. *Journal of Gerontology, 61A*(8), 832–838.

McAuley, E., Mihalko, S. L., & Rosengren, K. (1997). Self-efficacy and balance correlates of fear of falling in the elderly. *Journal of Aging and Physical Activity, 5*(4), 329-340.

Mirelman, A., Weiss, A., Buchman, A., Bennett, D., Giladi, N., & Hausdorff, J. (2014). Association between performance on Timed Up and Go subtasks and mild cognitive impairment: Further insights into the links between cognitive and motor function. *Journal of the American Geriatrics Society, 62*(4), 673-678.

Muir, S., Berg, K., Chesworth, B., & Speechley, M. (2008). Use of the Berg Balance Scale for predicting multiple falls in community-dwelling elderly people: A prospective study. *Physical Therapy, 88,* 449-459.

Noren, A., Bogren, U., Bolin, J., & Stenstrom, C. (2001). Balance assessment in patients with peripheral arthritis: Applicability and reliability of some clinical assessments. *Physiotherapy Research International, 6*(4), 193.

Podsiadlo, D., & Richardson S. (1991). The Timed "Up & Go": A test of basic functional mobility for frail elderly persons. *JAGS: Journal of American Geriatrics Society, 39*(2), 142-148.

Riddle, D., & Stratford, P. (1999). Interpreting validity indexes for diagnostic tests: An illustration using the Berg Balance Test. *Physical Therapy, 79*(10), 939-948.

Ries, J., Echternach, J., Nof, L., & Gagnon Blodgett, M. (2009). Test-retest reliability and minimal detectable change scores for the Timed "Up & Go" Test, the Six-Minute Walk Test, and gait speed in people with Alzheimer disease. *Physical Therapy, 89*(6), 569-579.

Rocque, R., Bartlett, D., Brown, J., & Garland, S. (2005). Influence of age and gender of healthy adults on scoring patterns on the Community Balance and Mobility Scale. *Physiotherapy Canada, 57*(4), 285-292.

Schepens, S., Sen, A., Painter, J. A., & Murphy, S. L. (2012). Relationship between fall-related efficacy and activity engagement in community-dwelling older adults: A meta-analytic review. *American Journal of Occupational Therapy, 66*(2), 137-148.

Shumway-Cook, A., Brauer, S., & Woollacott, M. (2000) Timed Up and Go Test. Graduate student association. University of Buffalo. Retrieved from http://gsa.buffalo.edu/DPT/tug_0109.pdf

Shumway-Cook, A., Matsuda, P. N., & Taylor, C. (2015). Research report. Investigating the validity of the environmental framework underlying the original and modified Dynamic Gait Index. *Physical Therapy, 95*(6), 864-870

Shumway-Cook, A., Taylor, C., Matsuda, P., Studer, M., & Whetten, B. K. (2013). Expanding the scoring system for the Dynamic Gait Index. *Physical Therapy, 93*(11), 1493-1506.

Stevenson, T. (2001). Detecting change in patients with stroke using the Berg Balance Scale. *Australian Journal of Physiotherapy, 47*(1), 29-38.

Stevenson, T., Connelly, D., Murray, J., Huggett, D., & Overend, T. (2010). Threshold Berg Balance Scale scores for gait-aid use in elderly subjects: A secondary analysis. *Physiotherapy Canada, 62*(2), 133-140.

Takacs, J., Garland, S. J., Carpenter, M. G., & Hunt, M. A. (2014). Validity and reliability of the Community Balance and Mobility Scale in individuals with knee osteoarthritis. *Physical Therapy, 94*(6), 866-874.

Tinetti, M., Mendes de Leon, D., Doucette, J., & Baker, D. (1994) Fear of falling and fall-related efficacy in relationship to functioning among community-living elders. *Journal of Gerontology, 49*(3), M140–M147.

Tinetti, M., Richman, D., & Powell, L. (1990). Falls efficacy as a measure of fear of falling. *Journal of Gerontology, 45*(6), P239-P243.

Tyson, S. (2004). *Brunel Balance Assessment (BBA)* (1st ed.). Salford, United Kingdom: Centre for Research and Human Performance Research, University of Salford.

Tyson, S., & DeSouza, L. (2004). Development of the Brunel Balance Assessment: A new measure of balance disability post stroke. *Clinical Rehabilitation, 18*(7), 801-810.

Tyson, S., Hanley, M., Chillala, J., Selley A., & Tallis, R. (2007). The relationship between balance, disability, and recovery after stroke: Predictive validity of the Brunel Balance Assessment. *Neurorehabilitation and Neural Repair,* (4), 341-346.

Whitney, S., Wrisley, D., & Furman, J. (2003). Concurrent validity of the Berg Balance Scale and the Dynamic Gait Index in people with vestibular dysfunction. *Physiotherapy Research International, 8*(4), 178-186.

Whitney, S., Marchetti G., Schadee, A., & Wrisley, D. (2004). The sensitivity and specificity of the Timed 'Up & Go' and the Dynamic Gait Index for self-reported falls in persons with vestibular disorders. *Journal of Vestibular Research, 14*, 397-409.

Yardley, L., Beyer, N., Hauer, K., Kempen, G., Piot-Ziegler, C., & Todd C. (2005). Development and initial validation of the Falls Efficacy Scale-International (FES-I). *Age Ageing, 34*(6), 614-619

IV

Caregiver Level of Burden

Bortnick, K.
*Occupational Therapy Assessments for Older Adults: 100 Instruments for
Measuring Occupational Performance* (pp. 61-68).
© 2017 Taylor & Francis Group.

Chapter 22: Caregiver Strain Index (CSI) and Modified Caregiver Strain Index (mCSI)

Description

The Caregiver Strain Index (CSI) by Robinson (1983) is a 13-item questionnaire originally created to screen for caregiver strain experienced after hospital discharge of a family member (Thornton & Travis, 2003). The CSI is both objective and subjective and examines three dimensions associated with the level of burden a person may be experiencing (perception of care-giving, care-recipient characteristics, and emotional status) as well as the following eight foundational concepts: (1) care recipient mental functioning, (2) physical functioning, (3) global functioning, (4) medication complexity, (5) age of caregiver, (6) age of care recipient, (7) length of time of caregiving, and (8) family caregiver medication administration issues (Thornton & Travis, 2003). During the assessment the subject is asked, through self-report or interview, to consider if they are experiencing strain along a 2-point dichotomous scale where 0=no and 1=yes for the 13 categories of questions. Scores range from 0 to 13 and higher scores suggest more perceived strain. A modified version developed Thornton and Travis (2003) is also available that uses the same original 13 categories; however, some clarifications were made to the wording which has resulted in increased sensitivity (Sullivan, 2007). Also, the scoring rubric was upgraded to a 3-point scale (0 to 2) where 0=no on a regular basis, 1=sometimes, and 2=yes. The maximum score of the modified CSI (mCSI) is 26 with a range of 0 to 26, and like the original, higher scores indicate more strain. Both version can be completed in less than 5 minutes.

Table 22-1
Question Categories on the Caregiver Strain Index and Modified Caregiver Strain Index
• Sleep disturbance
• Inconvenience
• Physical strain
• Feelings of confinement
• Family adjustments
• Changes in personal plans
• Feeling overwhelmed
• Demands on personal time
• Emotional adjustments
• Finances
• Work adjustments
• Changes from former self
• Upsetting behavior
Adapted from Thornton, M., and Travis, S. S. (2003). Analysis of the reliability of the modified caregiver strain index. *The Journals of Gerontology, 58B*(2), S129.

Psychometrics

Internal consistency (Cronbach's alpha) for the original 13-item CSI was found to be α = 0.86 among a sample of spouses, family, friends, and neighbors, aged 22 to 83 years, who provided varying degrees of care to recently hospitalized hip surgery and heart patients aged 65 years and over (Robinson, 1983). A convenience sample of 26 partners of stroke patients found reproducibility of the CSI to be very good at r= 0.93 with a range of 0.84 to 0.97 (Post, Festen, van der Port, & Visser-Meily, 2007). Another study of stroke patient spouses (n = 116) found that the median CSI score at both the 3- and 6-month interval was 5 and the correlation between those time frames was r = 0.86 (Blake, Lincoln, & Clarke, 2003). At 3 months, 45 (39%) spouses considered themselves strained and 71 (61%) as not strained, while at 6 months 46 (40%) spouses were strained and 70 (60%) were not strained with highest scores for feeling overwhelmed, having to change personal plans, and feelings of confinement (Blake et al., 2003). The internal reliability coefficient for the modified CSI, using a long-term caregiving sample, was 0.90, whereas 2-week retest data also resulted in a good test-retest reliability coefficient of r = 0.88 (Thornton & Travis, 2003). The same study found that caregiver age had a significant inverse correlation with caregiver strain (r = −0.33) suggesting that younger long-term caregivers experienced higher levels of caregiver strain. It was also determined that the age of the care recipient was significantly correlated with caregiver strain (r = 0.17), suggesting that the older the care recipient, the greater the level of caregiver strain (Thornton & Travis, 2003).

Advantages

Both the CSI and the mCSI are brief, easily administered, self-report/interview questionnaires that require no special training and can be used by various members of the treatment team (i.e., occupational therapists, nurses, social workers) to identify those individuals who may benefit from more in-depth assessment and follow-up between team members (Sullivan, 2007). Its results can be used to document the causes of strain and changes in strain over time, and the expanded scoring system of the mCSI has been shown to decrease floor/ceiling effects as well as improve the sensitivity and specificity of the original (Onega, 2008).

Disadvantages

Some have noted inconsistencies in how scores are interpreted as there is no breakdown of scores regarding low, moderate, or high perceived caregiver strain; thus, professional judgment is needed to evaluate the total score and level of caregiver strain (Sullivan, 2007). Others have noted that caregiver strain may vary depending on ethnic and cultural influences as well, making burden of care difficult to ascertain in some populations (Onega, 2008). Finally, there is some research to suggest the inclusion of positive aspects of caring when quantifying strain as a number of characteristics are associated with mediating the role of stress in caring not utilized in either CSI (Al-Janabi, Frew, Brouwer, Rappange, & Van Exel, 2010).

Administration

Testing for both versions of the CSI have clearly outlined basic instructions which require the person to consider each question and apply it to his or her own life circumstance. For example, during administration the subject reads or is told that items on the assessment include issues that other caregivers have found to be difficult and are asked to put a check mark for the answer that is most appropriate to them (i.e., 2 = yes on a regular basis, 1 = yes sometimes, or 0 = no for the mCSI, and either 1 = yes or 0 = no on the CSI). Each question then includes an example of what a caregiver may be experiencing to help the subject apply the question correctly. For instance, the question of "My sleep is disturbed" includes the illustration of "The person I care for is in and out of bed or wanders around at night."

Permissions

Each assessment is free to use in individual practice. Use of either the CSI or the mCSI in research, publication, or commercial purposes can be obtained by contacting the creators of the measure at the information following or contacting the publishers of the original work (for both tests it is the Gerontological Society of America). More information can be found in the following journal articles:

Robinson, B. C. (1983). Validation of a caregiver strain index. *Journal of Gerontology, 38*, 344-348.
Thornton, M., & Travis, S. S. (2003). Analysis of the reliability of the modified caregiver strain index. *The Journals of Gerontology, 58B*(2), S127-32.

Summary

POPULATION	Caregiver
TYPE OF MEASURE	Self-report or interview questionnaire
WHAT IT ASSESSES	Level of strain
TIME	<5 minutes
COST	Free

Contact

Shirley S. Travis, PhD, APRN, FAAN

Faculty—College of Health and Human Services

George Mason University

Fairfax, Virginia

Web: www.novahealthforce.com/about/steering/travis. html

CHAPTER 23: ZARIT BURDEN INTERVIEW (ZBI)

Description

The Zarit Burden Interview (ZBI), by Zarit and Zarit (1987) is a 22-item questionnaire designed to measure the extent to which a caregiver perceives his or her level of burden as a result of caring for a person with a particular diagnosis. Initially developed to measure strain associated with the care of community-dwelling older persons it has subsequently been validated across many patient populations and is a common measure of caregiver burden. Based on the original 29-item scale, the ZBI has undergone several modifications which has resulted in the current 22-item assessment. ZBI questions comprise 5 domains: (1) burden in the relationship (6 items), (2) emotional well-being (7 items), (3) social and family life (4 items), (4) finances (1 item), and (5) loss of control over one's life (4 items). Most of the items explore either personal strain (12 items) or role strain (6 items). The ZBI uses a 4-point ordinal scale which describes the degree of burden being experienced from 0 = never to 4 = almost always and takes about 10 minutes to complete. The maximum score is 88 with higher scores indicative of more burden. Example questions include the following: (1) do you feel stressed between caring for your relative and trying to meet other responsibilities for your family work; (2) do you feel embarrassed over your relative's behavior; and (3) do you feel that your relative asks for more help than he or she needs?

Psychometrics

A study of 152 dyads of community dwelling older adults with neurocognitive disorders (NCD) of the dementia type determined that the primary caregiver was typically a spouse (49.3%), an adult child (44.2%), other (niece, nephew, neighbor, friend; 4.3%), or regular home help (2.2%) of the care recipient. Study results showed the mean ZBI score for those caregivers to be 32.9, which according to established cutoff scores burden was *severe* for 13 caregivers (8.6%), *moderate to severe* for 32 caregivers (21%), *mild to moderate* for 72 caregivers (47.4%), and *absent to mild* for 35 caregivers or (23%) (Ankri, Andrieu, Beaufils, Grand, & Henrard, 2005). A study by Schreiner, Morimoto, Arai, and Zarit (2006) found that high scores on the ZBI were significantly related to a decrease in mental and physical health, as well as decreased vitality and social functioning, and determined that a cutoff score of 25 correctly identified 77% of high-burden stroke caregivers as having further need of assessment for depression, while a cutoff of 26 identified 64% of general disability caregivers with probable depression. A cutoff of 24 for the combined sample had a positive predictive value of 64% and a negative predictive value of 72%. Research

incorporating several studies found that the average estimate of internal consistency as measured by Cronbach's alpha was $\alpha = 0.86$ (Bachner & O'Rourke, 2007). Test-retest reliability was also found to be good at $r = 0.89$ among adult family caregivers (n = 149) of persons with NCD dementia (Seng et al., 2010).

Advantages

The ZBI is a relatively quick measure that is easy to administer and can be completed in less than 10 minutes. There is a significant amount of research in support of its use in clinical practice and it is considered by many to be the gold standard for determining level of caregiver burden. Hérbert, Bravo, and Préville (2000) argue that the ZBI is culturally neutral, as they found scores to be unrelated to age, gender, locale, language, living situation, marital status, or employment status, suggesting its appropriateness across many patient populations. A 12-item brief version is also available by Bédard et al. (2001). Based on the original, it consists of only items with the highest correlations as well as reflecting upon the original domains of personal strain and role strain, which has shown acceptable indices of internal consistency for both ($\alpha = 0.88$ and a 0.78) (O'Rourke & Tuokko, 2003).

Disadvantages

Wantz and Barker (2012) argue that the self-checklist format of the ZBI can be limiting, and similar to the disadvantages of the CSI discussed in Chapter 22, positive aspects of caregiving that might reduce feelings of burden are not explored. Wantz and Barker (2012) also suggest that a clinician could create a structured interview with the client that could be as effective in determining ongoing problems of caregiver stress.

Administration

The ZBI has standardized instructions and assessment requires the person to consider 22 objective and subjective statements and how they relate to the level of caregiver burden that they may or may not be experiencing. Example questions include: "Do you feel you should be doing more for your relative?" or "Do you feel you have lost control of your life since your relative's illness?" Where both would be scored as either (0) never, (1) rarely, (2) sometimes, (3) quite frequently, or (4) nearly always. Items are then summed and total scores are interpreted as follows: 0 to 21 little or no burden, 21 to 40 mild to moderate burden, 41 to 60 moderate to severe burden, and 61 to 88 severe burden.

Permissions

The ZBI can be accessed through the MAPI Research Trust education information dissemination website and can be used in clinical practice if requested first. A user agreement is necessary if it is to be used for commercial or research purposes. Distribution fees may be requested according to the study design and context of use of the questionnaire. More information can be found in the following publications:

Zarit, S. H., Reever, K. E., Bach-Peterson, J. (1980). Relatives of the Impaired elderly: Correlates of feelings of burden. *The Gerontologist, 20*(6), 649-55.

Zarit, S. H. & Zarit, J. M. (1990). *The Memory and Behavior Problems Checklist and the Burden Interview.* University Park, PA: Penn State Gerontology Center.

Summary

POPULATION	Caregiver
TYPE OF MEASURE	Self-report or interview questionnaire
WHAT IT ASSESSES	Level of burden
TIME	< 5 minutes
COST	Free

Contact

MAPI Research Trust

27, rue de la Villette

69003 Lyon, France

Phone: +33 (0) 472-13-65-75

Email: contact@mapi-trust.org

Website: www.mapi-trust.org

REFERENCES

Al-Janabi, H., Frew, E., Brouwer, W., Rappange, D., & Van Exel, J. (2010). The inclusion of positive aspects of caring in the Caregiver Strain Index: Tests of feasibility and validity. *International Journal of Nursing Studies, 47*, 984–993.

Ankri, J., Andrieu, S., Beaufils, B., Grand, A., & Henrard, J. C. (2005). Beyond the global score of the Zarit Burden Interview: Useful dimensions for clinicians. *International Journal of Geriatric Psychiatry, 20*(3), 254-260.

Bachner, Y., & O'Rourke, N. (2007). Reliability generalization of responses by care providers to the Zarit Burden Interview. *Aging & Mental Health, 11*(6), 678-685.

Bédard, M., Molloy, D., Squire, L., Dubois, S., Lever, J., & O'Donnell, M. (2001). The Zarit Burden Interview: A new short version and screening version. *The Gerontologist, 41*(5), 652-657

Blake, H., Lincoln, N., & Clarke, D. (2003). Caregiver strain in spouses of stroke patients. *Clinical Rehabilitation, 17*(3), 312-317.

Hérbert, R., Bravo, G., & Préville, M. (2000). Reliability, validity, and reference values of the Zarit Burden Interview for assessing informal caregivers of community-dwelling older persons with dementia. *Canadian Journal on Aging, 19*, 494-507.

O'Rourke, N., & Tuokko, H. (2003). Psychometric properties of an abridged version of the Zarit Burden Interview within a representative Canadian caregiver sample. *The Gerontologist, 43*(1), 121–127.

Onega, L. (2008). Helping those who help others: The modified Caregiver Strain Index. *American Journal of Nursing, 108*(9), 62-69.

Post, M., Festen, H., van der Port, I., & Visser-Meily, J. (2007). Reproducibility of the Caregiver Strain Index and the Caregiver Reaction Assessment in partners of stroke patients living in the Dutch community. *Clinical Rehabilitation, 21*(11), 1050-1055.

Robinson, B. C. (1983). Validation of a caregiver strain index. *Journal of Gerontology, 38*, 344-348.

Schreiner, A., Morimoto, T., Arai, Y., & Zarit, S. (2006). Assessing family caregiver's mental health using a statistically derived cut-off score for the Zarit Burden Interview. *Aging & Mental Health, 10*(2), 107-111.

Seng, B., Luo, N., Ng, W., Lim, J., Chionh, H., Goh, J., & Yap, P. (2010). Validity and reliability of the Zarit Burden interview in assessing caregiving burden. *Annals of the Academy of Medicine, Singapore, 39*(10), 758.

Sullivan, M. (2007). The Modified Caregiver Strain Index (CSI). The Hartford Institute for Geriatric Nursing. *Try This: Best Practices in Nursing Care to Older Adults, (14)*, 1-2.

Thornton, M., & Travis, S. (2003). Analysis of the reliability of the modified caregiver strain index. *The Journals of Gerontology, 58B*(2), S127-S132.

Wantz, R., & Barker, B. (2012). Memory and Behavior Problems Checklist and the Burden Interview. *Mental Measurements Yearbook with Tests in Print*, EBSCOhost (accessed February 6, 2014).

V

Cognitive Impairment

Bortnick, K.
Occupational Therapy Assessments for Older Adults: 100 Instruments for Measuring Occupational Performance (pp. 69-84).
© 2017 Taylor & Francis Group.

Chapter 24: Allen Cognitive Level Screen (ACLS)

Description

The Allen Cognitive Level Screen (ACLS) battery is a standardized assessment that requires the client to physically perform hand manipulation activities by stitching thin leather laces into various pieces of leather. The test is composed of three types of stitches: a running stitch (easiest), a whipstitch, and a single cordovan stitch (hardest), as well as two different sizes of leather to be stitched. It is thought that the somewhat complex activity of stitching has the ability to measure a person's attention, visuomotor control, and verbal performance that are considered important aspects of several occupational performance indicators. During assessment, the subject is graded according to his or her ability to cognitively understand and physically perform the activities relative to the amount and type of cues needed for successful task completion. The ACLS comprises seven scoring levels which can be used to predict a person's ability to engage in life tasks from (0) coma, (1) awareness, (2) gross body movements, (3) manual actions, (4) familiar activity, (5) learning new activities, and (6) planning new activities. Each level is further defined into sequential ascending abilities for more accurate scoring. For example, a person determined to be functioning at level 3.0 would be able to "grasp objects" and would require 24-hour nursing care to elicit habitual motions for activities of daily living (ADLs) and to complete motions for an acceptable level of hygiene, whereas a person functioning at level 3.8 would be able to "use all objects" with close supervision to get materials out that are needed to do ADLs, as well as to check results, and to remove dangerous objects (Allen, 1991). The assessment has no time limit but can typically be completed in less than 15 minutes.

Psychometrics

Early research found inter-rater reliability to be $r = 0.91$ among 20 subjects. (Howell, 1993). A study of the original 6 cognitive levels using 32 subjects found nearly perfect inter-rater reliability at $r = 0.99$ with levels ranging from 2 to 6 (Allen, 2000). A study of 71 persons admitted to a psychiatric unit found the mean score of the sample to be 4.9 with no significant correlations found between the ACLS, the Beck Depression Inventory, or the Minnesota Multiphasic Personality Inventory scales; however, a moderate correlation was found between the Symbol-Digit Modalities Test at $r = 0.520$ and subject age at $r = -0.424$ (David & Riley, 1990). A study of 31 persons post-stroke found a moderate positive correlation between the (large) ACLS activities (version 3 to 5.8) and the Assessment of Motor and Process Skills motor subtest (AMPS-M) at $r = 0.57$, as well as a moderate to high positive correlation between the AMPS-P process scale ($r = 0.66$) (Marom, Jarus, & Josman, 2006).

Advantages

The ACLS measures several domains such as cognitive, visuomotor, and hand/finger dexterity, and there is a fair amount of research in support of its use in clinical practice. It is easy to administer and no training or certifications are needed. Allen Conferences Inc. maintains a website devoted to the measure where it can be purchased along with other products offering insight into the ACLS.

Disadvantages

The test can be time consuming (> 30 minutes) and problematic for certain populations, such as those with major neurocognitive disorders or those individuals with advanced physical disability. Scoring may not accurately reflect ability for those clients with only hand or motor issues and no cognitive deficits.

Administration

The ACLS requires the subject to perform a leather lacing activity composed of lacing stitches of increasing complexity and includes a running stitch, whipstitch, and single cordovan stitch into two separate pieces of leather. The 7-level hierarchical scoring system of the ACLS has 27 separate scoring options or descriptors that are used to predict a subject's ability to engage in occupation and includes (2.4) Aimless Walking which is suggestive of the need for 24-hour nursing care to initiate and assist with all ADLs and to prevent wandering and getting lost (Allen, 1991). During assessment of the running and whipstitch various interventions and cueing may be used and scoring is relative to the amount and type of cues provided. When attempting the single cordovan stitch the task difficulty jumps from 4.4 to 5.8 as an outcome of creating an opportunity to observe learning without a demonstration (Allen, 2000)

Permissions

The ACLS can be purchased from several therapy supply companies as well as from the author's website for $60. To use in research or publication contacts its author at the information following. More information can be found in the following journal article:

Allen, C. (1991). Cognitive disability and reimbursement for rehabilitation and psychiatry. *Journal of Insurance Medicine, 23*(4), 245-247.

Summary

POPULATION	Suspected cognitive impairment
TYPE OF MEASURE	Activity based
WHAT IT ASSESSES	Ability to engage in occupations
TIME	<15 minutes for most populations
COST	$60

Contact

Allen Cognitive Level Screen

385 Coquina Ave

Ormond Beach, FL 32174

Phone: (800) 853-2472

Email: jim@allen-cognitive-levels.com

Web: www.allen-cognitive-levels.com

CHAPTER 25: FUNCTIONAL ASSESSMENT STAGING SCALE (FAST)

Description

The Functional Assessment Staging (FAST) by Reisberg (1988) is an observational rating tool developed to quantify the clinically identifiable stages of neurocognitive disorders (NCD) of the Alzheimer's and related types as well as age associated impairment. It is a procedure that describes a continuum of 16 successive stages and substages (from normal to severe) experienced by individuals with cognitive impairment through examination of the presence or absence of specific behaviors associated with decline. The concept of *staging* employed by FAST is unique in that it can identify pre-morbid and potentially manifest conditions associated with the evolution of the disease process, which is thought to follow a specific course, as well as the ability to track the latter stages of NCD dementias when most mental status assessments are no longer valid (Reisberg et al., 2011). FAST categorizes individuals into a 7-point rating scale (1 to 7) where a lower score is indicative of less impairment. Stages 6 and 7 are further divided into 11 subscales (6a to 6f and 7a to 7e) allowing the clinician to further enumerate the perceived phenomenon they are witnessing, thus allowing the clinician an important diagnostic and differential diagnostic tool (Auer & Reisberg, 1997). If the client is familiar, assessment can be as little as 5 minutes.

Psychometrics

FAST scale reliability studies have demonstrated rater consistency of $r = 0.86$ and rater agreement of $r = 0.87$, whereas the coefficient of reproducibility, a measure of uni-dimensionality, was 0.99 (a reproducibility higher than 0.9 indicates a valid scale; Sclan & Reisberg, 1992). When compared with the Ordinal Scales of Psychological Development (OSPD), FAST correlated significantly at −0.79 and levels ranged from −0.60 to −0.79 between individual FAST/OSPD subtests (Sclan & Reisberg, 1992). Another study found that the correlation between FAST and the Global Deterioration Scale (GDS) was 0.9 The correlation between the FAST and the Mini-Mental State Exam (MMSE) was observed to be 0.8 (Auer & Reisberg, 1997). A significant correlation between the FAST stage and the basic age (BA) value on the Tanaka–Binet intelligence scale (TB scale) was also observed ($r = 0.85$); however, the TB scale could not assess basic age through stage 7 because of floor effects (Masumi et al., 2003). A subsequent study by its authors suggest that the FAST staging procedure has the ability to account for more than twice the variance in temporal course explained by conventional mental status assessments and when used in conjunction with the GDS it can account

for approximately three times the variance explained by the MMSE alone (Auer & Reisberg, 1997). Finally, the predictive value of FAST was discussed by Komarova and Thalhauser (2011) where they noted the presence of large variations in disease progression in a cohort of 648 individuals and found that for stage 4 the typical amount of time person with NCD Alzheimer's spent was 2.1 years, stage 5, 1.8 years, and for 6 it was 4.3 years.

Advantages

The FAST scale is a simple observational tool that requires no special training and there is a good amount of research in support of its use in clinical practice. Another advantage of the FAST staging system is that it allows the assessment and staging of the various types of NCD throughout the entire range of the disablement process from normal aging to very severe, end-stage symptoms. This allows the designation of disease progress over time as well as the ability to determine if any changes in a person's condition are due to NCD or other conditions such as medication because NCD stages, as they relate to the FAST scale, are thought to occur in sequence (Komarova & Thalhauser, 2011). The FAST scale has shown to correlate well with other measures and is considered to be concordant with the GDS from which it was derived. Finally, the fact that FAST delineates 5 functional sub-stages between stage 6 and stage 7 is advantageous because many conventional measures experience floor/ ceiling effects in the final 6 to 8 substages of the disease process that FAST is able to differentiate.

Disadvantages

The FAST scale is not designed as a classical standardized assessment per se, and is dependent on skilled observation and knowledge of the disease process in order to correctly classify an individual along its continuum; thus, an understanding of each level's inclusion/exclusion criteria is necessary. The rater may find stages 6 and 7, which have 11 substages, particularly difficult when trying to evaluate the subtle nuances and markers of the disease toward the end stages.

Administration

The FAST scale is an observational tool in which a person's cumulative score is calculated by increasingly discerning the presence or absence of manifestations of neurocognitive impairment typical of that found in NCD of Alzheimer's and related types. Table 25-1 is an example of the 7 basic stages (excluding the 11 sub-stages between 6 and 7). More detailed scales and explanations can be found elsewhere or in Reisberg's 1988 article from *Psychopharmacology Bulletin*.

TABLE 25-1
THE 7 STAGES OF THE FUNCTIONAL ASSESSMENT STAGING SCALE
1. Normal adult: No functional decline.
2. Normal older adult: Personal awareness of some functional decline.
3. NCD Alzheimer and related type: Noticeable deficits in job and demanding situations.
4. Mild NCD: Requires assistance in complicated tasks such as handling finances, planning parties, etc.
5. Moderate NCD: Requires assistance in choosing proper attire.
6. Moderately severe NCD: Requires assistance dressing, bathing, and toileting. Experiences urinary and fecal incontinence
7. Severe NCD: Speech ability declines to about a half-dozen intelligible words. Progressive losses of abilities to sit up, smile, and hold head up.
Adapted from Reisberg, B. (1988). Functional Assessment Staging (FAST). *Psychopharmacology Bulletin, 24,* 653-659.

Permission

The FAST scale can be used freely in clinical practice. To use in research, publication, or for commercial purposes contact its developer. The FAST scale is wholly contained in the following article:

Reisberg, B. (1988). Functional Assessment Staging. (FAST). *Psychopharmacology Bulletin, 24*, 653-659.

Summary

POPULATION	NCD of the Alzheimer's and related types
TYPE OF MEASURE	Observational grading system
WHAT IT ASSESSES	Stage of the disease process presenting
TIME	<5 to 15 minutes
COST	Free

Contact

Barry Reisberg, MD

Department of Psychiatry

New York University Medical Center

New York, New York

CHAPTER 26: MINI-COG EXAM/CLOCK DRAWING TEST (CDT)

Description

The Mini-Cog is a quick screen for cognitive impairment that comprises two parts: a three-word registration and recall where the person is told three words that they must recall at a later time (0 to 2 points) and a clock-drawing task (0 or 2 points). The Mini-Cog can be completed in less than 5 minutes (less than 3-minutes in certain populations); thus, it can be effective in identifying those who require further investigation into their clinical presentation in fast paced settings such as emergency rooms or other settings that are time dependent (Thompson, 2008). During administration, the client is first asked to repeat three unrelated words, such as penny, apple, and chair, then he or she is asked to draw a clock with two hands denoting a specific time. The subject is then scored on his or her ability to complete each task where scores of 0, 1, or 2 denote probable impairment and 3, 4, or 5 indicate impairment is less likely.

Psychometrics

Research by the screen's creators found that when scores of those with "possible cognitive impairment" or "probably normal" were compared to the Mini Mental State Exam's (MMSE) cutoff score of 25, both batteries had similar sensitivity (0.76 vs 0.79) and specificity of 0.89 vs 0.88 (Borson, Scanlon, Chen, & Ganguli, 2003). Scores for both the Mini-Cog and MMSE were found to be comparable with that achieved using conventional neuropsychological batteries (0.75 sensitivity and 0.90 specificity) as well (Borson et al., 2003). A subsequent study, also by its creators, found that the Mini-Cog fared slightly better than the MMSE in accurately classifying impaired individuals at 83% for the Mini-Cog and 81% for the MMSE. The Mini-Cog was also found to be better at recognizing persons with neurocognitive disorders (NCD) of the Alzheimer type as opposed to other types such as Lewy body or vascular type. Costa, Severo, Fraga, and Barros (2012) had somewhat different results in their sample of 609 community dwelling Portuguese adults aged 60 years and over where they found that an MMSE cutoff score of 25 (6.2%) was considered impaired, whereas the Mini-Cog (at a cutoff score of 3) detected impairment in 11.3% of the sample. Research by Doerflinger (2007) found the Mini-Cog to have a sensitivity in detecting cognitive impairment ranging from 0.76 to 0.99, and specificity ranging from 0.89 to 0.93 at the 95% confidence interval.

A chi square test, which investigates the distribution of categorical variables, was reported at 234.4 for NCD of the Alzheimer's type and 118.3 for other NCD dementias, further highlighting its particular ability to detect NCD of the Alzheimer's type.

Advantages

The Mini-Cog is a simple screen that has a high sensitivity and acceptable specificity in the general practice setting (Kamenski et al., 2009). There is also evidence to suggest that the Mini-Cog has good predictive value in multiple clinical settings (Borson, Scanlan, Brush, Vitallano, & Dokmak, 2000; Borson et al, 2003). It is a quick screen (< 5 minutes to administer) and no training is needed. The assessment may be less stressful to clients than other longer mental status tests and when compared to the MMSE (which is arguably the gold standard), it showed close agreement with regard to sensitivity and negative predictive value, thus making the Mini-Cog a viable fast screen to decide if further testing is warranted (Doerflinger, 2007).

Disadvantages

Scoring for the CDT section can be difficult and is dependent on skilled observation; thus standardization of scoring could be somewhat problematic as it relies on a clinician's individual interpretation of a drawn clock which can be abundant. One study evaluating Mini-Cog cultural heterogeneity found that both its sensitivity (0.63) and specificity (0.59) were low among subjects with < 5 years of formal education when compared to subjects with 5 to 8 years of formal education where accuracy was better (Borson & Scanlan, 2006).

Administration

The Mini-Cog is composed of an interactive memory recall section in which a person is asked to recall three unrelated items. The client is then asked to complete a drawing-based activity in which a person is asked to draw a clock. The cumulative score is calculated by summing each item score where the test's maximum score is 5. A score of 0, 1, or 2 is suggestive of probable impairment and scores of 3, 4, or 5 suggests cognitive impairment is less likely.

Permission

The Mini-Cog is free to use in practice and can be downloaded at the website following, as well as others. Use of the assessment in research or publication can be obtained by contacting its creator. More information can be found in the following research article:

Borson, S., Scanlan, J. M., Watanabe, J., Tu, S. P., & Lessing, M. (2006). Improving identification of cognitive impairment in primary care. *International Journal of Geriatric Psychiatry, 21*, 349-355.

Summary

POPULATION	Suspected cognitive impairment (CI); general
TYPE OF MEASURE	Quick screen; cognitive recall and 1 clock-drawing activity
WHAT IT ASSESSES	Presence of CI
TIME	<5 minutes
COST	Free

Contact

Soo Borson, MD

Professor, Psychiatry and Behavioral Sciences

University of Washington

Seattle, Washington

Web: www.alz.org/documents_custom/minicog.pdf

CHAPTER 27: MINI-MENTAL STATE EXAMINATION (MMSE)

Description

The Mini-Mental State Examination (MMSE) by Folstein, Folstein, and McHugh (1975) is one of the most widely used scales for assessing cognitive ability and is considered by many to be the gold standard in its respective field. Designed as a brief quantitative measure of cognitive status, the MMSE can be used to screen for cognitive impairment (CI), estimate its severity, follow the course of cognitive changes over time, and document response to treatment (Monroe & Carter, 2012). The MMSE comprises 11 items across 6 domains and includes such items as recalling what year it is, correctly identifying a familiar object like a pencil, counting backward, and writing a sentence. The measure has clearly outlined scoring parameters that range from 0 to 30 with higher scores indicating less impairment. The MMSE can take up to 15 minutes to complete and the examiner's manual has well established norms across a number of age groups and populations.

TABLE 27-1
DOMAINS OF THE MINI MENTAL STATE EXAM
1. Orientation to time and place
2. Registration of three words
3. Attention and calculation
4. Recall of three words
5. Language
6. Visual construction

Psychometrics

Studies of reliability over a 24-hour period with single and multiple users found that the intra-rater reliability was r=0.88 when given by the same testers, and when using different testers, the inter-rater reliability was r=0.82 (Monroe & Carter, 2012). Research conducted as part of the larger QUALIDEM study of neurocognitive disorder (NCD) subjects found that the diagnostic values of a MMSE scores of ≤23 produced a sensitivity of 0.97 and specificity of 0.59 (Paquay, De Lepeleire, Schoenmakers, Ylieff, Fontaine, & Buntinx, 2006). A study of the oldest-old (n=435) established the sensitivity and specificity of the MMSE in identifying the various types of NCD in subjects aged 90 to 93 years with a college degree or higher found that at a cutoff score of ≤25 the sensitivity was 0.82 and specificity was 0.80; whereas in those aged 94 to 96 years with a college degree or higher at the suggested cutoff of ≤24, sensitivity was 0.85 and specificity was 0.80 (Kahle-Wrobleski, Corrada, Li, & Kawas, 2007). Research by Ala, Hughes, Kyrouac, Ghobrial, and Elble (2002) was able to differentiate between those individuals with NCD of the Lewy body (LB) and Alzheimer's type by examining differences between the attention and construction subtest scores where those with NCD LB fared worse than those with NCD Alzheimer's. For example, only 4/16 LB subjects were able to spell "world" backward correctly, whereas 18/26 Alzheimer's subjects spelled it correctly. Furthermore, only 1 LB subject was able to perform serial 7s correctly (counting backward by 7) and only 1 Alzheimer subject performed them incorrectly. The authors of the study determined that when the following mathematical equation was applied (Attention – 5/3 Memory + 5 x Construction) of the 3 sub-scores a score less than 5 points was associated with NCD LB with a sensitivity of 0.82 at a 95% confidence interval (CI) and a specificity of 0.81 also at a 95% CI (Ala et al., 2002). Finally, the following data published by Psychological Assessment Resources Inc. (PAR), the copyright holder, derived from a normative sample of more than 1500 individuals used to establish reliability and normal range of scores for the slightly modified MMSE-2, found that internal consistency ranged from α=0.66 to 0.79 with test-retest stability at ≥0.96 for all versions, while the interrater reliability of the measure ranged from 0.94 to 0.99 (PAR, 2011).

Advantages

There is a significant amount of research pertaining to the MMSE to support its use in clinical practice. It is also one of the most widely used cognitive batteries across numerous health professions. The MMSE is relatively quick and easy to administer and often can be completed in less than 10 minutes. It assesses a number of cognitive functions and does not require any specialized training. Several standardized versions of the measure are also available from PAR Inc, although the original is still the most established.

Disadvantages

Several researchers have argued that the utility of the MMSE decreases for persons with mild CI and one of the most frequently cited limitations is its poor sensitivity to mild cognitive decline, which may be due to the ease with which individuals perform most of the test items. Thus, it is argued that only severe impairment would prevent individuals from correctly answering most test items (Spencer et al., 2013). Other studies have noted the occurrence of floor/ceiling effects as well as an inability to differentiate between the various types of neurocognitive disorders (i.e., of the Alzheimer's or vascular type) (Monroe & Carter, 2012). Its cultural sensitivity has been questioned by some, as individuals with language, or sensory disorders or those with less than an eighth grade education may perform poorly (Monroe & Carter, 2012).

Administration

The MMSE is based mostly on client interview that consists of a series of questions and tasks grouped into 11 categories for which a maximum of 30 points can be obtained, and where a score of 23 or lower is widely accepted as the cutoff point, which suggests the presence of CI and a need for further evaluation (Albanese & Ward, 2003). Various scoring paradigms are available and a typical classification is as follows: 27 to 30, normal; 21 to 26, mild CI; 11 to 20, moderate CI; and 0 to 10, consistent with severe CI. The manual provides explicit instructions for administration and scoring and contains normative data based on a large sample of 18,056 individuals that are dissected by age and educational level to further aid in correctly classifying an individual's level of cognitive functioning (Albanese & Ward, 2003).

Permissions

Use of the original or modified versions of the MMSE can be obtained by contacting PAR Inc., who own the rights to the exam, where several versions such as the standard and expanded version of the test are available. The price for the standard full kit is roughly $200. PAR also handles requests by individuals or entities to use the measure in research, publication, or for commercial purposes. More information can found in the following original journal article:

Folstein, M. F., Folstein, S. E., & McHugh, P. R. (1975). Mini mental state: Practical method for grading the cognitive state of patients for the clinician. *Journal of Psychiatric Research, 12*, 189-198.

Summary

POPULATION	Suspected CI; general
TYPE OF MEASURE	Interview; cognitive-based activities
WHAT IT ASSESSES	Presence of or level of CI
TIME	≤15 minutes
COST	$200

Contact

PAR, Inc.

16204 North Florida Avenue

Lutz, FL 33549

Phone: (800) 331-8378

Web: www4.parinc.com/Search.aspx?q=mmse

Chapter 28: Montreal Cognitive Assessment (MoCA)

Description

The Montreal Cognitive Assessment (MoCA), developed by Nasreddine et al., (2005), is an interactive tool developed to detect mild cognitive dysfunction through the assessment of the cognitive domains of attention, concentration, executive function, memory, language, visuoconstructional skills, conceptual thinking, calculations, and orientation. The MoCA comprises 11 items and example items include drawing a line from a number to a letter in ascending order, copying a drawing of a cube as accurately as possible, and drawing a clock with hands at ten past eleven (11:10). The MoCA is similar to the Mini Mental State (MMSE; see Chapter 27) although it is somewhat more complex as it places greater emphasis on frontal executive function and attention tasks. Thus it is considered more sensitive in detecting mild cognitive impairment (MCI) as well as non-Alzheimer's neurocognitive disorder (NCD) when compared with the gold standard MMSE (Wong et al., 2013). The MoCA takes approximately 10 minutes to administer and the maximum possible score is 30. Higher scores are indicative of better executive functioning.

Table 28-1
Item Categories on the Montreal Cognitive Assessment
1. Alternating trail making
2. Visuoconstructional skills—cube
3. Visuoconstructional skills—clock
4. Sentence repetition
5. Abstraction
6. Delayed recall
7. Naming
8. Memory
9. Attention
10. Verbal fluency
11. Orientation

Adapted from Nasreddine, Z., Phillips, N., Bédirian, V., Charbonneau, S., Whitehead, V., Collin, I., Cummings, J., & Chertkow H. (2005). The Montreal Cognitive Assessment (MoCA©): A brief screening tool for mild cognitive impairment. *Journal of the American Geriatric Society 53*, 695–699.

Psychometrics

Preliminary studies of the reliability of the MoCA using 26 subjects over 35 days yielded high correlation coefficients at r = 0.92 for individual items (Nasreddine et al., 2005). Reliability, examined by Gill et al. (2008), using a sample of persons with Parkinson's disease, found that test-retest reliabilities were r = 0.79 while the inter-rater coefficient was 0.81. A convenience sample of 107 individuals with NCD of the Alzheimer's type and MCI found that the MoCA had moderate to significant correlations with the MMSE and the Dementia Rating Scale at 0.66 and 0.77, respectively (Lam et al., 2013). Smith, Gildeh, and Holmes (2007) found that using a MMSE cutoff score of 26, the assessment only had a sensitivity of 17% in detecting subjects with MCI whereas the MoCA's ability to detect MCI was 83%. Finally, a study of 185 veterans (mean age: 70 years) suggested a cutoff score of ≤ 20 should be considered rather than < 26 or 23 which others have argued as these cutoffs may have a tendency to "over pathologize" neurologically intact individuals (Waldron-Perrine & Axelrod, 2012).

Advantages

The MoCA is easy to administer and can be completed in ≤ 15 minutes; however, Olson, Chhanabhai, and McKenzie (2008) found that it could be completed in 10 minutes by 88% of TBI subjects. Some have also argued the MoCA to be superior to the MMSE at detecting mild cognitive changes. Several advantages it has over the MMSE are the fact that it incorporates more executive function and visuospatial items as well as the use of a five-word recall task to better probe subtle memory changes compared to the MMSE three-word task recall section (Lam et al., 2013). The MoCA is available in 34 languages and has been validated in many different cultural settings. Several versions of the assessment are available, including a 12-item short form. No special training or certifications are needed; however, they are available to the untrained clinician. Its creators maintain an informative interactive website where the measure can be downloaded and other relevant information, such as research updates, can be accessed as well.

Disadvantages

There is some research to suggest that the subtle differences between normal controls and MCI can be difficult to detect suggesting further testing may be warranted or that the MoCA exam may not have definitive prediction value. The problem was highlighted in research by Coen, Cahill, and Lawlor (2011) where they expressed concern that the MoCA may actually misclassify individuals as cognitively impaired. Others have raised questions about the measure's specificity which was only 0.50 in one study (Smith et al., 2007). Also, there is some evidence to suggest that the cutoff point recommended by the assessment's authors may be too high and that a lower cutoff point of 23 or below should be considered to increase specificity without compromising the sensitivity (Coen et al., 2011).

Administration

The MoCA has several activity components which encompass six subtests: visuospatial-executive functions, naming, attention, abstraction, recall, and orientation. Detailed instructions for testing and scoring can be obtained at the MoCA website. Example items include visuoconstructional skills or Cube administration, which requires the examiner to point to the cube and tell the subject to copy the drawing as accurately as possible in the space provided; while for the attention item the clinician reads to the person a list of five digits (i.e., 21854) and the subject then must repeat them in the correct ascending or descending order. Normative data established by the authors suggest that scores of 26 and above are considered normal, whereas those less than 26 are suggestive of MCI. A score of ≤22 is considered to be MCI, whereas those ≤16 are reflective of a NCD of the various types (Nasreddine et al., 2005; Wong et al., 2013). In order to increase cultural sensitivity for certain populations, one point is added for participants who have fewer than 12 years of education (Wong et al., 2013).

Permissions

The MoCA is free to use in private practice and may be used, reproduced, and distributed without permission to the following entities: universities, foundations, health professionals, hospitals, clinics, and public health institutes. Permission to use in research or publication can be obtained by contacting the copyright holder at the information following. More information can be found in the following journal article:

Nasreddine, Z., Phillips, N., Bédirian, V., Charbonneau, S., Whitehead, V., Collin, I.,…Chertkow H. (2005). The Montreal Cognitive Assessment (MoCA): A brief screening tool for mild cognitive impairment. *JAGS: Journal of the American Geriatric Society, 53*, 695–699.

Summary

POPULATION	Suspected MCI; general
TYPE OF MEASURE	Interview; cognitive-based activities
WHAT IT ASSESSES	Presence of or level of MCI
TIME	10 minutes
COST	Free

Contact

Z. Nasreddine, MD

CEDRA Center for Diagnosis and Research on Alzheimer's Disease

Email: info@mocatest.org

Web: www.mocatest.org/

Chapter 29: Short Orientation-Memory-Concentration Test or Short Blessed Test (SBT)

Description

The Short Orientation-Memory-Concentration Test, also known as the Short Blessed Test (SBT) or the Orientation–Memory–Concentration Test, developed by Katzman et al., (1983) is a weighted six-item instrument designed to identify those individuals with cognitive impairment. Derived from the original 26-item Blessed Test by Blessed (1968), the SBT evaluates orientation, registration, and attention. Initially validated on subjects in a skilled nursing facility and active community-dwelling senior citizens it has proved to be relevant across a number of patient populations as a quick screening tool that can be administered in less than 10 minutes. During the assessment, subjects are asked to answer items relating to the year and month, time of day, counting backward from 20, reciting the months backward, and to recall a queued memory phrase given by the clinician (Carpenter et al., 2011). Much like other assessments also discussed in this section, the SBT can be used to track changes in cognitive functioning over time and assess the effects treatment and medications may have on the person. The SBT employs a unique weighted scoring grid (0 to 28) where higher scores are indicative of more severe impairment.

Psychometrics

Analysis of the original 26-item Blessed Test revealed 5 items with high correlations. These items were then used to create the final 6 items of the SBT in which multiple $r = 0.96$ and $r^2 = 0.93$ were produced, respectively (multiple correlation r is equal to the correlation between the predicted scores and the actual scores and r^2 is the number that indicates how well the data fits the statistical model often represented by a line or curve; Katzman, et al., 1983). In a study of 133 patients referred to a department of neurology SBT was found to be significantly negatively correlated with the Mental Status Questionnaire (MSQ) at $r = -0.90$ as well as with the Mini Mental State Exam (MMSE) at $r = -0.93$ (Davous, Lamour, Debrand, & Rondot, 1987). Early research by Fillenbaum, Heyman, Wilkinson, and Haynes (1987) of 24 subjects with probable neurocognitive disorder of the Alzheimer's type compared the gold standard MMSE and the six-item SBT and found similar results as the negative correlation between the two was -0.83 with a test-retest correlation of $r = 0.89$ for the MMSE and $r = 0.77$ for the SBT, suggesting that the briefer measure SBT may be the preferred choice in many patient populations. In the Davous et al. (1987) study discussed prior, the

SBT displayed the ability to correctly identify impairment in 88% of persons vs 72% for MSQ and 81% for MMSE. In contrast, the MSQ and MMSE were able to correctly identify 97% of the subjects without impairment vs 94% for the SBT. The same study found that optimum sensitivity and specificity of 88% and 94% was achieved at a cutoff score of 10 or 11. Finally, a study by Carpenter et al. (2011) found that the SBT demonstrated a 95% sensitivity and had a specificity of 65% in detecting cognitive impairment in a geriatric emergency department and concluded that the SBT provided optimal overlap with the MMSE's cutoff score of ≤ 23.

Advantages

The SBT is a relatively quick outcome measure that can be completed in less than 10 minutes to test for cognitive impairment as well as to determine if further testing is warranted. Developed in 1983, there is a good amount of research in support of its use in clinical practice and requires no specialized training. It has also shown to correlate well with other outcome measures of cognitive impairment. Wade and Vergis (1999) argue that it is reasonably culture free in part because it assesses a relatively narrow area of cognition (i.e., is the person orientated; can the person concentrate on a short task; and can the person learn and recall some simple information), which may also be advantageous over other tests which cover wider areas that typically include perception and language (Wade & Vergis, 1999).

Disadvantages

Although research of subjects at a memory clinic found the SBT to be gender neutral, variation in scores were determined to be lower among persons with 8 years of education or less when compared with the other groups. No systematic difference was seen for other levels of education (i.e., high school or above) (Stuss, Meiran, Guzman, Lafleche, & Willmer, 1996). The same study also found education, and to a lesser extent, age to have a significant main effect (Stuss et al., 1996).

Administration

The SBT is administered in a standardized interview/interactive format and detailed instructions can be found for its administration which includes saying correct phrases for each item. The SBT uses a detailed weighted scoring grid for its 6 items (some items have multiple questions) and scores can range from 0 to 28, where higher scores are consistent with more cognitive impairment. Normative scoring data suggests 0 to 8 be considered normal to minimum impairment, while scores of 9 to 19 suggest minimal to moderate impairment, and 20 to 28 suggest severe impairment. The unique scoring system employed by the SBT includes individual test items being multiplied by a weighted factor allowing the measure to generate better sensitivity, specificity and discriminant ability in determining the presence of cognitive impairment.

TABLE 29-1

WEIGHTED SCORING SYSTEM OF THE SHORT BLESSED TEST

ITEM	NUMBER OF ERRORS (0 TO 5)	WEIGHTING FACTOR	SCORE
1			x 4
2			x 3
3			x 3
4			x 2
5			x 2
6			x 2
			Sum total =
			Range = 0 to 28

Permissions

The American Psychiatric Association (APA) holds the copyright for the SBT and it can be used freely for non-commercial purposes if requested first. It can be found in its entirety in numerous articles as well as the Internet. To use in research, publication, or for commercial purposes contact the APA. More information can be found in the following journal article:

Katzman, R, Brown, T., Fuld, P., Peck, A., Schechter, R., & Herbert Schimmel, (1983). Validation of a short orientation-memory concentration test of cognitive impairment. *American Journal of Psychiatry, 140*(6), 734-39.

Summary

POPULATION	Suspected cognitive impairment (CI); general
TYPE OF MEASURE	Interview; cognitive-based activities
WHAT IT ASSESSES	Presence of or level of CI
TIME	≤10 minutes
COST	Free

Contact

American Psychiatric Association

1000 Wilson Boulevard Suite 1825

Arlington, VA 22209

Phone: (888) 357-7924

Email: apa@psych.org

Web address: www.psych.org

Example of the SBT: http://alzheimer.wustl.edu/adrc2/Images/SBT.pdf

REFERENCES

Ala, T. A., Hughes, L. F., Kyrouac, G. A., Ghobrial, M. W., & Elble, R. J. (2002). The Mini-Mental State Exam may help in the differentiation of dementia with Lewy bodies and Alzheimer's disease. International *Journal of Geriatric Psychiatry, 17*(6), 503-509.

Albanese, M., & Ward, S. (2003). Review of the Mini-Mental State Examination. In B. Plake, J. Impara, & R. Spies. (Eds.). *15th mental measurements yearbook*. Lincoln, NE: Buros Institute of Mental Measurements.

Allen, C. (1991). Cognitive disability and reimbursement for rehabilitation and psychiatry. *Journal of Insurance Medicine, 23*(4), 245-247.

Allen, C. (2000) Allen Cognitive Level Screen and the Allen Battery. Allen Conferences Inc. Retrieved from www.allencognitivelevels.com/acls.htm

Auer, S., & Reisberg, B. (1997). The GDS/FAST staging system. *International Psychogeriatrics, 9*(S1), 167-171.

Borson, S., & Scanlan, J. (2006). The accuracy of the Mini-Cog in screening low-educated elderly for dementia. *Journal of the American Geriatrics Society, 54*(2), 376-378.

Borson, S., Scanlan, J. M., Brush, M., Vitallano, P., & Dokmak, A. (2000). The Mini-Cog: A cognitive 'vital signs' measure for dementia screening in multilingual elderly. *International Journal of Geriatric Psychiatry, 15*(11), 1021-1027.

Borson, S., Scanlan, J., Chen, P., & Ganguli, M. (2003). The Mini-Cog as a screen for dementia: Validation in a population-based sample. *Journal of the American Geriatrics Society, 51*(10), 1451-1454.

Carpenter, C., Bassett, E., Fischer, G., Shirshekan, J., Galvin, J., & Morris, C. (2011). Four sensitive screening tools to detect cognitive dysfunction in geriatric emergency department patients: Brief Alzheimer's Screen, Short Blessed Test, Ottawa 3DY, and the Caregiver-completed AD8. *Academic Emergency Medicine, 18*(4), 374-384.

Coen, R., Cahill, R., & Lawlor, B. (2011). Things to watch out for when using the Montreal Cognitive Assessment (MoCA). *International Journal of Geriatric Psychiatry, 26*(1), 107-108.

Costa, D., Severo, M., Fraga, S., & Barros, H. (2012). Mini-cog and Mini-Mental State Examination: Agreement in a cross-sectional study with an elderly sample. *Dementia and Geriatric Cognitive Disorders, 33*(2-3), 118-24.

David, S., & Riley, W. (1990). The relationship of the Allen Cognitive Level Test to cognitive abilities and psychopathology. *American Journal of Occupational Therapy, 44*(6), 493-497.

Davous, P., Lamour, Y., Debrand, E., & Rondot, P. A. (1987). Comparative evaluation of the Short Orientation Memory Concentration Test of cognitive impairment. *Journal of Neurology and Neurosurgery Psychiatry, 50*, 1312-17.

Doerflinger, D. (2007). Mental status assessment of older adults: The Mini-Cog. Try this: Best practices in nursing care to older adults. Retrieved from http://consultgerirn.org/uploads/File/try this/try_this_3.pdf

Fillenbaum, G., Heyman, A., Wilkinson, W., & Haynes, C. (1987). Comparison of two screening tests in Alzheimer's disease. The correlation and reliability of the Mini-Mental State Examination and the modified Blessed test. *Archives of Neurology, 44*(9), 924-927.

Folstein M., Folstein S., & McHugh P. (1975) Mini-Mental State: A practical method for grading the cognitive state of patients for the clinician. *Journal of Psychiatry Research 12*, 189-198.

Gill, D., Freshman, A., Blender, J., & Ravina, B. (2008). The Montreal Cognitive Assessment as a screening tool for cognitive impairment in Parkinson's disease. *Movement Disorders, 23*(7), 1043-1046.

Howell, R. F. (1993). *The Allen Cognitive Level Test–1990: Reliability studies with the depressed population*. Unpublished Master's Thesis, University of Florida. Gainesville, FL.

Kahle-Wrobleski, K., Corrada, M., Li, B., & Kawas, C. (2007). Sensitivity and specificity of the Mini-Mental State Examination for identifying dementia in the oldest-old: The 90+ Study. *JAGS: Journal of the American Geriatrics Society, 55*, 284-289.

Kamenski, G., Dorner, T., Lawrence, K., Psota, G., Rieder, A., Schwarz, F.,...Strotzka, S. (2009). Detection of dementia in primary care: Comparison of the original and a modified Mini-Cog assessment with the Mini-Mental State Examination. *Mental Health in Family Medicine, 6*(4), 209-217.

Katzman, R., Brown, T., Fuld, P., Peck, A., Schechter, R., & Schimmel, H. (1983). Validation of a Short Orientation-Memory-Concentration test of cognitive impairment. *American Journal of Psychiatry, 140*, 734-39.

Komarova, N., & Thalhauser, C. (2011). High degree of heterogeneity in Alzheimer's disease progression patterns. *PloS Computational Biology, 7*(11), 1-6.

Lam, B., Middleton, L., Masellis, M., Stuss, D., Harry, R., Kiss, A., & Black, S. (2013). Criterion and convergent validity of the Montreal Cognitive Assessment with screening and standardized neuropsychological testing. *JAGS: Journal of the American Geriatrics Society, 61*, 2181-2185.

Marom, B., Jarus, T., & Josman, N. (2006). The relationship between the Assessment of Motor and Process Skills (AMPS) and the Large Allen Cognitive Level (LACL) test in clients with stroke. *Physical and Occupational Therapy in Geriatrics, 24*(4), 33-50.

Masumi, S., Hayat, J., Meguro, K., Jafri, S., Atsushi, Y., & Reisberg, B. (2003). Correlation between functional assessment staging and the 'Basic Age' by the Binet Scale supports the retrogenesis model of Alzheimer's disease: A preliminary study. *Psychogeriatrics, 3*(2), 82.

Monroe, T., & Carter, M. (2012). Using the Folstein Mini Mental State Exam (MMSE) to explore methodological issues in cognitive aging research. *European Journal of Ageing, 9*(3), 265-274.

Nasreddine, Z., Phillips, N., Bédirian, V., Charbonneau, S., Whitehead, V., Collin, I.,...Chertkow H. (2005). The Montreal Cognitive Assessment (MoCA©): A brief screening tool for mild cognitive impairment. *Journal of the American Geriatric Society 53*, 695-699.

Olson, R., Chhanabhai, T., & McKenzie, M. (2008). Feasibility study of the Montreal Cognitive Assessment (MoCA) in patients with brain metastases. *Supportive Care in Cancer, 16*(11), 1273-1278

Paquay, L., De Lepeleire, J., Schoenmakers, B., Ylieff, M., Fontaine, O., & Buntinx, F. (2007). Comparison of the diagnostic accuracy of the Cognitive Performance Scale (Minimum Data Set) and the Mini-Mental State Exam for the detection of cognitive impairment in nursing home residents. *International Journal of Geriatric Psychiatry, 22*(4), 286-293.

Psychological Assessment Resources Inc. (2011). *Mini-Mental State Examination* (MMSE-2) (2nd ed.). Retrieved from www4.parinc.com/Products/Product.aspx?ProductID=MMSE-2

Reisberg, B. (1988). Functional Assessment Staging (FAST). *Psychopharmacology Bulletin, 24*, 653-659.

Reisberg, B., Jamil, I. A. Sharjeel Khan, S., Monteiro, I., Torossian, C., Ferris, S.,...Wegiel, J. (2011). *Staging Dementia. Principles and practice of geriatric psychiatry* (3rd ed., pp. 163-170). Hoboken, NJ: John Wiley & Sons.

Sclan, S., & Reisberg, B. (1992). Functional Assessment Staging (FAST) in Alzheimer's disease: reliability, validity and ordinality. *International Psychogeriatrics, 4*(Suppl. l), 55-69.

Smith, T., Gildeh, N., & Holmes, C. (2007). The Montreal Cognitive Assessment: Validity and utility in a memory clinic setting. *Canadian Journal of Psychiatry, 52*(5), 329-332.

Spencer, R., Wendell, C., Giggey, P., Katzel, L., Lefkowitz, D. Siegel, E., & Waldstein, S. (2013). Psychometric limitations of the Mini-Mental State Examination among nondemented older adults: An evaluation of neurocognitive and magnetic resonance imaging correlates. *Experimental Aging Research, 39*(4), 382-397.

Stuss, D., Meiran, N., Guzman, A., Lafleche, G., & Willmer, J. (1996). Do long tests yield a more accurate diagnosis of dementia than short tests? A comparison of 5 neuropsychological tests. *Archives of Neurology, 53*(10), 1033-1039.

Thompson, N. (2008). Mini-Cog: A screening tool for early mental decline. *BAMI. U.S. Bay Area Medical Information.* Retrieved from www.bami.us/Neuro/MiniCog.html

Wade, D., & Vergis, E. (1999). The Short Orientation Memory-Concentration Test: A study of its reliability and validity. *Clinical Rehabilitation, 13*(2), 164-170.

Waldron-Perrine, B., & Axelrod, B. (2012). Determining an appropriate cutting score for indication of impairment on the Montreal Cognitive Assessment. *International Journal of Geriatric Psychiatry, 27*(11), 1189-1194.

Wong, G., Lam, S., Wong, A., Ngai, K., Poon, W., & Mok, V. (2013). Comparison of Montreal Cognitive Assessment and Mini-Mental State Examination in Evaluating cognitive domain deficit following aneurysmal subarachnoid hemorrhage. *PloS One, 8*(4), 1-7.

VI

Levels of Consciousness

Bortnick, K.
Occupational Therapy Assessments for Older Adults: 100 Instruments for Measuring Occupational Performance (pp. 85-100).
© 2017 Taylor & Francis Group.

Chapter 30: Glasgow Coma Scale (GCS)

Description

The Glasgow Coma Scale (GCS), by Teasdale and Jennet (1974), is an interactive observation-based tool designed to describe the level of consciousness in patients with head injuries in order to facilitate the assessment and grading of brain dysfunction severity after a trauma. Developed to be a quick screen to determine if further examination is warranted, it measures three components: (1) eye opening, (2) motor, and (3) verbal response to various basic stimuli, as it is thought that the measurement of these allows the clinician to assess the function of the cerebral cortex, the upper brainstem, and the reticular activating system, where the eye-opening response measures the arousal mechanism of the brainstem; motor response; the integrity of cerebral cortex and spinal cord; and the verbal response, the integration of cerebral cortex and brainstem (Zuercher, Ummenhofer, Baltussen, & Walder, 2009). The GCS can be used as a tool to assist in the decision to intubate as well, and has been shown to be a better predictor of the need to intubate than the gag reflex (Holdgate, Ching, & Angonese, 2006). GCS scores range from 15 to 3 with lower scores indicating more severe impairment. A score of 14 to 15 is considered mild, 9 to 13 moderate, and 3 to 8 severe impairment. A modified scoring system was created based on several studies including the Canadian Computed Tomography Head Rule Study which suggest that a score of 13 be placed within the mild category of traumatic brain injury (TBI; mild, 13 to 15). However, results from a study by Mena, et al. (2011) question that decision where they plotted the odds of mortality after a TBI with GCS scores and found that a score of 13 was closer to score of 12 rather than a score of 14 (Mena et al., 2011). The following is a testing example of the eye opening response in which the person is scored as either (4) spontaneous-open with blinking at baseline, (3) to verbal stimuli, command, speech, (2) to pain only (not applied to face), and (1) no response. The GCS can be completed in less than 15 minutes.

Psychometrics

Results reporting agreement between GCS scores across a number of disciplines have shown only moderate inter-rater agreement; however, in persons with high GCS scores, inter-rater agreement has been shown to be excellent (Zuercher et al., 2009). Davis et al. (2006) suggested that "on-scene" GCS scores were strongly correlated with hospital admission and in more than 9000 non-intubated moderate to severe TBI patients a correlation coefficient of 0.67 was observed. A study of 538 persons admitted to the ICU found that those with GCS scores of 13 to 15 had a favorable outcome 93% of the time, which decreased to 83% in persons with scores of 10 to 12, 37% in scores of 7 to 9, and 10 % for scores of 3 to 6 where the mortality rate was 45% (Leitgeb et al., 2013). Those with scores of 3 to 6 found that as scores decreased mortality was 24%, 5%, and 3% with worsening GCS scores (Leitgeb et al., 2013). Finally, a study by Kevric, Jelinek, Knott, and Weiland (2011; n = 217) found that the GCS was strongly positively correlated with the Full Outline of Unresponsiveness Scale (FOUR) among 2 raters (r = 0.87 and r = 0.87); however, the inter-rater reliability for total FOUR Scale was superior to that of the GCS (0.76 and 0.59).

Advantages

The GCS is a relatively quick cognitive outcome measure that can be completed in less than 15 minutes and requires no special training or certifications. There is a good amount of research in support of its use in clinical practice and is considered by some to be a gold standard assessment. The GCS is also a component of several larger assessments such as the Acute Physiology and Chronic Health Evaluation II score, the (Revised) Trauma Score, the Trauma and Injury Severity Score, and the Circulation, Respiration, Abdomen, Motor, Speech Scale, demonstrating the widespread adoption of the scale (Majerus, Gill-Thwaites, Andrews, & Laureys, 2005). The Institute of Neurological Sciences and the Coma Science Group maintain websites devoted to the scale where one can obtain relevant information as well as downloads.

Disadvantages

Bazarian, Eirich, and Salhanick (2003) suggest that GCS has poor discriminant ability among those with scores in the moderate range. In addition, inter-rater reliability has been shown to be low for the motor component in some studies. Others have suggested that due to its ease of use, misinterpretations have occurred whereas others have argued that the application of painful stimuli (i.e., peripheral vs central) to elicit a particular response remains obscure and ill defined (McLernon, 2014). Another limitation of the scale is the fact that the GCS assesses verbal response; therefore, it is difficult to apply to a number of patient populations. However, a study found that many clinicians had a poor understanding of this, with only 46% agreeing with the statement that the GCS cannot be used on intubated patients (Kevric et al., 2011).

Administration

Both the GCS and modified version are interactive observational tools in which the clinician denotes the presence or absence of certain patient responses as well as the ability to perform rudimentary tasks and respond to specific stimuli relative to the eyes' ability to respond spontaneously to sound or pressure; a person's ability to respond to verbal cues to assesses if the person is orientated or confused; if he or she can respond to words or sounds; and finally, motor response, which examines if the person can obey commands and if he or she have localized normal flexion, abnormal flexion, or extension. Scores range from 0 to 15 with lower scores suggestive of more impairment.

TABLE 30-1	
EXAMPLE SCORING OF THE GLASGOW COMA SCALE	
EYE OPENING	**RATING**
Open before stimulus	Spontaneous
After spoken or shouted request	To sound
After fingertip stimulus	To pressure
No opening at any time	None
Closed by local factor	Untestable
Adapted from Teasdale, G. (2015) *Glasgow Coma Scale: Do it this way. GCS at 40.* Glasgow, Scotland: Institute of Neurological Sciences NHS Greater Glasgow and Clyde.	

Permissions

The GCS is free to use in clinical practice and can be downloaded at http://glasgowcoascale.org. Authorization to use the GCS outcome measure in research or publication can be obtained by contacting its authors or the Institute of Neurological Sciences at the information following. More information can be found in the following journal articles:

Jennett, B. (2002). The Glasgow Coma Scale: History and current practice. *Trauma, 4*(2), 91-103.

Teasdale, G., & Jennett, B. (1974). Assessment of coma and impaired consciousness. A practical scale. *Lancet, 2,* 81-84.

Summary

POPULATION	TBI; coma; trauma; disorders of consciousness
TYPE OF MEASURE	Rating scale; ability to respond to stimuli; rudimentary motor
WHAT IT ASSESSES	Level of neurobehavioral function
TIME	< 15 minutes
COST	Free

Contact

Paul Brennan, BSc (Hons), MB BChir MRCS (Ed), PhD

Edinburgh Cancer Research Centre

Edinburgh, Scotland

Web: www.ecrc.ed.ac.uk/Researchers/item/Dr-Paul-Brennan.html

Download the GCS at GCS at 40

Web: http://glasgowcomascale.org/

Email: http://glasgowcomascale.org/contact-us/

CHAPTER 31: JFK COMA RECOVERY SCALE-REVISED (CRS-R)

Description

The JFK Coma Recovery Scale (CRS) by Giacino et al. (1991) is a standardized instrument designed to measure the neurobehavioral function in persons with disorders of consciousness and was developed to more fully characterize and monitor patients functioning at level I (generalized response) to level IV (confused-agitated response) on the Rancho Los Amigos Levels of Cognitive Functioning Scale (Giacino & Kalmar, 2004; Giacino, Kalmar, & Whyte, 2004). Revised in 2005 by Giacino and Kalmar, modifications included the addition of new items, merging of items found to be statistically similar in terms of their ability to differentiate patients' neuro-behavioral status, the deletion of some items demonstrating poor fit, and renaming of items to provide better face validity for the behaviors they represent. The current CRS-Revised (CRS-R) comprises 6 subscales that quantify such things as auditory function and visual function where during assessment the individual is graded on their ability to react to specific stimuli such as localization to sound, object recognition, localization to noxious stimulation, oral reflexive movement, and attention (Wilde, Whiteneck, et al., 2010). There are a total of 23 scoring choices and each of the 6 subscales uses a Likert scale where scores can range from 0 to 6. The lowest score on each subscale typically represents basic reflexive activity while the highest items suggesting cognitively mediated behaviors (Giacino & Kalmar, 2005). The assessment takes approximately 10 minutes to complete where higher scores suggest increased cerebral ability/activity.

Psychometrics

A convenience sample of 80 subjects in a specialized coma intervention program found inter-rater reliability to be high (r = 0.84) with the lowest score for the visual subtest at 0.80 (Giacino et al., 2004). Test-retest reliability for the total score was also high (r = 0.94) with the lowest reliability for the oromotor/verbal subscale at 0.70, while total scores on the CRS-R were shown to correlate well with total scores on the original CRS at 0.97 as well as with the Disability Rating Scale (0.90) (Giacino et al., 2004). A study by Kalmar and Giacino (2005) of 20 subjects determined inter-rater reliability to be r = 0.84, test–retest reliability to be r = 0.94, and internal consistency to be α = 0.83. A convenience sample of 31 subjects found that inter-rater and test-retest reliabilities had a range of r = 0.65 to 0.82 with

2 raters over a 3-day period (Lovstad et al., 2010). A study of 44 patients who were clinically diagnosed as being in a vegetative state (VS), the CRS-R detected signs of awareness in 18 patients (41%) suggesting that they were actually in a minimally conscious state not VS (Schnakers et al., 2009). Misdiagnosis was greater for chronic patients than for acute patients and the behavioral signs detected in those misdiagnosed primarily included purposeful eye movements such as visual fixation and visual pursuit (Schnakers et al., 2009).

Advantages

The CRS-R is a relatively brief/simple assessment to administer. There is a fair amount of research in support of its use in clinical practice and it is an excellent way to track change in a person's consciousness level over time. The CRS-R is based on the first 4 levels of the Rancho Los Amigos Levels of Cognitive Functioning Scale thereby making it more sensitive to a person's level of consciousness across the levels pertaining to generalized response up to the confused–agitated response. No certifications are required and administration time is less than 10 minutes. CRS-R has also been translated to 11 languages suggesting it is a culturally relevant outcome measure.

Disadvantages

The detection of slight degrees of brain activity (i.e., an auditory startle or visual startle) required at the lowest levels of the assessment may be difficult for some individuals, which can lead to misdiagnosis or poor inter-rater reliability between clinicians.

Administration

During assessment, the client is presented with a stimuli and is scored on their ability to perform or react to that stimuli which typically occurs based on their level of consciousness. The assessment comprises 6 subtests that gauge a person's (1) auditory, (2) visual, (3) motor, (4) oromotor/verbal, (5) communication, and (6) arousal functioning. Each subtest uses a variable Likert scale ranging from 0 to 6, in which higher scores indicate increasing levels of consciousness. Total scores range from 0 to 23. Example items include eye movement commands where the clinician asks the subject to look at object #1 then look at object #2, as well as limb movement commands in which the clinician asks the subject to take object #1 and #2 and then kick object #1 and #2.

TABLE 31-1
EXAMPLE SCORING DOMAINS OF THE COMA RECOVERY SCALE-REVISED
MOTOR FUNCTION SCALE
6—Functional object use
5—Automatic motor response
4—Object manipulation
3—Localization to noxious stimulation
2—Flexion withdrawal
1—Abnormal posturing
0—None/flaccid
OROMOTOR/VERBAL FUNCTION SCALE
3—Intelligible verbalization
2—Vocalization/oral movement
1—Oral reflexive movement
0—None
Adapted from Giacino, J. T., & Kalmar, K. (2004). *CRS-R Coma Recovery Scale-Revised: Administration and Scoring Guidelines* (p. 1). Edison, NJ: Center for Head Injuries: JFK Johnson Rehabilitation Institution.

Permissions

The CRS-R is free to use in clinical practice. Consent to use in research or publication can be obtained by contacting the creators of the measure or its publishers at the information following. More information can be found in the following article:

Giacino, J. T., & Kalmar, K. (2005). The JFK Coma Recovery Scale—Revised. *Neuropsychological Rehabilitation. 15*(3/4), 454–460.

Summary

POPULATION	Traumatic brain injury; coma; disorders of consciousness
TYPE OF MEASURE	Rating scale; ability to respond to stimuli; basic cognitive and motor
WHAT IT ASSESSES	Level of neurobehavioral function
TIME	< 10 minutes
COST	Free

Contact

Joseph Giacino, PhD

Spaulding Rehabilitation Hospital

Harvard Medical School

Boston, Massachusetts

Kathleen Kalmar, PhD

JFK Johnson Rehabilitation Institute

Institute at JFK Medical Center

Brain Trauma Unit 3 ER/Neuropsychology

Edison, New Jersey

Examiner's manual: www.tbims.org/combi/crs/CRS%20Syllabus.pdf

Chapter 32: Neurological Outcome Scale for Traumatic Brain Injury (NOS-TBI)

Description

The Neurological Outcome Scale for Traumatic Brain Injury (NOS-TBI) is a standardized assessment tool of neurological function that is based on the National Institutes of Health Stroke Scale (NIHSS) that has been uniquely modified to take into account the specific neurological deficits that may occur with head injury (Rosenfeld, 2012). The scale contains domains that are similar to the NIHSS such as level of consciousness, best gaze, visual field, facial palsy, motor arm and motor leg assessment; as well the inclusion of new items such as olfaction, pupillary response, and auditory functioning (McCauley et al., 2013). The NOS-TBI contains 15 items which have 23 components (i.e., some items have multiple modules) and takes approximately 15 minutes to complete. During assessment the clinician notes the presence or absence of certain responses to varying stimuli. An example item includes level of consciousness in which the subject is observed through examination, his or her level of arousal is then scored as (0) alert, (1) not alert, but arousable with minimal stimulation, (2) not alert, requires repeated stimulation to attend, or (3) coma—responds only with reflex motor or autonomic effects or totally unresponsive. Each item is rated by level of impairment from 0 to 5 (varies) with higher scores representing more impairment (Wilde, McCauley, Kelly, Levin, et al., 2010).

Psychometrics

Statistical properties of the NOS-TBI were established by Boake et al., (2010) in which test-retest reliability scores obtained over 2 consecutive days performed by the same rater were significant at $r = 0.97$. Internal consistency for all items was also significant at $\alpha = 0.94$; however, several test items had low correlations from 0.34 to 0.84. Convergent validity displayed moderate to significant correlations with the Disability Rating Scale at 0.75, the Supervision Rating Scale at 0.59, and the Rancho Los Amigos Scale at −0.60. A research study of individuals who had sustained a TBI (n = 50) with a mean Glasgow Coma Scale score of 6 (which only tests for rudimentary eye, verbal, and motor responses) found that the most common anomalies discovered using the NOS-TBI were impaired olfaction, present in 76% of subjects, language impairment (46%), disorientation (42%), impairment in gross motor functioning (30% to 38%), facial paresis (30% to 34%), and sensory functioning (14% to 28%) (Wilde, McCauley,

Kelly, Weyand, et al., 2010). Another study demonstrated good-to-excellent concurrent validity with other outcome measures at 3, 6, and 12 months post-injury where correlations ranged from 0.44 to 0.70 with the Glasgow Outcome Scale and its extended version, the Disability Rating Scale, and the Neurobehavioral Rating Scale-Revised (McCauley et al., 2013). The same study showed that NOS-TBI scores changed significantly between 3 and 6 months, which was contrary to the Glasgow measures, suggesting that the NOS-TBI was more sensitive to change over the 3- to 6-month time period (McCauley et al., 2013).

Advantages

The NOS-TBI is a relatively quick outcome measure that has a fair amount of research in support of its use in clinical practice. Adapted from the NIHSS, it can be completed in less than 15 minutes. The NOS-TBI incorporates elements of a clinical neurological examination not seen in other TBI-specific assessments and due to its increased complexity, may play an important contribution when used in conjunction with other scales such as the Glasgow Coma Scale for initial stratification of injuries based on severity as well as for outcome assessment (Rosenfeld, 2012). The NOS-TBI is also included as part of several larger measures such as the National Institute of Neurological Disorders and Stroke and the Federal Interagency Common Data Elements Initiative for TBI also suggesting widespread use and acceptance (McCauley et al., 2013).

Disadvantages

Administration of the measure to severely injured or those in the sub-acute phase of recovery can be difficult and although there is a fair amount of research supporting the assessment, the NOS-TBI lacks an amount of peer-reviewed literature especially not involving the authors, directly or indirectly (Wilde, McCauley, Kelly, Levin, et al., 2010).

Administration

During assessment the clinician assess gross neurological functioning relative to an individual's motor and sensory function where each of the 23 items are rated on the subject's ability to respond to certain stimuli or perform basic movements. Test items are scored along a variable scale (0 to 5) where 0 represents alert or no impairment and 5 represents coma. The total score for the NOS-TBI is the sum of the scores for items 1 to 13, whereas items

14 and 15 are considered supplemental and do not factor into the total score, a UN item score is also possible which is considered as untestable (i.e., limb is missing or joint is fused) (McCauley et al., 2010).

TABLE 32-1
ITEMS ASSESSED ON THE NEUROLOGICAL OUTCOME SCALE FOR TRAUMATIC BRAIN INJURY

1A to 1C	Level of consciousness—arousal, orientation, commands
2	Gaze
3A and 3B	Visual field— right and left
4	Pupillary response
5A and 5B	Hearing— right and left
6A and 6B	Facial paresis— right and left
7A and 7B	Motor upper extremity (UE)—right and left
8A and 8B	Motor lower extremity (LE)—right and left
9A and 9B	Sensory UE—right and left
9C and 9D	Sensory LE—right and left
10	Language
11	Dysarthria
12	Neglect—extinction
13	Olfaction
14	Gait ataxia
15A and 15B	Limb ataxia—right and left

Adapted from Wilde, E., McCauley, S., Kelly, T., Levin, H., Pedroza, C., Clifton, G.,…Moretti, P. (2010). Feasibility of the Neurological Outcome Scale for Traumatic Brain Injury (NOS-TBI) in adults. *Journal of Neurotrauma, 27*(6), 975–981.

Permissions

The NOS-TBI is located in the public domain, thus free to use in clinical practice. Its use in research or publication can be obtained by contacting the creators of the scale or its publishers at the information that follows. The assessment is wholly contained in the following journal article:

Wilde, E. A., McCauley, S. R., Kelly, T. M., Levin, H. S., Pedroza, C., Clifton, G. L.,…Moretti, P. (2010). Feasibility of the Neurological Outcome Scale for Traumatic Brain Injury (NOS-TBI) in adults. *Journal of Neurotrauma, 27*(6), 975–981.

Summary

POPULATION	TBI; disorders of consciousness
TYPE OF MEASURE	Rating scale; ability to respond to stimuli; basic motor ability
WHAT IT ASSESSES	Level of neurobehavioral and motor function
TIME	< 15 minutes
COST	Free

Contact

Elisabeth A. Wilde, PhD

Cognitive Neuroscience Laboratory

Baylor College of Medicine

Houston, Texas

Chapter 33: Rancho Los Amigos Levels of Cognitive Functioning Scale (RLAS)—Third Edition

Description

The Rancho Los Amigos Levels of Cognitive Functioning Scale (RLAS) by Hagen, Malkmus, and Durham (1972), is an outcome measure used to describe an individual's cognitive functioning after a traumatic brain injury (TBI) and is commonly used as a descriptive tool to track a person's level of recovery following TBI (Zollman, 2011). Revised several times, its development is based on the assumption that if recovery is possible, a patient would regain cognitive functioning in a definable and predictable pattern and that, over time, changes in the patient's behavior would provide indices of those changes in recovery of cognitive function. (Flannery, 1998). The current version contains 10 levels designed to describe a person's conscious state as well as his or her level of participation in activities of daily living (ADLs) as he or she begins to regain function following injury. Levels on the scale include (1) no response (total assistance), (2) generalized response (total assistance), and (3) localized response (total assistance). Each level comprises several descriptors that the clinician can use to gauge whether or not the patient is to be scored at a particular level; for example, in level 3, localized response, total assistance criteria include the following: (1) demonstrates withdrawal or vocalization to painful stimuli, (2) turns toward or away from auditory stimuli, (3) blinks when strong light crosses visual field, (4) follows moving object passed within visual field, (5) responds to discomfort by pulling tubes or restraints, (6) responds inconsistently to simple commands, (7) responds directly related to type of stimulus, and (8) may respond to some persons (especially family and friends) but not to others. The assessment can be completed in less than 15 minutes where a higher level score is considered to be better performance.

TABLE 33-1		
LEVELS OF THE RANCHOS LOS AMIGOS SCALE		
LEVEL	RESPONSE	AMOUNT OF ASSISTANCE
1	No response	Total assistance
2	Generalized response	Total assistance
3	Localized response	Total assistance
4	Confused, agitated	Maximum assistance
5	Confused, inappropriate, non-agitated	Maximum assistance
6	Confused, appropriate	Moderate assistance
7	Automatic, appropriate	Minimal assistance for ADLs
8	Purposeful, appropriate	Stand by assistance
9	Purposeful, appropriate	Stand by assistance on request
10	Purposeful, appropriate	Modified independent

Adapted from Stenberg, M., Godbolt, A. K., Boussard, C. N., Levi, R., & Stalnacke, B. M. (2014). Cognitive impairment after severe traumatic brain injury, clinical course and impact on outcome: A Swedish-Icelandic study. *Behavioural Neurology*, 2015, Article ID 680308, p. 3.

Psychometrics

Gouvier, Blanton, and LaPorte (1987) found early test-retest reliabilities to be good (r = 0.82) while inter-rater reliability was also good, ranging from r = 0.87 to 0.94. Concurrent validity was established where predictive validity of the scale was assessed by correlations with discharge scores of the Glasgow Outcome Scale (0.57) and expanded Glasgow Outcome Scale (0.68) in 40 TBI patients admitted to an acute rehabilitation facility. A later study by Beauchamp et al. (2001) found inter-rater reliability to be high (r = 0.91). The same study found correlations between the scores of different pairs of observers to be high as well at 0.84. A regression analysis of 219 severe TBI subjects' long-term oropharyngeal dysphagia (> 6 weeks) revealed that low RLAS scores were associated with being discharged from an acute-care hospital with a feeding tube as 96 subjects with a mean score of 3.7 (1.6) received a feeding tube which was contrary to 123 patients who had a mean RLAS score of 5.1 (1.8) who did not (Mandaville, Ray, Robertson, Foster, & Jesser, 2014).

Advantages

The RLAS is a relatively quick measure that can be completed in less than 15 minutes and requires no special training or certifications. It has also gained widespread acceptance in clinical practice with several other accepted assessments based on its unique levels and terminology.

Disadvantages

There is a limited amount of available research pertaining to the RLAS.

Administration

The RLAS battery is an interactive/observational tool in which the clinician denotes the presence or absence of particular abilities in response to certain stimuli as well as the patient's capacity to engage in functional performance as his or her functioning begins to improve. The assessment contains 10 categories ordered along an ascending scale with higher scores indicative of less impairment. Administration time is < 15 minutes. Further examples of the measure include level 9: purposeful, appropriate: stand-by assistance on request, which would be achieved if the person is able to shift between tasks for 2 hours, may require some assistance to adjust to life demands and emotional and behavioral issues may be of concern; and level 10: purposeful, appropriate: modified independent is attained if the subject is goal directed, handling multiple tasks and independently using assistive strategies; however, he or she may be prone to breaks in attention and may require additional time to complete tasks.

Permissions

The RLAS can be accessed through the Ranchos Los Amigos Medical Center website as well as other places such as the Centre for Neuro Skills where detailed information about the measure can also be found. Authorization to use in research or publication can be obtained by contacting its creators or where it has been published. More information can be found in the following publication:

Hagen, C, Malkmus D., & Durham, P. (1979). Levels of cognitive functioning. In *Rehabilitation of the head injured adult: Comprehensive physical management*. Professional Staff Association of Rancho Los Amigos Hospital, Inc. Downey, CA.

Summary

POPULATION	TBI; disorders of consciousness
TYPE OF MEASURE	Rating scale; observed re-acquisition of skills
WHAT IT ASSESSES	Conscious state; level of participation in ADLs
TIME	< 15 minutes
COST	Free

Contact

Ranchos Los Amigos Medical Center

Communication Disorders Department

7601 East Imperial Highway

Downey, California 90242

Email: Inquiry@rancho.org

Web: www.neuroskills.com/resources/rancho-los-amigos-revised.php

CHAPTER 34: WESSEX HEAD INJURY MATRIX (WHIM)

Description

The Wessex Head Injury Matrix (WHIM), by Shiel et al. (2000) was developed to assess subjects in and emerging from coma as well as those in vegetative and minimally conscious states. It is a 62-item observational matrix that collects data by observation as well as the person's reaction to specific stimuli with regard to his or her arousal level and concentration, visual consciousness (visual pursuit), communication, cognition (memory and spatiotemporal orientation), and social behaviors by observing those behaviors that occur spontaneously or in response to stimulation (Schnakers, 2012). Use of the WHIM can give the clinician an opportunity to (1) monitor all of the stages of recovery from TBI, starting from coma to emerging post-traumatic amnesia; (2) monitor subtle changes in slow to recover persons; (3) reflect performance in activities of daily living; (4) help identify short-term objectives and realistic goals for those with TBI; and lastly, (5) specify a sequence of recovery (Majerus, Van der Linden, & Shiel, 2000). WHIM employs a unique scoring system in which the 62 items are categorized into 6 subscales (communication, attention, social behavior, concentration, visual awareness, and cognition) and are ordered in a hierarchical ascending scale reflecting a statistically derived order of recovery from coma such that the person's ability to achieve item 1 should appear before item 2, item 2 before item 3, etc.; thus the WHIM score represents the rank order of the most advanced ability or item observed (rather than adding the different items observed) (Laureys, 2007a). Administration times can vary from less than 40 minutes to several hours.

Psychometrics

Original research by Shiel et al. (2000) concluded that correlation between the WHIM and Glasgow Coma Scale (GCS) was highly significant at $r = 0.94$, whereas inter-rater agreement was also excellent at 0.98. Validation of a French version of the WHIM scales showed good inter-rater agreement for 93% of the items and very good test-retest reliability at $r = 0.98$ (Laureys, 2007a). A final study explored the extent to which outcomes following sudden onset of a vegetative state or minimally conscious state could be predicted from baseline data of age, time since onset, length of observation period, or admission WHIM ratings and it was determined that only WHIM ratings had significant correlations for *most advanced behavior* at 0.49, while correlations for the most advanced behavior excluding 2 items was 0.58 and for total number of different behavior items

0.46, respectively (Turner-Stokes, Bassett, Rose, Stephen Ashford, & Thu, 2015).

Advantages

The WHIM is a relatively simple assessment to administer and has shown to have greater sensitivity than the GCS upon an individual's exit from coma, the post-coma period, and the vegetative state; although, the GCS was more sensitive than the WHIM for the deep coma period, suggesting a greater sensitivity in detecting changes across the minimally conscious state not captured by other assessments (Majerus et al., 2000). Also, most standardized assessments have ordinal scoring, which is a behavioral description of a phenomenon where scores are summed across several dimensions that may not necessarily correlate with each other, whereas the hierarchical approach used by the WHIM allows for the more exact identification and assessment of a person's abilities observed during recovery from one of the many TBI states (Shiel et al., 2000).

Disadvantages

There is a limited amount of supporting research outside of that involving its creators and the subtle gradations between each item of the scale can also be difficult to discern at times. Administration time is not standardized and may vary from a few minutes to several hours; however, Turner-Stokes et al. (2015) found that it was typically 20 to 40 minutes. Their research also noted that items 26 (frowning and grimacing) and 43 (smiles for any reason) may potentially be out of order where a stepwise regression analysis, excluding those two items, was able to account for 68% of the variance and along with total numbers of behaviors charted accounted for a further 5% of the variance, suggesting that at least some of the items are out of order.

Administration

WHIM is an interactive observational tool where the clinician discerns the presence or absence of the operational defined abilities of an individual outlined in an ascending hierarchical scale in the form of a checklist. WHIM has 62 items divided into 6 subtests where the final score is representative of the most advanced ability observed in the subject. The clinician can also study the most advanced behavior observed as well as the total number of different behaviors to gain further insight into functional performance. The following are example items of the matrix.

TABLE 34-1
EXAMPLE HIERARCHY OF ITEMS ON THE WESSEX HEAD INJURY MATRIX
1. Eyes open briefly
2. Eyes open for an extended period
3. Eyes open and move but do not focus on object/person
4. Attention held momentarily by dominant stimulus
5. Looks at person briefly
6. Volitional vocalization to express feelings
7. Distressed when cloth put on face
8. Makes eye contact
9. Looks at person talking
10. Expletive utterance

Adapted from Shiel, A., Horn, S., Wilson, B. A., McLellan, D. L., Watson, M., & Campbell, M. (2000). The Wessex Head Injury Matrix (WHIM) main scale: A preliminary report on a scale to assess and monitor patient recovery after severe head injury. *Clinical Rehabilitation, 14,* 413.

Permissions

The WHIM assessment can be purchased from Pearson Inc. for $105. Consent to use in research or publication can be obtained by contacting the creators of the measure, its publishers, or Pearson at the information following. More information can be found in the following article:

Shiel, A., Horn, S., Wilson, B. A., McLellan, D. L., Watson, M., & Campbell, M. (2000) The Wessex Head Injury Matrix main scale: A preliminary report on a scale to assess and monitor patients' recovery after severe head injury. *Clinical Rehabilitation, 14,* 408-416.

Summary

POPULATION	TBI; disorders of consciousness
TYPE OF MEASURE	Hierarchical rating scale
WHAT IT ASSESSES	Conscious state; basic cognitive and motor ability
TIME	20 to 40 minutes; up to several hours
COST	$105

Contact

Agnes Shiel, PhD

Occupational Therapy—Head of Discipline

National University of Ireland—Galway

Galway, Ireland

Pearson Inc.

P.O. Box 599700

San Antonio, TX 78259

Phone: (800) 627-7271

Email: clinicalcustomersupport@pearson.com

Web: www.pearsonclinical.com/psychology/ products/100000602/wessex-head-injury-matrix- the-whim.html

Chapter 35: Western Neuro Sensory Stimulation Profile (WNSSP)

Description

The Western Neuro Sensory Stimulation Profile (WNSSP), by Ansel and Keenan, (1989), was developed to assess cognitive function in severely impaired head-injured adults as well as to monitor and predict change over time. Designed as a measure of responsiveness to structured stimuli, the WNSSP was created in response to the need for an objective measure of both cognitive and communicative function relative to the Rancho Los Amigos Levels of Cognitive Functioning (RLAS) levels 2 to 5, as well as slow to recover individuals such as those who remain at RLAS levels 2 and 3 for extended periods of time. Focused on its ability to identify the emergence from the disorders of consciousness or from a minimally conscious state, the WNSSP presents items with a hierarchy of weighted scores in which higher levels of function receive higher scores suggestive of a recovery sequence (Lannin, Cusick, McLachlan, & Allaous, 2013). The WNSSP has 33 items and is composed of 9 subscales: arousal attention (4 items), auditory response (2 items), auditory comprehension (6 items), expressive communication (3 items), visual tracking (7 items), visual comprehension (5 items), tactile response (2 items), object manipulation (3 items), and olfactory response (1 item). Scoring is based on type of stimulation (general or specific), latency of reaction, as well as the need for cueing (Cusick, Lannin, Hanssen, & Allaous, 2014). Total scores range from 0 to 113 where lower scores indicate poorer function. The assessment takes approximately 45 minutes to complete.

Psychometrics

Original research involving slow to recover traumatic brain injury (TBI) subjects (n = 57) determined the WNSSP to be an ecologically valid assessment in which results showed that internal consistency for the total score was α = 0.95, whereas internal consistency for the subscales of auditory comprehension was 0.87, visual comprehension 0.87, visual tracking 0.95, object manipulation 0.94, arousal/attention 0.73, while for tactile/olfactory it was only 0.59 (Ansell & Keenan, 1989). Inter-rater reliability results using 3 different raters involving 23 subjects found that total and subscales ranged from r = 0.94 to 0.99 except for arousal/attention and tactile/olfactory subscales where correlations ranged from 0.78 to 0.90 and 0.64 to 0.86, respectively (Ansell & Keenan 1989). Later work by Cusick et al. (2014) found internal consistency

reliability to be high at α = 0.93 among 33 subjects with severe TBI. The same study found concurrent validity in relation to the Functional Independence Measure (FIM) Scale at discharge to have a modest relationship with the motor subscale (0.37), and the FIM cognition subscale (0.41) but not with FIM total scale, while concurrent validity, in relation to the RLAS scale, was both strong at admission (0.60) and at discharge (0.79). Other studies found the WNSSP to correlate significantly with the Wessex Head Injury Matrix scale at r = 0.87 and the Post-Acute Level of Consciousness scale at 0.88 to 0.93 involving 29 brain-injured comatose patients aged 21 to 83 years who were followed longitudinally (Eilander et al., 2009; Schnakers, Laureys, & Majerus, 2004). Whereas, a study by Gill-Thwaites and Munday (2004) of 60 subjects diagnosed in vegetative state on admission and assessed at 2 60-day intervals found the correlation between WNSSP total score and the Sensory Modality Assessment total scores was significant at 0.70. Finally, a retrospective medical chart audit design of 38 subjects with an RLAS score between 2 and 3 showed that at admission the mean total-score WNSSP was 38 and at discharge it was 70, suggesting an ability to detect meaningful change (Allaous, McLachlan, Cusick, & Lannin, 2011).

Advantages

The WNSSP is based in part on the RLAS levels 2 to 5 and is designed to be a particularly sensitive instrument relative to levels 2 and 3 of that scale (generalized response, localized response, confused, agitated, and confused, inappropriate, non-agitated state) as well as those individuals who are slow to recover in general, thus it is considered more sensitive to change between levels 2 through 5 of the RLAS. Also, items on the WNSSP use an ordered hierarchy similar in some ways similar to that of the Wessex Head Injury Matrix scale discussed in Chapter 34, making it a unique assessment tool.

Disadvantages

The WNSSP can take up to 45 minutes to complete and requires the use of various items. The amount of peer-reviewed literature is also limited. A systematic review by Seel et al. (2010) noted poor internal consistency for some subscales (α = 0.35 to 0.59) as well as not being sensitive to change in low-functioning individuals and argue that overall, the scale's validity remains unproven.

Administration

The WNSSP is an observational test of 33 that are items administered bedside and scored on the type of stimulation (general or specific), the latency of reaction, and need for cueing (Lannin et al., 2013). Tools needed include a handheld mirror, an object for manipulation, cologne or other olfactory stimulus, a type of "read and do what it says" card, cotton swab, spoon, comb, and a pencil, among others. Each test section has several items and includes a communication section which examines the presence of a yes/no response and the ability to vocalize or mouth words; an auditory section that rates the perception of voice and nonverbal sound and response to auditory commands; a visual response section that assesses tracking behavior and subject response to written commands; a tactile response section that judges perception of touch and the use of common objects; and finally, an olfactory response section used to rate the subject's perception of various odors.

Permissions

The assessment is free to use in clinical practice. Use of the WNSSP in research or publication can be obtained by contacting the creators of the measure or its publishers at the information that follows. More information can be found in the following article:

Ansell, B., & Keenan, J. (1989). The Western Neuro Sensory Stimulation Profile: A tool for assessing slow-to-recover head-injured patients. *Archives of Physical Medicine and Rehabilitation, 70*(2), 104-108.

Summary

POPULATION	TBI; disorders of consciousness
TYPE OF MEASURE	Hierarchical rating scale
WHAT IT ASSESSES	Emergence from coma and the minimally conscious state
TIME	45 minutes
COST	Free

Contact

Natasha A. Lannin, PhD

Associate Professor—Occupational Therapy

Faculty of Health Sciences

La Trobe University

Melbourne, Victoria, Australia

Barbara J. Ansell

Retired faculty

University of Wisconsin

Madison, Wisconsin

Web: www.coma.ulg.ac.be/medical/chronic.html

TABLE 35-1
EXAMPLE ITEMS OF THE WESTERN NEURO SENSORY STIMULATION PROFILE
VISUAL RESPONSE
Horizontal Tracking
0. No response
1. Follows (from midline)—left or right
2. Follows (from midline)—left and right
3. Follows across midline—either side
OBJECT MANIPULATION
0. No response
1. Grasps/releases object
2. Moves object incorrectly
3. Reaches for/pushes away object
4. Uses appropriately—with cueing
5. Uses appropriately
Adapted from Laureys, S. (2007b). Western Neuro Sensory Stimulation Profile (WNSSP). Coma Science Group. Retrieved from www.coma.ulg.ac.be/images/wnssp.pdf

REFERENCES

Allaous, J., McLachlan, R., Cusick, A., & Lannin, N. (2011). Patterns of recovery observed in patients in vegetative or minimally conscious states following severe traumatic brain injury: What determines rehabilitation readiness? In D. Sansonetti. (2011). Evaluating cognitive assessment in occupational therapy: The clinical reasoning around cognitive assessment for individuals post stroke and TBI... Occupational Therapy Australia, 24th National Conference and Exhibition, 29 June - 1 July 2011. *Australian Occupational Therapy Journal*, 5831-5832.

Ansell, B., & Keenan, J. (1989). The Western Neuro Sensory Stimulation Profile: A tool for assessing slow-to-recover head-injured patients. *Archives of Physical Medicine and Rehabilitation, 70*(2), 104-108.

Bazarian, J., Eirich, M., & Salhanick, S. (2003). The relationship between pre-hospital and emergency department Glasgow Coma Scale Scores. *Brain Injury, 17*(7), 553-560.

Beauchamp, K., Baker, S., McDaniel, C., Moser, Zalman, D. C., Balinghoff, J.,...Stecker, M. (2001). Reliability of nurses' neurological assessments in the cardiothoracic surgical intensive care unit. *American Journal of Critical Care, 10*(5), 298-305.

Boake, C., Kelly, T., Levin, H., McCauley, S., Moretti, P., Pedroza, C.,....Yallampalli, R. (2010). The Neurological Outcome Scale for Traumatic Brain Injury (NOS-TBI): II. Reliability and convergent validity. Journal of Neurotrauma, 27(6), 991-997.

Cusick, A., Lannin, N. A., Hanssen, R., & Allaous, J. (2014). Validating the Western Neuro Sensory Stimulation Profile for patients with severe traumatic brain injury who are slow-to-recover. *Australian Occupational Therapy Journal, 61*(4), 276-283.

Davis, D., Serrano, J., Vilke, G., Sise. M., Kennedy F., Eastman. A.,... Hoyt, D. (2006). The predictive value of field versus arrival Glasgow Coma Scale score and TRISS calculations in moderate-to-severe traumatic brain injury. *Journal of Trauma, 60*, 985–990.

Eilander, H., van de Wiel, M., Wijers, M., van Heugten, C., Buljevac, D., Lavrijsen, J.,...Prevo, A. (2009). The reliability and validity of the PALOC-S: A post-acute level of consciousness scale for assessment of young patients with prolonged disturbed consciousness after brain injury. *Neuropsychological Rehabilitation, 19*(1), 1-27.

Flannery, J. (1998). Using the Levels of Cognitive Functioning Assessment Scale with patients with traumatic brain injury in an acute care setting. *Rehabilitation Nursing, 23*, 88–94.

Giacino, J. T., & Kalmar, K. (2004). *CRS-R Coma Recovery Scale-revised: Administration and scoring guidelines*. Edison, NJ: Center for Head Injuries: JFK Johnson Rehabilitation Institution..

Giacino, J. T., & Kalmar, K. (2005). The JFK Coma Recovery Scale—Revised. *Neuropsychological Rehabilitation, 15*(3/4), 454–460.

Giacino, J. T, Kalmar, K., & Whyte, J. (2004). The JFK Coma Recovery Scale—Revised: Measurement characteristics and diagnostic utility. *Archives of Physical Medicine and Rehabilitation, 85*, 2020-2029.

Gill-Thwaites, H., & Munday, R. (2004). The Sensory Modality Assessment and Rehabilitation Technique (SMART): A valid and reliable assessment for vegetative state and minimally conscious state patients. *Brain Injury, 18*(12), 1255-1269.

Gouvier, W., Blanton, P., & LaPorte, K. (1987). Reliability and validity of the Disability Rating Scale and the Levels Of Cognitive Functioning scale in monitoring recovery from severe head injury. *Journal of Head Trauma Rehabilitation, 2*(4), 91.

Hagen C., Malkmus D., & Durham P. (1972). *Rancho Los Amigos Levels of Cognitive Functioning Scale*. Downey, CA: Rancho Los Amigos Hospital.

Holdgate, A., Ching, N., & Angonese. L. (2006). Variability in agreement between physicians and nurses when measuring the Glasgow Coma Scale in the emergency department limits its clinical usefulness. *Emergency Medicine Australasia, 18*, 379–384.

Kalmar, K., & Giacino, J. T. (2005). The JFK Coma Recovery Scale—revised. *Neuropsychological Rehabilitation, 15*(3), 454-460.

Kevric, J., Jelinek, G., Knott, J., & Weiland, J. (2011). Validation of the Full Outline of Unresponsiveness (FOUR) Scale for conscious state in the emergency department: Comparison against the Glasgow Coma Scale. *Emergency Medicine Journal, 28*, 486-490.

Lannin, N., Cusick, A., McLachlan, R., & Allaous, J. (2013). Observed recovery sequence in neurobehavioral function after severe traumatic brain injury. *American Journal of Occupational Therapy, 67*(5), 543-549.

Laureys, S. (2007a). Consciousness scales employed in the chronic setting. Coma Science Group: Université de Liège. Retrieved from:www.coma.ulg.ac.be/medical/chronic.html

Laureys, S. (2007b). Western Neuro Sensory Stimulation Profile (WNSSP). Coma Science Group. Retrieved from www.coma.ulg.ac.be/images/wnssp.pdf

Leitgeb, J., Mauritz, W., Brazinova, A., Majdan, M., Janciak, I., Wilbacher, I., & Rusnak, M. (2013). Glasgow Coma Scale score at intensive care unit discharge predicts the 1-year outcome of patients with severe traumatic brain injury. *European Journal of Trauma and Emergency Surgery, 39*(3), 285-292

Lovstad, M., Froslie, K. F., Giacino, J. T., Skandsen, T., Anke, A., & Schanke, A. (2010). Reliability and diagnostic characteristics of the JFK Coma Recovery Scale-revised: Exploring the influence of rater's level of experience. *Journal of Head Trauma Rehabilitation, 25*(5), 349-356.

Majerus, S., Gill-Thwaites, H., Andrews, K., & Laureys, S. (2005). *Behavioral evaluation of consciousness in severe brain damage*. Liege, Belgium: Cyclotron Research Center University of Liege.

Majerus, S., Van der Linden, M., & Shiel, A. (2000) Wessex Head Injury Matrix and Glasgow/Glasgow-Liège Coma Scale: A validation and comparison study. *Neuropsychological Rehabilitation, 10*, 167-184.

Mandaville, A., Ray, A., Robertson, H., Foster, C., & Jesser, C. (2014). A retrospective review of swallow dysfunction in patients with severe traumatic brain injury. *Dysphagia, 29*, 310–318.

McCauley, S., Wilde, E., Kelly, T., Weyand, A., Yallampalli, R., Waldron, E.,...Moretti, P. (2010). The Neurological Outcome Scale for Traumatic Brain Injury (NOS-TBI): II. Reliability and convergent validity. *Journal of Neurotrauma, 27*(6), 991–997.

McCauley, S., Wilde, E., Moretti, P., MacLeod, M., Pedroza, C., Drever, P.,...Clifton, G. (2013). Neurological Outcome Scale for Traumatic Brain Injury: III. Criterion-related validity and sensitivity to change in the NABIS hypothermia-II clinical trial. *Journal of Neurotrauma, 30*(17), 1506–1511.

McLernon, S. (2014). The Glasgow Coma Scale 40 years on: A review of its practical use. *British Journal of Neuroscience Nursing, 10*(4), 179-184

Mena, J., Sanchez, A., Rubiano, A., Peitzman, A., Sperry, J., Gutierrez, M., & Puyana, J. (2011). Effect of the Modified Glasgow Coma Scale score criteria for mild traumatic brain injury on mortality prediction: Comparing Classic and Modified Glasgow Coma Scale score model scores of 13. *Journal of Trauma, 71*(5), 1185–1193.

Rosenfeld, J. (2012). *Practical management of head and neck injury* (1st ed.). Chatswood, Australia: Elsevier Australia.

Schnakers, C. (2012). Clinical assessment of patients with disorders of consciousness. *Archives Italiennes de Biologie, 150*, 36-43.

Schnakers, S., Laureys, S., & Majerus, S. (2004). A comparison of a behavioural assessment tool and electrophysiological measures of recovery from coma. *Critical Care, 8*(Suppl 1), 313.

Schnakers, C., Vanhaudenhuyse, A., Giacino, J., Ventura, M., Boly, M., Majerus, S.,... Laureys, S. (2009). Diagnostic accuracy of the vegetative and minimally conscious state: Clinical consensus versus standardized neurobehavioral assessment. *Neurology, 9*(35), 1-5.

Seel, R., Sherer, M., Whyte, J., Katz, D., Giacino, J., Rosenbaum, A.,... Zasler, N. (2010). Assessment scales for disorders of consciousness: Evidence-based recommendations for clinical practice and research. *Archives of Physical Medicine and Rehabilitation, 91*(12), 1795-1813. In A. Cusick, N. A. Lannin, R. Hanssen, & J. Allaous. (2014). Validating the Western Neuro Sensory Stimulation Profile for patients with severe traumatic brain injury who are slow-to-recover. *Australian Occupational Therapy Journal, 61*(4), 276-283.

Shiel, A., Horn, S., Wilson, B. A., McLellan, D. L., Watson, M., & Campbell, M. (2000) The Wessex Head Injury Matrix main scale: A preliminary report on a scale to assess and monitor patients' recovery after severe head injury. *Clinical Rehabilitation, 14*, 408-416.

Stenberg, M., Godbolt, A. K., Boussard, C. N., Levi, R., & Stalnacke, B. M. (2014). Cognitive impairment after severe traumatic brain injury, clinical course and impact on outcome: A Swedish-Icelandic study. *Behavioural Neurology, 2015*, Article ID 680308.

Teasdale, G. (2015). *Glasgow Coma Scale: Do it this way. GCS at 40.* Glasgow, Scotland: Institute of Neurological Sciences NHS Greater Glasgow and Clyde.

Teasdale G., & Jennett B. (1974). Assessment of coma and impaired consciousness. A practical scale. *Lancet, 2*, 81–84.

Turner-Stokes, L. Bassett, P., Rose, H., Stephen Ashford, S., & Thu, A. (2015). Wessex Head Injury Matrix in the diagnosis of patients in vegetative and minimally conscious states: A cohort analysis. *BMJ Open, 5*(4), e006051. doi:10.1136/bmjopen-2014-006051

Wilde, E., McCauley, S., Kelly, T., Levin, H., Pedroza, C., Clifton, G.,... Moretti, P. (2010). Feasibility of the Neurological Outcome Scale for Traumatic Brain Injury (NOS-TBI) in adults. *Journal of Neurotrauma, 27*(6), 975–981.

Wilde, E., McCauley, S., Kelly, T., Weyand, A., Pedroza, C., Levin, H. S.,...Moretti, P. (2010). The Neurological Outcome Scale for Traumatic Brain Injury (NOS-TBI): I. Construct validity. *Journal of Neurotrauma, 27*(6), 983-989.

Wilde, E., Whiteneck, G., Bogner, J., Bushnik, T., Cifu, D., Dikmen. S.,...von Steinbuechel N. (2010). Recommendations for the use of common outcome measures in traumatic brain injury research. *Archives of Physical Medicine and Rehabilitation, 91*,1650-60.

Zollman, F. S. (2011). *Manual of traumatic brain injury management.* New York, NY: Demos Medical Pub.

Zuercher, M., Ummenhofer, W., Baltussen, A., & Walder, B. (2009). The use of Glasgow Coma Scale in injury assessment: A critical review. *Brain Injury, 23*(5), 371–384.

VII

Cerebrovascular Accident (CVA) and Parkinson's Disease Specific Assessment

Bortnick, K.
Occupational Therapy Assessments for Older Adults: 100 Instruments for Measuring Occupational Performance (pp. 101-116).
© 2017 Taylor & Francis Group.

CHAPTER 36: HOEHN AND YAHR STAGING SCALE OF PARKINSON'S DISEASE (HY SCALE)

Description

The Hoehn and Yahr Staging Scale of Parkinson's Disease (HY scale) by Hoehn and Yahr (1967), is a standard clinical measure of the progression of Parkinson's disease (PD) designed to measure the signs and symptoms associated with functional impairment such as postural instability, rigidity, tremor, or bradykinesia, as well as other symptoms accompanying PD (Quelhas & Costa, 2009). The HY scale is a descriptive staging system, similar to the Functional Assessment Staging Scale for neurocognitive disorders, in which the clinician estimates the presence of functional deficits (disability) and objective signs (impairment) seen in subjects with PD by employing a 5-point descriptive scale (1 to 5) where increasing impairment is charted from unilateral disease (stage 1), to bilateral disease without balance difficulties (stage 2), to the presence of postural instability (stage 3), loss of physical independence (stage 4), and being wheelchair or bed bound (stage 5) (Goetz et al., 2004). A modified version was developed in the 1990s that adds 0.5 point increments to the scoring scale to increase its descriptive value and sensitivity. Administration for each version requires the clinician to gather information against the inclusion/exclusion criteria of the 5 descriptive levels by observing the client as he or she performs activities. Both HY scales can be completed in less than 5 minutes.

Psychometrics

A study by Muller et al. (2000) found the HY scale to have good discriminant ability as subjects with PD (n = 18) showed significantly longer latencies in each HY stage than patients with atypical Parkinsonian disorder (APD; n = 63). Results of the study determined that no subject with PD progressed to stage HY-3 within 1 year, whereas 72% of those with APD did. A subsequent study of 43 PD subjects by Quelhas and Costa (2009) revealed that an HY score together with the Hospital Anxiety and Depression Scale score accounted for 42% of the variance of global quality-of-life scores, which confirmed previous studies that noted that the HY scale had stronger correlations with quality-of-life scores than other more detailed clinical assessments such as the Unified Parkinson's Disease Rating Scale (UPDRS). A falls study by Thomas, Rogers, Amick, and Friedman (2010) of 102 persons with a median HY score of 2.5 found that the HY scale had a positive correlation with Tinetti's Falls Efficacy Scale (FES) of 0.48 and concluded that those subjects whose gait froze more frequently used an assistive walking device, such as a cane or walker, or had more severe PD by HY stage, and exhibited greater fear of falling as measured by FES scores. A similar study of 38 men with PD found that Berg Balance Scale scores were inversely correlated with modified HY scale scores (2.48, SD 0.61; range 2 to 4) at −0.45, while the UPDRS motor scores (23.05, SD 8.48; range 9 to 43) correlated somewhat better at −0.58 (Qutubuddin et al., 2005). Finally, a study of 98 persons with PD and 31 healthy controls determined that strong correlations existed between the original HY scale and the Trunk Mobility Scale at 0.72, whereas correlations with the UPDRS motor were again somewhat better at 0.84. Both HY scales take less than 5 minutes to complete, whereas the UPDRS takes 30 minutes (Franco, Leao, Townsend, Carlos, & Rieder, 2011).

Advantages

There is a fair amount of research in support of the HY scale as a unique staging tool that can measure PD across the disease continuum. It requires no training or certifications to use in practice and its general acceptance throughout the health professions has increased communication by supporting a common language to classify the particular phenomenon witnessed in PD, thereby eliminating some barriers to treatment and participation.

	TABLE 36-1
	MODIFIED HOEHN AND YAHR STAGING SCALE
1.0	Unilateral involvement
1.5	Unilateral and axial involvement
2.0	Bilateral involvement—balance unimpaired
2.5	Mild bilateral disease with recovery on pull test
3.0	Mild to moderate bilateral disease—postural instability independent
4.0	Severe disability—walk/stand unassisted
5.0	Wheelchair bound or bedridden unless aided

Adapted from Goetz, C., Poewe, W., Rascol, O., Sampaio, C., Stebbins, G., Counsell, C.,…Seidl. L. (2004). Movement Disorder Society task force report on the Hoehn and Yahr Staging Scale: Status and recommendations. *Movement Disorders, 19*(9), 1021.

Disadvantages

The Movement Disorder Society (MDS) critique of the HY scale noted that it is weighted heavily toward postural instability as the primary index of disease severity and may not capture the essence of impairments or disability from other impairment areas such as non-motor problems (Goetz et al., 2004). For example, cognitive impairment often occurs in both early and advanced stages of the disease and it has been proposed that as many as 25% of persons with PD fulfill criteria for mild cognitive impairment, which may include decreased attention, reduced executive function, as well as visuospatial and memory dysfunctions (Santangelo, Barone, Abbruzzese, Ferini-Strambi, & Antonini, 2014). The MDS critique also found that psychometric testing of the modified HY scale, which includes 0.5 increments, to be limited and suggested that without such testing the original 5-point scale should be maintained (Santangelo et al., 2014).

Administration

During assessment the clinician judges a person's functional as well as motor performance against the inclusion/exclusion criteria of the HY scoring systems.

TABLE 36-2	
HOEHN AND YAHR STAGING SCALE STAGE PROGRESSION	
STAGE PROGRESSION	**MEDIAN TIME (MONTHS)**
1 to 2	20
2 to 2.5	62
2.5 to 3	25
3 to 4	24
4 to 5	25
n=695 mean age=65 years	

Adapted from Zhao, Y. J., Wee, H. W., Chan, Y-H., Seah, S. H., Au, W. L., Lau, P. N.,...Tan, L. (2010). Progression of Parkinson's disease as evaluated by Hoehn and Yahr stage transition times. *Movement Disorders, 25*(6), 710.

Permissions

The HY scale is free to use in clinical practice and is available in its entirety in several journal articles as well as on the web. Use of the HY scale in research or publication can be obtained by contacting its creators or where it has been published. Information can also be obtained by contacting the International Parkinson and Movement Disorder Society as well as through the following publications:

Goetz, C., Poewe, W., Rascol, O., Sampaio, C., Stebbins, G., Counsell, C.,...Seidl. L. (2004). Movement Disorder Society task force report on the Hoehn and Yahr Staging Scale: Status and recommendations. *Movement Disorders, 19*(9), 1020–1028.

Hoehn, M., & Yahr, M. (1967). Parkinsonism: Onset, progression and mortality. *Neurology, 17*, 427–442.

Summary

POPULATION	Suspected PD
TYPE OF MEASURE	Descriptive staging system
WHAT IT ASSESSES	Disease progression
TIME	<5 minutes
COST	Free

Contact

Christopher G. Goetz, MD

Rush University Medical Center

Chicago, Illinois

MDS International Secretariat

555 East Wells Street, Suite 1100

Milwaukee, WI 53202-3823 USA

Phone: (414) 276-2145

Email: info@movementdisorders.org

Web: www.movementdisorders.org/MDS/Search-Results.htm?Search_Keywords=hoehn%20%26yahr

Chapter 37: Modified Rankin Scale (MRS)

Description

The Modified Rankin Scale (MRS) is a quick screen staging tool considered to be a single-item global outcome scale for use with stroke populations. The scale describes 6 grades of disability that are common to stroke patients (0 to 5) with 0 being no symptoms and 5 considered severe disability. During assessment, information about the client is obtained through observation and interview. The practitioner then uses that information to quantify an individual's level of participation as well as functional mobility against the inclusion/exclusion criteria of the 5 stages. The original scale, developed by Rankin (1950), was later modified by Warlow et al. (1988) to include a grade 0, as well as further refinements to grade 1 to include "no significant disability: able to carry out all usual duties," as well as to grade 2 to encompass "slight disability: unable to carry out some of previous activities" (Van Swieten, Koudstaal, Visser, Schouten, & van Gijn, 1988). The MRS can be completed in less than 5 minutes.

TABLE 37-1	
THE MODIFIED RANKIN SCALE	
LEVEL	DESCRIPTION
0	No symptoms
1	No significant disability, despite symptoms; able to perform all usual duties and activities
2	Slight disability; unable to perform all previous activities but able to look after own affairs without assistance
3	Moderate disability; requires some help, but able to walk without assistance
4	Moderately severe disability; unable to walk without assistance and unable to attend to own bodily needs without assistance
5	Severe disability; bedridden, incontinent, and requires constant nursing care and attention

Adapted from Van Swieten, J., Koudstaal, P., Visser, M., Schouten, H., & van Gijn, J. (1988). Interobserver agreement for the assessment of handicap in stroke patients. *Stroke, 19*(5), 605.

Psychometrics

A systematic review by Quinn Dawson, Walters, and Lees (2009) found that the inter-rater reliabilities of the MRS varied from near perfect (r = 0.95) to poor (0.25) with overall scores considered moderate. The same study found three articles that established good to very good intra-rater reliability (r = 0.94). A second systematic review of 50 articles also found several studies with robust test-retest reliability scores that ranged from r = 0.81 to 0.95 with inter-rater reliability improving with the use of structured interviews from 0.56 vs 0.78. A study by Sulter, Steen, and De Keyser (1999) calculated individual intra-rater variability for 7 raters and found overall, positive results for rater 1 (0.86), rater 2 (0.89), rater 3 (0.75), rater 4 (0.40), rater 5 (0.63), rater 6 (1.0), and rater 7 (0.91). Uyttenboogaart, Stewart, Vroomen, De Keyser, and Luijckx (2005) examined how scores of the Barthel Index (BI) and the MRS related by establishing corresponding cutoff scores between the two instruments. For MRS grade 1 (no significant disability, despite symptoms; able to perform all usual duties and activities) the optimal cutoff score on the BI was 95, with a sensitivity of 85.6% and a specificity of 91.7%. For MRS grade 2 (slight disability; unable to perform all previous activities but able to look after own affairs without assistance) a BI score of 90 had a sensitivity of 90.7% and a specificity of 88.1%. At the MRS level 3 (moderate disability; requires some help, but able to walk without assistance) a BI score of 75, had a sensitivity of 95.7% and a specificity of 88.5%.

Advantages

The MRS is a quick and easy outcome measure that has a good amount of research in support of its use in clinical practice. No special training or certifications are needed to administer the assessment and, like the Hoehn and Yahr scale discussed previously, its widespread use has fostered increased communication throughout the various health professions. The MRS is located in the public domain, and is both free to use and considered relevant across number of settings. A 9-item modified version is also available.

Disadvantages

The simple staging design suggest that its best use may be as a quick screen to determine if further investigations into the client's condition is warranted.

Administration

During assessment the clinician observes and compares the subject's functional performance against the inclusion/exclusion criteria of the clearly outlined 5 MRS stages, which is done by using clinical judgment or other means, such as testing, when deciding which level is the most appropriate placement.

Permissions

The van Swieten modified version of the Rankin scale is located in the public domain and is free to use in clinical practice, research, or publication. A free training program developed by the University of Glasgow is also available to certify health professionals in its use which consists of a series of digital video recordings, written material for self-paced instruction, a demonstration module, and certification modules available at the information that follows. More information can be found in the following publications:

Rankin, J. (1957). Cerebral vascular accidents in patients over the age of 60. *Scott Medical Journal, 2,* 200-215.

Van Swieten, J., Koudstaal, P., Visser, M., Schouten, H., & van Gijn, J. (1988). Interobserver agreement for the assessment of handicap in stroke patients. *Stroke, 19*(5), 604-607.

Summary

POPULATION	Stroke; cerebrovascular accident
TYPE OF MEASURE	Descriptive staging system
WHAT IT ASSESSES	Disease progression
TIME	<5 minutes
COST	Free

Contact

Kennedy Lees, MD, FRCP

University of Glasgow

Glasgow, Scotland

Web: www.rankinscale.org

Chapter 38: Movement Disorder Society-Unified Parkinson's Disease Rating Scale (MDS-UPDRS)

Description

The Movement Disorder Society-Unified Parkinson's Disease Rating Scale (MDS-UPDRS) by Fahn et al. (1987) is a widely used comprehensive assessment of the severity of Parkinson's disease (PD). Delivered through both an interview and self-report questionnaire, it is considered by many to be a gold standard of PD assessment. Revised in 2008 by the Movement Disorder Society (MDS), it assesses motor and non-motor experiences of daily living as well as motor complications which are thought to be hallmark symptoms of the disablement process posed by PD (Martínez-Martín et al., 2014). The MDS-UPDRS is composed of four subscales: (1) non-motor experiences of daily living (nMEDL); (2) motor experiences of daily living (M-EDL); (3) motor examination (MEx); and (4) motor complications (MCompl). The measure has 50 items scored along a 5-point Likert scale (0 to 4) with scoring descriptors varying for each item (Martínez-Martín et al., 2014). An example question relating to cognitive impairment is, "Over the past week have you had problems remembering things, following conversations, paying attention, thinking clearly, or finding your way around the house or in town?" which would be scored from (4) normal or no cognitive impairment to (0) severe cognitive dysfunction such that it precludes the patient's ability to carry out normal activities and social interactions (Goetz et al., 2008). The MDS-UPDRS can be completed in 30 minutes with lower scores indicative of better performance.

Psychometrics

A study establishing the validity of the original version using 37 community-dwelling adults with PD found that test-retest reliability intra-class coefficients for all subtests as well as total scores were high with a range of $r = 0.89$ to 0.93, while internal consistency, as measured over 2 days, was moderate to good ranging from $\alpha = 0.66$ to 0.89 (Steffen & Seney, 2008). Development research of the MDS-UPDRS using 877 subjects with PD showed high internal consistency across its parts with Cronbach's alpha's ranging from $\alpha = 0.79$ to 0.93, while further results found a significant correlation with the original at 0.96 (Goetz et al., 2008). A study by Shulman et al. (2010) measuring the clinically important differences (CID), which is the amount of change in score needed for a client or clinician to recognize value, found that for minimal detectable change to occur 2.3 to 2.7 points were needed for the motor score and 4.1 to 4.5 was needed for the total score. A moderate

change was considered 4.5 to 6.7 points (motor) and for the total score it was 8.5 to 10.3. A large CID was considered 10.7 to 10.8 points (motor) and 16.4 to 17.8 for the total score. Another study that involved an analysis of a sample of 435 Parkinson patients identified the following 3 factors that explained 70% of the variance of total scores:

1. Factor 1: The non-motor experiences of daily living composed of both rater and patient scores, as well as motor experiences of daily living (M-EDL) and its fluctuations.

2. Factor 2: Scores related to rigidity, bradykinesia and axial signs.

3. Factor 3: Included tremor and dyskinesia scores (Martínez-Martín et al., 2014).

The same study also found that the M-EDL domain was the most powerful determinant of health-related quality of life

Advantages

There is a good amount of research in support of the MDS-UPDRS assessment for use in both research as well as clinical practice and it can be obtained free of charge. The MDS also has a helpful interactive website devoted to this and other Parkinson assessments that the clinician may find useful.

Disadvantages

Although no special training is required, specific knowledge, skills, and terminology associated with PD are necessary where problems associated with those issues were highlighted in a study of inter-rater agreement between nurses and physicians using the original version that showed only moderate agreement between the two fields with an overall intra-class coefficient of 0.65 (Palmer et al., 2010). As for the question of whether all UPDRS-ME (motor exam) items were normal, there was agreement of only 0.53, suggesting that the UPDRS batteries may be complex to both administer and score (Palmer et al., 2010).

Administration

The MDS-UPDRS questionnaire has detailed instructions for scoring and administration provided in the examiner's manual. The 50 questions that include elements of both rater and self-report items are scored along a 5-point scale (0 to 4) using various descriptors that roughly equate to (0) normal; (1) slight symptoms/signs with sufficiently low frequency or intensity to cause no impact on function; (2) mild symptoms/signs of frequency or intensity sufficient to cause a modest impact on function; (3) moderate symptoms/signs sufficiently frequent or intense to impact considerably, but not prevent, function; or (4) severe symptoms/signs that prevent function (Goetz et al., 2008).

TABLE 38-1
EXAMPLE ITEMS AND DOMAINS OF THE MOVEMENT DISORDER SOCIETY-UNIFIED PARKINSON'S DISEASE RATING SCALE
PART I: NON-MOTOR ASPECTS OF EXPERIENCES OF DAILY LIVING
• Apathy
• Sleep problems
• Daytime sleepiness
• Pain and other sensation
PART II: MOTOR EXPERIENCES OF DAILY LIVING
• Dressing
• Handwriting
• Turning in bed
• Tremor impact on activities
PART III: MOTOR EXAMINATION
• Facial expression
• Rigidity
• Hand movements
• Freezing of gait
PART IV: MOTOR COMPLICATIONS
• Dyskinesias
• Motor fluctuations
Adapted from Goetz, C. G., Fahn, S., Martínez-Martín, P., Poewe, W., Sampaio, C., Stebbins, G.,…LaPelle, N. (2007). Movement Disorder Society-sponsored revision of the Unified Parkinson's Disease Rating Scale (MDS-UPDRS): Process, format, and clinimetric testing plan. *Movement Disorders, 22*(1), 44.

Permissions

The MDS-UPDRS is owned by the Movement Disorder Society and can be obtained from their International Parkinson and Movement Disorder website at the information that follows. It is free to use in clinical practice with no financial support; however, different fees are outlined for industry, government, research, and publication. More information can be found in the following journal article:

Goetz, C., Tilley, B., Shaftman, S., Stebbins, G., Fahn, S., Poewe, W.,…LaPelle, N. (2008). Movement Disorder Society-sponsored revision of the Unified Parkinson's Disease Rating Scale (MDS-UPDRS): Scale presentation and clinimetric testing results. *Movement Disorders, 23*(15), 2129-2170.

Summary

POPULATION	Suspected PD
TYPE OF MEASURE	Interview and self-report questionnaire
WHAT IT ASSESSES	Global rating of PD effect
TIME	30 minutes
COST	Free

Contacts

Movement Disorder Society (MDS)

International Secretariat

555 East Wells Street, Suite 1100

Milwaukee, WI 53202-3823 USA

Phone: (414) 276-2145

Email: info@movementdisorders.org

Web: www.movementdisorders.org/MDS/Education/ Rating-Scales/Rating-Scales.htm

Christopher G. Goetz, MD

Rush University Medical Center

Chicago, Illinois

Chapter 39: National Institutes of Health Stroke Scale (NIHSS)

Description

The National Institutes of Health Stroke Scale (NIHSS) is a standardized assessment designed to measure stroke severity and is considered unique in that it assesses the spectrum of neurological deficits that present following a stroke rather than simply concentrating on motor deficits like many other outcome measures (Dewey et al., 1999). Both an interactive and observational tool, it allows the clinician to evaluate and document neurological status, determine treatment options, anticipate discharge planning, as well as measure patient outcomes across several domains such as level of consciousness, extra-ocular movements, visual fields, facial muscle function, extremity strength, coordination, sensory function, language, speech, and hemi-attention (neglect) (Dancer, Brown, & Yanase, 2009). First designed as a 15-item scale in 1989, it has been modified to include 13- and 11-item versions; however, the original remains the most commonly used. An example item of the assessment is facial palsy, where the subject is encouraged, often through pantomime, to show their teeth or raise their eyebrows and close their eyes, which is scored as (0) normal symmetrical movements, (1) minor paralysis (flattened nasolabial fold, asymmetry on smiling), (2) partial paralysis (total or near-total paralysis of lower face), or (3) complete paralysis of one or both sides (absence of facial movement in the upper and lower face) (Appelros & Terent, 2004). The NIHSS can be administered as early as 1 hour after the onset of symptoms as well as >3 months post-cerebrovascular accident (CVA) and has a scoring range from 0 to 42, where 0 indicates no clinically relevant neurological abnormality and a score of 20 or higher is suggestive of dense paralysis with impaired consciousness (Jain, Van Houten, & Sheikh, 2016). The NIHSS can be completed in less than 10 minutes.

Psychometrics

A study using 2 series of 4 patients rated at baseline and 3 months by 30 physicians and 29 non-physician study coordinators determined that intra-class correlation coefficients to be high at r=0.93 and 0.95, respectively, reflecting both high levels of intra-rater and inter-rater reliability (Goldstein & Samsa, 1997). A similar reliability study between neurologists and nurses found moderate to excellent agreement for the majority of the NIHSS items except for the sensory component, which only had an agreement range of 0.37 to 0.47 between the 2 health professions

(Dewey et al., 1999). A study by Appelros and Terent (2004) established health outcomes by examining scores at baseline and 1 year following a stroke (n=377) found that the median score of all subjects was 6 (range 3 to 12) at baseline, whereas at follow up it was 1 (range 0 to 3), suggesting good discriminant ability and ability to document change and of the patients that scored less than 4 at baseline 75% were functionally independent after 1 year. Jain et al. (2016) found similar results as NIHSS scores were found to be a strong predictor of both patient discharge disposition and ambulatory status and with every 1-point increase in the stroke scale at baseline, there was a 2.3 times increased likelihood of mortality and 3 times increased likelihood in worsening of ambulatory function.

Advantages

There is a considerable amount of research in support of the NIHSS for use in clinical practice and it is considered to be a gold standard of stroke assessment. The NIH has an excellent interactive website devoted to the assessment where one can find training and certification programs as well as videos and written study material devoted to the measure. Training in use of the NIHSS is also offered by the American Heart Association. Finally, the cross cultural adaptation of the scale has been well established.

Disadvantages

Specialized training may be required for some due to the unique and highly specific stroke and neurologic terminology associated with the measure.

Administration

The NIHSS is typically performed bedside in which the clinician notes the presence, absence, and/or grade of disability relative to items on the assessment. Each question uses variable rating scales (range: 0 to 4) and has detailed instructions. All items are administered in a specific order. The level of instruction is highlighted in the following example of the visual fields item where both the upper and lower quadrants are tested by confrontation, using finger counting or visual threat as appropriate (NIHSS, 2003). The clinician is told that patients may be encouraged, but if he or she is able to look at the side of the moving fingers appropriately, he or she can be scored as normal, whereas if there is unilateral blindness or enucleation, visual fields in the remaining eye are tested and are scored 1 only if there is a clear-cut asymmetry, including if quadrantanopia is present (NIHSS, 2003). If the patient is blind from any cause he or she is scored 3, in which double simultaneous stimulation is then performed. If there is extinction the patient receives a score of 1 (NIHSS, 2003).

Permissions

The NIHSS assessments can be obtained from the NIH website and is free to use in clinical practice. To use in research or publication contact the NIH directly. More information can be found in the following journal article:

Appelros, P., & Terent, A. (2004). Characteristics of the National Institute of Health Stroke Scale: Results from a population-based stroke cohort at baseline and after one year. *Cerebrovascular Diseases, 17*(1), 21-7.

Summary

POPULATION	CVA
TYPE OF MEASURE	Rating scale
WHAT IT ASSESSES	Neurological status
TIME	< 10 minutes
COST	Free

Contact

NIH Neurological Institute

P.O. Box 5801

Bethesda, MD 20824

Phone: (800) 352-9424

Web: http://stroke.nih.gov/resources/scale.htm

Pamphlet: http://stroke.nih.gov/documents/NIH_ Stroke_Scale_Booklet.pdf

Training manual: www.ninds.nih.gov/doctors/stroke_ scale_training.htm

CHAPTER 40: ORPINGTON PROGNOSTIC SCALE (OPS)

Description

The Orpington Prognostic Scale (OPS) is an impairment-based scale developed by Kalra and Crome (1993) to be a quick screen to estimate early survival, basic activities of daily living (ADLs), level of dependence, and the need for long-term care of stroke survivors (Studenski, Wallace, Duncan, Rymer, & Lai, 2001). The OPS is considered a consolidation of the Edinburgh Prognostic Score and the Hodkinson's Mental Test and assesses motor deficit, proprioception, balance, and cognition (Rieck & Moreland, 2005). During administration the subject is graded on his or her ability to flex the shoulders to 90° with resistance while lying supine, locate his or her affected thumb with the opposite hand while the eyes are closed, sit, stand, and walk, as well as answer several cognitive recall questions. The OPS can be completed in less than 5 minutes and its scores range from 1.6 (lowest level of disability) to 6.8 (highest level of disability) (Rieck & Moreland, 2005) with higher scores suggesting more impairment.

Psychometrics

A study by 2 physical therapists of 94 subjects post-stroke found that inter-rater reliability as measured by intra-class correlation coefficients was high at r = 0.99 (Rieck & Moreland, 2005). Test-retest reliability was high as well (r= 0.95), whereas the accuracy for predicting discharge to home was 65% (Rieck & Moreland, 2005). A study by Celik, Aksel, and Karaoglan (2006) of 25 subjects 7 days post-cerebrovascular accident (CVA) found that the OPS significantly correlated with the National Institute of Health Stroke Scale (NIHSS) at 0.76. A longitudinal study by Shoemaker, Mullins-MacRitchie, Bennet, Vryhof, and Boettcher (2006) of 22 subjects with acute stroke found a significant negative correlation with the Functional Independence Measure (FIM) motor subscale at admission and discharge at r = -0.74 and r = -0.81, respectively. Lai, Duncan, and Keighley (1998) showed that the OPS balance subscale was able to explain 51% of the variance in ADL outcomes and when compared to the NIHSS it was able to explain more variance in individuals with a higher level of physical function than the NIHSS. Another study explored the predictive value of the OPS given at 48 hours post-CVA (OPS-1) and given at 2 weeks (OPS-2) where results showed that the sensitivity, specificity, and positive predictive values (PPV) of those with a good OPS (score < 3.2) at 6 months were 85%, 92%, and 85% for OPS-1 vs 63%, 87%, and 92% for OPS-2 (Pittock, Meldrum, Ni Dhuill, Hardiman, & Moroney, 2003). The sensitivity, specificity, and PPV of poor subjects (i.e., those with scores >5.2) were 100%, 93%, 100% for OPS -1 vs 48%, 35%, 97% for OPS-2 suggesting that the OPS, when given at 48 hours, is a good predictor of outcome after ischemic stroke and allows for early identification of patients most likely to benefit from intensive rehabilitation (Pittock et al., 2003).

Advantages

The OPS is easy to administer and can be completed in less than 5 minutes. No special training or certifications are needed and there is a good amount of research in support of its use in clinical practice. It is also located in the public domain and thus free to use in practice, research, or publication. The OPS has also shown to correlate well with other outcome measures such as the FIM scale, Barthel Index and the NIHSS.

Disadvantages

There is some evidence to suggest that its use may be limited to those with mild and moderate CVA.

Administration

During testing the clinician rates client performance as the client engages in basic physical and cognitive activities outlined on the assessment. Each of the 4 domains has unique scoring criteria and a total score of <3.2 is suggestive of minor impairment, whereas a score between >3.2 and ≤5.2 would be considered moderate, and scores >5.2 would be considered major impairment.

TABLE 40-1
EXAMPLE ITEMS OF THE ORPINGTON PROGNOSTIC SCALE
PROPRIOCEPTION: LOCATES AFFECTED THUMB WITH OPPOSITE HAND
• Accurately
• Slight difficulty
• Finds thumb via arm
• Unable to find thumb
BALANCE
• Walks 10 feet without help
• Maintains standing position (unsupported for 1 minute)
• Maintains sitting position (unsupported for 1 minute)
• No sitting balance
COGNITION (EX. 10 ITEMS SCORED 1 POINT FOR EACH)
• Age of patient
• A year of the Second World War (1939 to 1945)
• Name of the president
• Count backwards (20 to 1)
Adapted from Stroke Prevention Exercise Program. (n.d). *SPEP Orpington Prognostic Scale.* Madison, WI: UW Health: University of Wisconsin Hospital and Clinics.

Permissions

The OPS is located in the public domain and is free to use in clinical practice, research, or publication. More information can be obtained by contacting its copyright holders or creators of the measure at the information following. The OPS scale can be found in its entirety in the following journal articles:

Kalra, L., & Crome, P. (1993). The role of prognostic scores in targeting stroke rehabilitation in elderly patients. *Journal of the American Geriatric Society, 41,* 396-400.

Rieck, M., & Moreland, J. (2005). The Orpington Prognostic Scale for patients with stroke: Reliability and pilot predictive data for discharge destination and therapeutic services. *Disability and Rehabilitation, 27*(23), 1425-1433.

Summary

POPULATION	CVA
TYPE OF MEASURE	Rating scale; physical and cognitive activities
WHAT IT ASSESSES	Neurological, physical status
TIME	<5 minutes
COST	Free

Contact

Lalit Kalra, MD

King's College

London, United Kingdom

Web: https://kclpure.kcl.ac.uk/portal/en/persons/lalit-kalra%288b580f28-c45d-420e-8465-57dfa216eb24%29.html

CHAPTER 41: STROKE IMPACT SCALE (SIS)

Description

The Stroke Impact Scale (SIS), developed by Duncan et al. (1999), is a comprehensive measure of health outcomes for stroke populations that incorporates meaningful dimensions of function and health related to quality of life into a single questionnaire that is completed as either a self-report or by proxy (Lai, Studenski, Duncan, & Perera, 2002). Several versions are available. The most recent, SIS 3.0, comprises 59 items that assess the following 8 domains of performance: (1) strength, (2) hand function, (3) mobility, (4) activities of daily living (ADLs), (5) emotion, (6) memory, (7) communication, and (8) social participation, as well as a physical domain that combines the first 4 domains to better examine the person's physical attributes affected by stroke. A 16-item version is also available that was developed on the basis of the 2.0 version and consists of 7 ADL/instrument ADL (IADL) items, 8 mobility items, and a single hand function item that was designed to quickly address the physical aspects of stroke (Edwards & O'Connell, 2003). Each item of the SIS measures is scored according to 3 possible 5-point Likert scales (1 to 5), where higher scores suggest better performance. The assessment employs a unique scoring algorithm where the maximum raw score (295) is computed through a mathematical equation to give a final score where both can be completed in less than 15 minutes.

Psychometrics

A study of 229 stroke patients found good internal consistency of the SIS 3.0 subscales for hand function ($\alpha = 0.82$), mobility subscale (0.86), ADL (0.79), emotion (0.79), memory (0.87), communication (0.87), and participation (0.75) with the lowest being strength at 0.63 (Nichols-Larsen, Clark, Zeringue, Greenspan, & Blanton, 2005). Instrument reliability of the 2.0 version found that Cronbach coefficients of internal consistency were also good with a range of $\alpha = 0.83$ to 0.90 and when stroke impact was measured over time internal consistency of all domains ranged from $\alpha = 0.70$ to 0.92, with the exception of emotion at 0.57, suggesting that the SIS in its present form is a stable instrument (Duncan et al., 1999). The same study showed that each of the 8 domain scales had good criterion validity and that the measures of disability (i.e., mobility and ADL/IADL), in particular, had good correlation coefficients in the range of 0.82 to 0.84 with other established measures such as the Barthel

Index (BI) and Functional Independence Measure scale (Duncan et al., 1999). Multiple regression analysis showed that three factors, physical function, emotion, and participation, explained 45% of the variance of the patient's global assessment of recovery (Duncan et al., 1999). Research by Lai et al (2002) showed that the SIS 3.0 was able to capture persisting difficulties in the performance of stroke patients who otherwise might have been considered functionally independent according to measures such as the BI or the modified Rankin Scale. For example, individuals with BI scores of 95 are usually considered recovered, however, Lai et al. (2002) showed that stroke patients who achieved a BI score of 95 continued to have residual disability and impaired quality of life as noted by SIS scores, highlighting its ability to detect impairment where other global assessments cannot.

Advantages

The assessment is available in several formats as well as proxy and self-administered versions. There is also a good amount of research in support of its use in clinical practice. No special training or certifications are needed to administer the exam and there is an excellent interactive website maintained by the University of Kansas Medical Center pertaining to the measure where one can download a copy as well as supporting material along with access to exclusive SIS databases of statistical and scoring information.

Disadvantages

A study of 377 subjects found that proxy-rated assessors tended to score patients as more severely affected than patients scored themselves on the SIS-16 version and in 7 of 8 domains of the full SIS 3.0. Five of those domain scores were considered statistically significant and although, intra-class correlation coefficients between proxy and patient ranged from 0.50 to 0.83 it was shown that this bias tended to increase as the severity of the patient's condition increased (Duncan et al., 2002).

Administration

During assessment the subject is asked to evaluate how stroke has impacted their health by rating questions relative to three possible scales depending on the question such as (5) a lot of strength to (1) no strength at all; (5) not difficult at all to (1) extremely difficult; or (5) none of the time to

(1) all of the time. An analog scale that explores the subjective level of recovery where (0) is no recovery to (100) full recovery is also completed. The SIS scoring algorithm is as follows:

$$\frac{[(\text{Actual raw score-lowest possible raw score})] \times 100}{\text{Possible raw score range}}$$

TABLE 41-1
EXAMPLE ITEM OF THE STROKE IMPACT SCALE
In the past 2 weeks, how difficult was it to use your hand that was most affected by your stroke to…
A. Carry heavy objects (i.e., bag of groceries)
B. Turn a doorknob
C. Open a can or jar
D. Tie a shoe lace
E. Pick up a dime

Permissions

Once registered as a user on the University of Kansas website, the SIS can be downloaded and is free to use in clinical practice as well as not for profit entities. To use in research or publication contact the copyright holders of the assessment at the information following. More information can be found in the following journal articles:

Duncan, P. W., Wallace, D., Lai, S. M., Johnson, D., Embretson, S., & Laster, L. (1999). The stroke impact scale version 2.0: Evaluation of reliability, validity, and sensitivity to change. *Stroke, 30*(10), 2131-40.

Lin, K., Fu, T., Wu, C., Hsieh, Y., Chen, C., & Lee, P. (2010). Psychometric comparisons of the Stroke Impact Scale 3.0 and Stroke-Specific Quality of Life Scale. *Quality of Life Research, 19*(3), 435-443.

Summary

POPULATION	Cerebrovascular accident
TYPE OF MEASURE	Rating scale
WHAT IT ASSESSES	Global effect of impairment
TIME	< 15 minutes
COST	Free

Contact

Sue M. Lai, PhD

University of Kansas Medical Center

Kansas City, Kansas

Web: www.kumc.edu/school-of-medicine/preventive-medicine-and-public-health/research-and-community-engagement/stroke-impact-scale.html

REFERENCES

Appelros, P., & Terent, A. (2004). Characteristics of the National Institute of Health Stroke Scale: Results from a population-based stroke cohort at baseline and after one year. *Cerebrovascular Diseases, 17*(1), 21-27.

Celik, C., Aksel, J., & Karaoglan, B. (2006). Comparison of the Orpington Prognostic Scale (OPS) and the National Institutes of Health Stroke Scale (NIHSS) for the prediction of the functional status of patients with stroke. *Disability and Rehabilitation, 28*(10), 609-612.

Dancer, S., Brown, A., & Yanase, L. (2009). National Institutes of Health Stroke Scale reliable and valid in plain English. *Journal of Neuroscience Nursing, 41*(1), 2-5.

Dewey, H., Donnan, G., Freeman, E., Sharples, C., Richard A., Macdonell, R.,...Thrift, A. (1999). Interrater reliability of the National Institutes of Health Stroke Scale: Rating by neurologists and nurses in a community-based stroke incidence study. *Cerebrovascular Diseases, 9*(6), 323-327.

Duncan, P., Lai, S., Tyler, D., Perera, S., Reker, D., & Studenski, S. (2002). Evaluation of proxy responses to the Stroke Impact Scale. *Stroke, 33*(11), 2593-2599.

Duncan, P., Wallace, D., Lai, S. M., Johnson, D., Embretson, S., & Laster, L. (1999). The Stroke Impact Scale version 2.0: Evaluation of reliability, validity, and sensitivity to change. *Stroke, 30*(10), 2131-2140.

Edwards, B., & O'Connell, B. (2003). Internal consistency and validity of the stroke impact scale 2.0 (SIS 2.0) and SIS-16 in an Australian sample. *Quality of Life Research, 12*(8), 1127-1135.

Franco, C. R. C., Leao, P., Townsend, R., Carlos, R. M., & Rieder, C. R. M. (2011). Reliability and validity of a scale for measurement of trunk mobility in Parkinson's disease *Arquivos de Neuro-Psiquiatria 69*(4), 636-641.

Goetz, C. G., Fahn, S., Martínez-Martín, P., Poewe, W., Sampaio, C., Stebbins, G.,...LaPelle, N. (2007). Movement Disorder Society-sponsored revision of the Unified Parkinson's Disease Rating Scale (MDS-UPDRS): Process, format, and clinimetric testing plan. *Movement Disorders, 22*(1), 41–47.

Goetz, C., Poewe, W., Rascol, O., Sampaio, C., Stebbins, G., Counsell, C.,...Seidl. L. (2004). Movement Disorder Society task force report on the Hoehn and Yahr Staging Scale: Status and recommendations. *Movement Disorders, 19*(9), 1020–1028.

Goetz, C., Tilley, B., Shaftman, S., Stebbins, G., Fahn, S., Poewe, W.,...LaPelle, N. (2008). Movement Disorder Society-sponsored revision of the Unified Parkinson's Disease Rating Scale (MDS-UPDRS): Scale presentation and clinimetric testing results. *Movement Disorders, 23*(15), 2129-2170.

Goldstein, L., & Samsa, G. (1997). Reliability of the National Institutes of Health Stroke Scale extension to non-neurologists in the context of a clinical trial. *Stroke, 28*, 307-310.

Hoehn, M., & Yahr, M. (1967). Parkinsonism: Onset, progression and mortality. *Neurology, 17*, 427–442.

Jain, A., Van Houten, D., & Sheikh, L. (2016). Retrospective study on National Institutes of Health Stroke Scale as a predictor of patient recovery after stroke. *Journal of Cardiovascular Nursing, 31*(1), 69-72.

Kalra, L., & Crome, P. (1993). The role of prognostic scores in targeting stroke rehabilitation in elderly patients. *Journal of the American Geriatric Society, 41*, 396-400.

Lai, S., Duncan, P., & Keighley, J. (1998). Prediction of functional outcome after stroke comparison of the Orpington Prognostic Scale and the NIH Stroke Scale. *Stroke, 29*, 1838-1842.

Lai, S., Studenski, S., Duncan, P., & Perera, S. (2002). Persisting consequences of stroke measured by the stroke impact scale. *Stroke, 33*(7), 1840-1844.

Martínez-Martín, P., Rodríguez-Blázquez, C., Forjaz, M. J., Álvarez-Sánchez, M., Arakaki, T., Bergareche-Yarza, A.,...Goetz, C. G. (2014). Relationship between the MDS-UPDRS domains and the health-related quality of life of Parkinson's disease patients. *European Journal of Neurology, 21*(3), 519-524.

Muller, J., Wenning, G., Jellinger, K., McKee, A., Poewe, W., & Litvan, I. (2000). Progression of Hoehn and Yahr stages in Parkinsonian disorders: A clinicopathologic study. *Neurology, 55*(6), 888-891.

National Institutes of Health Stroke Scale. (2003). *Know stroke.* Bethesda, MD: National Institute of Health.

Nichols-Larsen, D., Clark, P. C., Zeringue, A., Greenspan, A., & Blanton, S. (2005). Factors influencing stroke survivors' quality of life during subacute recovery. *Stroke, 36*, 1480-1484.

Palmer, J., Coats, M., Roe, C., Hanko, S., Xiong, C., & Morris, J. (2010). Unified Parkinson's disease Rating Scale-Motor exam: Inter-rater reliability of advanced practice nurse and neurologist assessments. *Journal of Advanced Nursing, 66*(6), 1382-1387

Pittock, S., Meldrum, D., Ni Dhuill, C., Hardiman, O., & Moroney, J. (2003). The Orpington Prognostic Scale within the first 48 hours of admission as a predictor of outcome in ischemic stroke. *Journal of Stroke and Cerebrovascular Diseases, 12*(4), 175–181.

Quelhas, R., & Costa, M. (2009). Anxiety, depression, and quality of life in Parkinson's disease. *The Journal of Neuropsychiatry and Clinical Neurosciences, 21*(4), 413-419.

Quinn, T., Dawson, J., Walters, M., & Lees, K. (2009). Reliability of the Modified Rankin Scale: A systematic review. *Stroke, 40*, 3393-3395.

Qutubuddin, A. A., Pegg, P. O., Cifu, D. X., Brown, R., McNamee, S., & Carne, W. (2005). Validating the Berg Balance Scale for patients with Parkinson's disease: A key to rehabilitation evaluation. *Archives of Physical Medicine and Rehabilitation, 86*(4), 789-792

Rieck, M., & Moreland, J. (2005). The Orpington Prognostic Scale for patients with stroke: Reliability and pilot predictive data for discharge destination and therapeutic services. *Disability and Rehabilitation, 27*(23), 1425–1433.

Santangelo, G., Barone, P., Abbruzzese, G., Ferini-Strambi, L., & Antonini, A. (2014). Validation of the Italian version of Parkinson's Disease-Cognitive Rating Scale (PD-CRS). *Neurological Sciences, 35*(4), 537-544.

Shoemaker, M., Mullins-MacRitchie, M., Bennett, J., Vryhof, K., & Boettcher, I. (2006). Predicting response to rehabilitation in elderly patients with stroke using the Orpington Prognostic Scale and selected clinical variables. *Journal of Geriatric Physical Therapy, 29*(2), 69-73.

Shulman, L., Gruber-Baldini, A., Anderson, K., Fishman, P., Reich, S., & Weiner, W. (2010). The clinically important difference on the Unified Parkinson's Disease Rating Scale. *Archives of Neurology, 67*(1), 64-70.

Steffen, T., & Seney, M. (2008). Test-retest reliability and minimal detectable change on balance and ambulation tests, the 36-Item Short-Form Health Survey, and the Unified Parkinson Disease Rating Scale in people with Parkinsonism. *Physical Therapy, 88*(6), 733-746.

Stroke Prevention Exercise Program. (n.d.). *SPEP Orpington Prognostic Scale*. Madison, WI: UW Health: University of Wisconsin Hospital and Clinics.

Studenski, S., Wallace, D., Duncan, P. W., Rymer, M., & Lai, S. M. (2001). Predicting stroke recovery: Three and six-month rates of patient-centered functional outcomes based on the Orpington Prognostic Scale. *Journal of the American Geriatrics Society, 49,* 308–312.

Sulter, G., Steen, C., & De Keyser, J. (1999). Use of the Barthel Index and Modified Rankin Scale in acute stroke trials. *Stroke, 30*(8), 1538-1541.

Thomas, A., Rogers, J., Amick, M., & Friedman, J. (2010). Falls and the Falls Efficacy Scale in Parkinson's disease. *Journal of Neurology, 257*(7), 1124-1128.

Uyttenboogaart, M., Stewart, R., Vroomen, P., De Keyser, J., & Luijckx, G. (2005). Optimizing cutoff scores for the Barthel Index and the Modified Rankin Scale for defining outcome in acute stroke trials. *Stroke, 36*(9), 1984-1987.

Van Swieten, J., Koudstaal, P., Visser, M., Schouten, H., & van Gijn, J. (1988). Interobserver agreement for the assessment of handicap in stroke patients. *Stroke, 19*(5), 604-607.

Zhao, Y. J., Wee, H. W., Chan, Y-H., Seah, S. H., Au, W. L., Lau, P. N.,... Tan, L. (2010). Progression of Parkinson's disease as evaluated by Hoehn and Yahr stage transition times. *Movement Disorders, 25*(6), 710-716.

VIII

Dexterity Assessment

Bortnick, K.
Occupational Therapy Assessments for Older Adults: 100 Instruments for Measuring Occupational Performance (pp. 117-135).
© 2017 Taylor & Francis Group.

CHAPTER 42: BOX AND BLOCK TEST (BBT)

Description

The Box and Block Test (BBT) is a standardized measure of unilateral gross manual dexterity as well as various hand/finger grip functions such as the pincer grasp, three jaw chuck, pad to pad, and lateral prehension. The BBT is appropriate for a number of developmental and other conditions, such as stroke, where a person's grasp or his or her ability crossing the midline may be of concern. During assessment, the subject is asked to pick up as many small, square, 2.5-cm blocks as possible from one compartment of a box and place them into another compartment in a 60 second time frame. The box, explained in detail by Mathiowetz, Volland, Kashman, and Weber (1985), when open forms two compartments with a partition in the middle that is high such that the subject must reach over the partition to place the blocks into the other side. The unit is typically constructed of plywood (1 cm) that in its open state is roughly 53 x 53 cm with 8.5-cm sides. In the middle of the open box is a 15-cm high partition. The box is designed to fold into an easy-to-use carrying case. The assessment comes with 150 cubes that are 2.5-cm squares, made of wood and colored blue, green, red, and yellow. Scoring involves the number of cubes moved from one compartment to the other in 60 seconds. The BBT can be completed and scored in less than 5 minutes.

Psychometrics

A study of test-retest reliabilities of 35 able-bodied subjects ranged from r = 0.90 right hand and 0.89 left; whereas reliabilities of 34 impaired subjects were r = 0.97 right and 0.96 left (Desrosiers, Bravo, Hébert, Dutil, & Mercier, 1994). A study of 27 occupational therapy student subjects found inter-rater reliability, using 2 raters, to be nearly identical for the right hand at 1.0 and for left hand 0.99 (Mathiowetz et al., 1985). Another inter-rater and intra-rater reliability study of subjects with rheumatoid arthritis (RA; n = 60), using 2 raters, ranged from r = 0.92 to 0.97 and r = 0.91 to 0.95, respectively. The same study found dexterity scores of those with RA were lower when compared to controls for the dominant hand (54.87 vs 68.18), contralateral hand (52.65 vs 65.6), as well as with population-based normative scores; dominant hand (54.87 vs 80.02) contralateral hand (52.65 vs 77.23) (Ranjan, Raj, Kumar, Sandhya, & Danda, 2015). A study of 104 subjects aged 60 to 94 years found that correlations between the BBT and the Action Research Arm Test were significant (0.80; right hand and 0.82; left); whereas correlations between the BBT and the Functional Autonomy Measurement System—activities of daily living subsection and total score were moderate at 0.42 right and 0.54 left and 0.47 right and 0.51 left (Desrosiers et al., 1994). Standardized norms have been established for the BBT using a sample of 628 20- to 94-year-old subjects, which noted that test scores typically decrease with age evidenced by scores of the 20- to 24-year-old age group were 88.0 right and 83.4 left compared to the 70- to 74-years-old age group (68.6 right and 68.3 left) (Mathiowetz et al., 1985). A similar study of 360 subjects aged 60 years or older, also to establish standardized norms, obtained a mean score of 66.9 for the right hand and a mean of 66.3 for the left (Desrosiers et al., 1994).

Advantages

There is a significant amount of literature in support of its use in clinical practice and no special training or certifications are required to administer the BBT. There are also well-established norms available for the assessment across the lifespan in a number of studies. The assessment has remained relatively unchanged from its original description in 1957 and administration time is less than 5 minutes.

Disadvantages

The box when closed may be considered by some to be awkward. The BBT is also more expensive than some of the pegboard assessments described later in this section and its availability may be limited to only a few therapy outlets. The inherent reward from moving blocks from one place to another may be limited as well, and because the test requires rapid movements, may add a stress component not found in more routine tasks (Canny, Thompson, & Wheeler, 2009).

Administration

During assessment the subject is asked to pick and place as many blocks as possible from one box compartment into another over a small partition in 60 seconds. The individual is scored on how many blocks can be placed in the allotted time. The examiner's manual has detailed instructions as well as standardized norms. Alternative scoring norms are available elsewhere.

NORMS FOR THE BOX AND BLOCK TEST (NUMBER OF BLOCKS PLACED)			
MALE	**N**	**RIGHT HAND**	**LEFT HAND**
55 to 59 years old	21	75.2	73.8
60 to 64 years old	24	71.3	70.5
65 to 69 years old	27	68.4	67.4
70 to 74 years old	26	66.3	64.3
75 years old or older	25	63.0	61.3
FEMALE	**N**	**RIGHT HAND**	**LEFT HAND**
55 to 59 years old	25	74.7	73.6
60 to 64 years old	25	76.1	73.6
65 to 69 years old	28	72.0	71.3
70 to 74 years old	29	68.6	68.3
75 years old or older	27	65.0	63.6

TABLE 42-1

Adapted from Mathiowetz, V., Volland, G., Kashman, N., & Weber, K. (1985). Adult norms for the Box and Block Test of manual dexterity. *American Journal of Occupational Therapy, 39*(6), 389-390.

Permissions

The BBT can be purchased from various therapy supply companies. Cost for the BBT varies from $220 to $300. To use in research or publication contact where purchased or where published at the information following. More information can be found in the following journal article:

Mathiowetz, V., Volland, G., Kashman, N., & Weber, K. (1985). Adult norms for the Box and Block Test of manual dexterity. *American Journal of Occupational Therapy, 39*(6), 386-391.

Summary

POPULATION	Suspected upper extremity limb or hand injury; work rehabilitation; general
TYPE OF MEASURE	Activity-based functional performance
WHAT IT ASSESSES	Gross, fine dexterity
TIME	<5 minutes
COST	$220 to $300

Contact

4MD Medical Solutions

315B 4th Street

Lakewood, NJ 08701

Phone: (877) 753-5426

Web: www.4mdmedical.com/box-block-test.html#.VdaDmH1GNf1

Chapter 43: Functional Dexterity Test (FDT)

Description

The Functional Dexterity Test (FDT; 1983) is designed to purvey information regarding a person's ability to use the hand for functional tasks requiring the use of gross prehension patterns (Aaron & Stegink-Jansen, 2003). During assessment the subject is required to turn over pegs from a pegboard starting from the opposite corner of the hand being tested in a zigzag fashion until all rows are overturned. The pegboard is a square wooden board that contains places for 16 pegs that are larger than typical pegboard assessments (i.e., 2.2 cm in diameter and 4 cm long), thus large enough for the client to exhibit the need for gross motor grasp such as three jaw chuck prehension between the fingers and thumb. The board's dimensions are roughly 20 cm x 20 cm and 4 cm deep and contains rows, 4 x 4 to accommodate the 16 pegs. While administering the test the clinician examines for unusual movements and the subject is scored according to the time it takes to turn over all pegs. Various time infractions can be incurred such as when a peg is dropped or if the person completely supinates their hand. Two scores are possible (1) total time and (2) total time plus penalties. Higher scores (in seconds) indicate more impairment and a score over 55 seconds is considered non-functional. The FDT can be completed in less than 5 minutes.

Psychometrics

Using 3 raters, Aaron and Stegink-Jansen (2003) found that for score 1 (total time) inter-rater reliability was excellent (r= 0.99); however, for score 2, which takes into account penalties, intra-class correlation coefficients were lower for the uninjured hand at $r = 0.88$ and for the injured hand it was 0.73. The same developmental study established validity by comparing FDT scores with the ability to complete four functional activities of daily living (buttoning a button, tying shoe laces, screwing a nut and bolt, and lacing yarn) with the injured hand where subjects were considered functional for those activities where for FDT scores between 16 and 25 seconds they were considered functional; scores between 26 to 33 seconds they were considered moderately functional; and at 34 to 50 seconds they were considered minimally functional. A subsequent study by Sartorio et al. (2013) of 324 healthy volunteers displayed excellent test-retest reliabilities of the FDT with values higher than $r = 0.90$.

TABLE 43-1							
REFERENCE NORMS SHOWN AS PERCENTILE RANK, NET TIME IN SECONDS FROM A HEALTHY SAMPLE							
		NON-DOMINANT			DOMINANT		
Age	*Sex*	*50th*	*84th*	*97.5*	*50th*	*84th*	*97.5*
50 to 59 years old	M	27.1	34.7	40.7	24.5	31.9	38.7
	F	32.3	37.4	43.9	27.4	34.3	43.8
60 to 69 years old	M	31.7	40.0	47.2	30.4	38.1	43.7
	F	33.8	40.6	46.8	31.2	35.9	42.9
70 to 79 years old	M	38.2	51.0	57.8	31.2	42.6	50.2
	F	38.3	45.3	48.9	37.0	42.0	43.3
n = 698; age = 20 to 79 years old							

Adapted from Sartorio, F., Bravini, E., Vercelli, S., Ferriero, G., Plebani, G., Foti, C., & Franchignoni, F. (2013). The Functional Dexterity Test: Test-retest reliability analysis and up-to date reference norms. *Journal of Hand Therapy, 26*(1), 65.

Advantages

No special training or certifications are needed and the FDT is relatively quick and easy to administer, at less than 5 minutes. The assessment is unique in that it is narrowly focused on more gross motor capabilities of the fingers and hand such as the dynamic prehension needed for grasping somewhat larger objects, which is unique when compared to other pegboards that typically assess fine motor skills.

Disadvantages

The amount of supporting literature pertaining to the measure is somewhat limited and cost of the FDT can range from $115 to $225.

Administration

The pegboard is placed 10 cm from the end of the table, the client is then instructed to turn over all of the pegs with the non-injured hand starting at the top row away from client (i.e., right hand would start at the upper left corner) turning pegs left to right (Aaron & Stegink-Jansen, 2013). When the top row is completed the subject drops down a row until complete, creating a zigzag pattern until all pegs are overturned. Specific verbal instructions as well as cueing are in the examiner's manual. For example, the person is told not to fully supinate the hand or touch the board with the other hand as these carry 5 second penalties. If a peg is dropped a 10 second penalty is added to the score. Two scores are obtained from the FDT, time it takes to complete and combined time, which includes any penalties (Aaron & Stegink-Jansen, 2013). A score over 55 seconds is considered non-functional and the test is stopped after 2 minutes. Standardized norms are available in the manual and elsewhere.

Permission

The FDT can be purchased from several therapy supply companies. Price varies from $115 to $225. To use in research or publication contact where purchased or published at the information that follows. More information can be found in the following journal article:

Aaron, D. & Stegink-Jansen, C. (2003). Development of the Functional Dexterity Test (FDT): Construction, validity, reliability, and normative data. *Journal of Hand Therapy, 16*(1), 12–21.

Summary

POPULATION	Suspected upper extremity limb or hand injury; work rehabilitation; general
TYPE OF MEASURE	Activity-based functional performance
WHAT IT ASSESSES	Gross prehension patterns
TIME	<5 minutes
COST	$115 to $225

Contact

Dorit Aaron, MA, OTR, CHT

Aaron & Winthrop Hand Therapy Services

Houston, Texas

Website: www.AaronWinthropHand.com

CHAPTER 44: GROOVED PEGBOARD TEST (GPT)

Description

The Grooved Pegboard Test (GPT) is a test of finger dexterity that assesses both psychomotor speed and fine motor control and has shown to be relevant in gauging the performance of assembly and machine-operating type of jobs, work hardening programs, and a number of health conditions in which hand and finger performance is of primary concern. During assessment the subject is required to place 25 keyed pegs into an array of 25 slotted holes as quickly as possible (Strenge, Niederberger, & Seelhorst, 2002). The GPT is a unique dexterity assessment in that each peg has a ridge on one side and therefore must be oriented correctly to fit into a hole on the pegboard; thus the GPT requires a level of complex visual-motor coordination for successful completion not seen in other pegboard batteries (Howell & Yancosek, 2009). During assessment both hands are tested separately, with the dominant hand tested first. The clinician records in seconds the length of time required to perform the task of putting all of the pegs in the slots on the board. Other scoring entails correctly placed pins as well as the number of drops. The GPT can be completed in less than 10 minutes.

Psychometrics

Reliability of the GPT has been addressed in several studies. Ruff and Parker (1993) reported test-retest coefficients ranging from r=0.69 to 0.76 for the dominant hand and r=0.68 to 0.78 for the non-dominant hand over a 6-month period (Mitrushina, 2005). A study by Wang et al. (2011) of 340 subjects ages 3 to 85 years old determined that the GPT had good test–retest reliability at r=0.91 and 0.85 for right and left hands, respectively and that it was moderately to significantly correlated with the Purdue Pegboard Test at −0.73 to −0.78. Results also found that the GPT was both longer and more challenging for the youngest children and oldest adults. Another investigation of healthy adults (n=66) revealed a significant main effect for gender; however, no significant interaction was observed with regard to the influence of left-hand peg placement direction (right-to-left vs left-to-right) (Fouty et al., 2015). A study by Schubert et al. (2013) found that those with olfactory impairment, which can occur after traumatic brain injury, took significantly longer to perform the GPT than those without impairment at 85.1 seconds compared with 72.2 for the unimpaired group. An examination of GPT scores of 49 medical students found that mean score for the right hand was 54.2 seconds (range 41 to 74 seconds) and for the left hand it was 57.9 seconds (range

44 to 68 seconds) (Strenge et al., 2002) Another study found moderate correlations between GPT performance and a subject's *level of alertness* (i.e., tonic or phasic for both the right and left hands) at tonic 0.25 (right) and 0.10 (left) while phasic correlations were 0.31 (right) and 0.30 (left), suggesting that alertness (either tonic or phasic) plays an important role in the performance of tasks demanding attention (Strenge et al., 2002). No significant effects of age or sex were noted in that study. A sample of 191 subjects with Parkinson's disease comparing the GPT with the Unified Parkinson's Disease Rating Scale (UPDRS) found the strongest relationships between the place phase (both limbs) and total UPDRS motor score (affected: r=0.60 and less-affected: r=0.59), whereas the GPT remove phase had weak positive relationships with total UPDRS scores (affected: r=0.31, less-affected r=0.31) (Sage, Bryden, Roy, & Almeida,2012), suggesting that the act of placing a keyed peg may require more motor as well as other abilities.

TABLE 44-1
REFERENCED GROOVED PEGBOARD TEST NORMS FOR SELECTED AGE GROUPS

Age	N	DOMINANT		NON-DOMINANT	
		Mean	SD	Mean	SD
50 to 59 years old	134	68.10	9.42	74.70	10.51
60 years old or older	100	82.70	18.70	87.85	26.20

Adapted from Lafayette Instrument Company. (2002). *Grooved Pegboard Test user instructions* (p. 8). Lafayette, IN.

Advantages

There is a good amount of evidenced in support of the GPT for use in clinical practice. It is also a simple assessment to administer requiring no special certifications or permissions. The examiner's manual has detailed instructions as well as established norms for age groups across the lifespan and like the Nine Hole Peg Test is smaller than other pegboard tests increasing its portability. Finally, the

GPT is unique in that each peg has a ridge on one side and therefore must be oriented correctly if it is to fit into the hole on the pegboard, requiring an added visuomotor component to the test, thus necessitating visual attention to the task as well as thumb and index finger manipulation of the peg, making it of interest to many investigators and clinicians (Howell & Yancosek, 2009).

Disadvantages

Persons who have corticospinal pathway or similar injuries are likely to have a more difficult time with this test.

Administration

Assessment requires the pegboard to be placed in midline with the person and the subject is then told to begin by putting the pegs into the board as fast as he or she can. For the right hand trial, the pegs are placed from the subject's left to right, and for the left hand trial pegs are placed from his or her right to left. The dominant hand trial is administered first, followed by the non-dominant. The subject must fill the top row completely from side to side, then go on to the next row without skipping any rows or dropping any pegs. The GPT includes 3 scores: (1) the time in seconds, (2) number of drops, and (3) number of correct pegs placed. Standardized norms for ages 5 to 60 years old or older are available in the manual and elsewhere.

Permission

The GPT is a standardized measure that can be purchased from a number of therapy supply companies where the cost can vary from $95 to $145. To use in research or publication contact where purchased or where published. More information can be found in the following article:

Ruff, R., & Parker, S. (1993). Gender- and age-specific changes in motor speed and eye-hand coordination in adults: Normative values for the Finger Tapping and Grooved Pegboard Tests. *Perceptual and Motor Skills*, *76*(3c), 1219-1230.

Summary

POPULATION	Suspected hand injury; work rehabilitation; general
TYPE OF MEASURE	Activity-based functional performance
WHAT IT ASSESSES	Fine motor dexterity
TIME	< 10 minutes
COST	$95 to$145

Contact

Lafayette Instrument Company

P.O. Box 5729

Lafayette, IN 47903

Phone: (800) 428-7545

E-mail: info@lafayetteinstrument.com

Web: www.lafayetteevaluation.com/product_detail. asp?itemid=167

CHAPTER 45: MINNESOTA MANUAL DEXTERITY TEST (MMDT) AND MINNESOTA RATE OF MANIPULATION TEST (MRMT)

Description

The Minnesota Manual Dexterity Test (MMDT) and the Minnesota Rate of Manipulation Test (MRMT) are considered large board assessments typically used to measure eye-hand coordination as well as gross motor arm quality and hand dexterity opposed to the fine motor quality of some of the pegboard assessments discussed prior. Both are relatively quick outcome measures that utilize similar hardware (i.e., a long board with holes in which blocks must be placed or displaced from the holes using various techniques). In particular, the original version MRMT consists of 2 wooden boards, 81.2-cm long, 22.9-cm wide, and 2.7-cm thick that rest on top of each other (Surrey et al., 2003). Each board has 60 holes, 3.8 cm in diameter and 1.3 cm deep and designed to fit inside the holes are 60 cylindrical blocks, 3.5 cm in diameter and 2.2 cm high (Surrey et al., 2003). The cylindrical blocks are yellow on one side and orange on the other side. The newer MMDT dimensions consist of one plastic accordion-style collapsible board that is 85.4-cm long, 22.8-cm wide only 0.5-cm thick (Surrey et al., 2003). The collapsible board also has 60 holes, 3.9 cm in diameter and 0.5-cm deep. The same number of cylindrical blocks (60) fit into the holes and measure 3.7 cm in diameter and 1.9-cm high (Surrey et al., 2003). The cylindrical blocks are red on one side and black on the other side. During assessment of both boards the person's abilities are scored relative to speed and correctness in completing a combination of 3 basic tasks: (1 to 2) placing or displacing the discs and (3) variations of turning the discs, such as, how quickly a subject can pick up each disc with one hand, turn them over into the other hand and replace them back into the hole on the board (Tajmir & Carnahan, 2013). The older MRMT has 5 distinct subtests with well-established referenced norms for placing, turning, displacing, one-hand turning and placing, and two-hand turning and placing. The newer MMDT manual only formally has directions for the placing and turning tests; however, the manual makes numerous references to the original MRMT and its norms, thus it is assumed that the 5 tests can be completed with the newer MMDT board as well. Time to complete all of the subtests is less than 15 minutes

Psychometrics

An MRMT study of 118 subjects treated surgically by a hand surgeon found that inter-rater reliability using 2 independent raters was moderate at r=0.75 (Gloss & Wardle, 1982). Whereas a study by Jurgensen, (1943) showed that a 2 trial test-retest reliability for placing was r=0.87, turning 0.91, 1-hand turning and placing 0.95, and 2-hand turning and placing 0.94; while a 4 trial reliability for placing was r=0.93, turning 0.95, 1-hand turning and placing 0.98, and 2-hand turning and placing 0.97 representing highly significant consistencies. Desrosiers, Hébert, and Bravo (1997) found that test-retest reliability of the MMDT subtests ranged from r=0.79 to 0.88 and correlation coefficients with the Box and Block Test and the Purdue Pegboard Test were moderate at −0.63 and −0.67, respectively. The same study, using only the common placing and turning test when comparing the MMDT with MRMT, found that the 2 were highly correlated at 0.85, 0.95, and 0.95 for right hand, left hand, and turning tests; however, it was also determined that the time required to complete MMDT tasks were longer than that of the MRMT. A study by Surrey et al. (2003) generally concurred with those results of 233 subjects aged 18 to 70 years that yielded statistically significant longer performance times for the MMDT (i.e., placing: MMDT 49.96 seconds vs. MRMT 45.58 seconds and turning subtests: MMDT 62.58 seconds and MRMT 61.23 seconds).

Advantages

There is a large amount of research pertaining to the subtests of both the MRMT and MMDT assessments and available normative data has been derived from large cohorts of people across the lifespan. Testing procedures and scoring have remained stable and relatively unchanged since the 1940s for the MRMT subtests which are often used in the newer MMDT as well. Alas, the MMDT may be considered more refined because it is made of plastic, is sleeker, and is able fold like an accordion into a briefcase. Neither test requires any special training.

Disadvantages

The original MMRT, constructed of wood, can be large and awkward and both tests require a lot of space due to the size of the boards when opened, 81 cm by 22 cm (31 inches x 9 inches) or greater, and since the test is completed in the standing position taller/shorter people may have difficulty with the recommended table height of 28 to 32 inches found in both assessments. Finally, there is less direct research pertaining to the newer MMDT.

Administration

The examiner's manual provides for standardized instruction as well as scoring norms, which are also available elsewhere. Each subtest is completed in the standing position and can include a placing test which measures the speed with which the subject can put the blocks into the holes with one hand; a displacing test that measures the speed with which blocks can be removed; a one-hand turning and placing test, which measures the speed with which a subject can manipulate the blocks, as well as put them into holes with one hand; and a two-hand turning and placing test that measures the speed with which the subject can manipulate two blocks, one with each hand, as well as put them into the holes.

Permissions

Both the MMDT and MRMT can be purchased from various therapy supply companies; however, the original wooden version may be difficult to find. Price for the readily available MMDT vary from $185 to $250. To use in research or publication contact where purchased or where published. More information can be found in the following article:

Surrey, L., Nelson, K., Delelio, C., Mathie-Majors, D., Omel-Edwards, N., Shumaker, J., & Thurber, G. (2003). A comparison of performance outcomes between the Minnesota Rate of Manipulation Test and the Minnesota Manual Dexterity Test. *Work, 20*(2), 97-102.

Summary

POPULATION	Suspected upper extremity (UE) limb or hand injury; work rehabilitation; general
TYPE OF MEASURE	Activity-based functional performance
WHAT IT ASSESSES	Gross motor UE; hand dexterity
TIME	< 15 minutes
COST	$185 to $250

Contact

Lafayette Instrument Company

P.O. Box 5729

Lafayette, IN 47903

Phone: (800) 428-7545 (Toll free US Only)

Email: info@lafayetteinstrument.com

Web: www.lafayetteevaluation.com/product_ detail. asp?itemid=164

Chapter 46: Nine Hole Peg Test (NHPT)

Description

The Nine Hole Peg Test (NHPT) is commonly used measure of finger dexterity that is a relatively quick standardized assessment designed to quantify the manual dexterity of an individual. During assessment the subject is asked to place pegs into holes on a specially designed board. The standardized equipment consists of 9 pegs (7-mm diameter, 32-mm length), a 100 cm x 100 cm x 10 cm container for the pegs, and a wooden board slightly smaller than the container with 9 holes evenly spaced and slightly wider than the pegs to be placed 32 mm apart. During assessment the subject is asked to pick up the pegs one at a time and put them into the holes as fast as possible using only one hand and starting with the unaffected hand or, if not affected on either side, with the dominant hand (Sommerfeld, Eek, Svensson, Widén Holmqvist, & von Arvin, 2004). The assessment typically takes less than 5 minutes to complete with the actual test taking less than 2 minutes. The person is scored on how fast it takes to complete the task. Several activities can be measured as well, such as the placement of pegs in, putting pegs both in and out, and how many pegs placed within a set time (i.e., 50 seconds or 100 seconds).

Psychometrics

A study by Mathiowetz, Weber, Kashman, and Volland (1985) found very high inter-rater reliability for the right hand ($r=0.97$) and for the left ($r=0.99$) from a cohort of 26 female occupational therapy students; however, test-retest reliability was reported to be only moderate ($r=0.69$; right and $r=0.43$; left). Concurrent validity of the NHPT was also explored with the Purdue Pegboard Test where observed correlations were $r=-0.61$ right and $r=-0.53$ left. An analogous designed study by Oxford-Grice et al. (2003) produced similar results from a cohort of 26 occupational therapy students with very high inter-rater reliability ($r=0.98$; right and $r=0.99$; left), whereas test–retest reliability produced only low to moderate coefficients for both the right and left hand at $r=0.46$ and $r=0.44$, respectively. A study of 262 individuals with Parkinson's disease (PD) found that the average time to complete the NHPT was 31.4 ± 15.7 seconds with the dominant hand and 32.2 ± 12.4 seconds with the non-dominant hand (Earhart et al., 2011). The same study found test-retest reliabilities to be high also ($r=0.88$; dominant and $r=0.91$; non-dominant) and that performance times were generally better among participants at Hoehn and Yahr Stage 1 relative to those at more advanced stages, and on average, people with PD took approximately 50% longer than healthy adults to complete the battery (Earhart et al., 2011). Gender (W) was also found to be a significant predictor, but for the non-dominant hand only (Earhart et al., 2011). Normative data from a cohort of 618 subjects aged 20 to 94 years established by Mathiowetz et al. (1985) demonstrated a high correlation between NHPT scores and age with the 20- to 24-year-old age group producing the best scores and those in the 75-years-old or older age group producing the worst, supporting the theory that dexterity gradually decreases with age. Outcomes also found that females performed slightly better than males and right-hand scores were typically better than left-hand scores. Normative data from the 2003 study by Oxford-Grice et al. of 703 subjects aged 21 to 70 years or older discussed earlier generally supports those conclusions, and as expected, a high correlation was found between performance on the NHPT and age (for males at $r=0.91$; right hand, $r=0.92$; left hand and females: $r=0.89$; right hand and $r=0.90$; left hand).

Advantages

There is a good amount of research in support of its use in clinical practice and the test can be administered throughout the adult age range as well as for a number of conditions in which hand/finger dexterity is of concern. No special training is needed and the time to complete is less than 5 minutes. The NHPT is a standardized tool with well-established norms that is commercially available and is portable for use in a variety of settings and is relatively inexpensive.

Disadvantages

There are several different commercial versions of the test available on the market and some researchers have found statistical differences in performance times between these various versions.

Administration

The NHPT has standardized instructions for the clinician to follow as well as score interpretations located in the examiner's manual. During assessment, the subject is asked to complete various tasks related to the placing and removing of pegs from the recessed container at the bottom portion of the board. Results are expressed in correct placements/removal as well as time in seconds.

TABLE 46-1

SCORING NORMS OF THE
NINE HOLE PEG TEST IN SECONDS

MALE	AGE	N	MEAN RIGHT HAND	MEAN LEFT HAND
	51 to 55 years old	25	18.93	19.84
	56 to 60 years old	25	20.90	21.64
	61 to 65 years old	24	20.87	21.60
	66 to 70 years old	14	21.23	22.29
	71 years old or older	25	25.79	25.95
FEMALE	AGE	N	MEAN RIGHT HAND	MEAN LEFT HAND
	51 to 55 years old	42	17.38	18.92
	56 to 60 years old	31	17.86	19.48
	61 to 65 years old	29	18.99	20.33
	66 to 70 years old	31	19.90	21.44
	71 years old or older	31	22.49	24.11

Subjects aged 46 to 71 years

Adapted from Oxford-Grice, K., Vogel, K. A., Le, V., Mitchell, A., Muniz, S., & Vollmer, M. A. (2003). Brief report: Adult norms for a commercially available Nine Hole Peg Test for finger dexterity. *American Journal of Occupational Therapy, 57,* 572.

Permissions

The NHPT can be purchased from a number of different therapy supply stores where the cost can range from $40 to $80. To use in research or publication contact where purchased or where published. More information can be found in the following journal articles:

Mathiowetz, V., Weber, K., Kashman, N., & Volland, G. (1985). Adult norms for the Nine Hole Peg Test of Finger Dexterity. *Occupational Therapy Journal of Research, 5,* 24-33.

Oxford-Grice, K., Vogel, K. A., Le, V., Mitchell, A., Muniz, S., & Vollmer, M. A. (2003) Brief report: Adult norms for a commercially available Nine Hole Peg Test for finger dexterity. *American Journal of Occupational Therapy, 57,* 570–573.

Summary

POPULATION	Suspected hand injury; work rehabilitation; general
TYPE OF MEASURE	Activity-based functional performance
WHAT IT ASSESSES	Hand dexterity
TIME	<5 minutes
COST	$40 to $80

Contact

Kimatha Oxford-Grice, MOT, OTR, CHT
Department of Occupational Therapy
University of Texas Health Science Center
Houston, Texas
Web: http://uthscsa.edu/ot2/oxford.html

4MD Medical Solutions
315B 4th Street
Lakewood, NJ 08701
Phone: (877) 753-5426
Web: www.4mdmedical.com

CHAPTER 47: O'CONNOR FINGER AND TWEEZER DEXTERITY TESTS

Description

The O'Connor Dexterity Battery by O'Connor (1926) is a standardized assessment of hand-eye coordination as well as fine motor control and consists of activities involving a finger test and a tweezer test. In both, the client is asked to place pins into a single hole on a board using only his or her fingers or by using a set of tweezers. The equipment for each subtest is separate, so the battery includes two separate boards. The main differences between the boards is the diameter of the hole and its ability to accommodate 1 or 3 pins at a time. Both boards consist of 100 holes arranged in 10 rows of 10 holes each spaced 0.5 inch apart. Above the holes at the top of the board is a well that holds the metal pins residing in a tray whose cover slides open and closed. Each pin is 1-inch long and 1/16 of an inch in diameter (Kirby, 1979). During the finger test, the subject is required to pick up and place 3 pins in 1 hole (x 100) on the board, thus the diameter of the holes can accommodate 3 pins at roughly 3/16 of an inch; whereas the tweezer test requires only 1 pin to be picked up at a time with tweezers and placed into each of the 100 holes that are roughly 1/16 of an inch. The time required, in seconds, to fill the 100 holes is the basis for the score for both batteries. Administration time is less than 20 minutes for each.

Psychometrics

Original test-retest reliability scores for the finger test were r=0.60 however, the research was completed under employment conditions which may account for low correlative scores where the fastest speed for both men and woman was 5.70 minutes with a median of 7.70 minutes (Hines & O'Connor, 1926). A later article by Fleishman (1953) noted studies by Darley (1934) and Blum (1940) that showed test-retest reliabilities to be r=0.90 and 0.89, respectively; whereas Fleishman's own work produced test-retest reliabilities ranging from 0.71 to 0.86 under various conditions such as time constraint and work limit (i.e., using full and half boards). A subsequent factor analysis determined that the O'Connor Finger Test was most heavily loaded on manual dexterity (0.62), followed by finger dexterity (0.28), visual acuity (−0.09), then depth perception (0.05); whereas factor analysis of the Tweezer test was 0.46 for manual dexterity, followed by finger dexterity (0.04), tweezer dexterity (0.32), and visual acuity (−0.23) (Bourassa & Guion, 1959). Candee and Blum (1937) were able to stratify people using the finger test into superior workers with a mean score of 6.55 (range 5.56 to 8.06) and mediocre workers with a mean score of 7.32 (range 5.57 to 9.49). Lundergan, Soderstrom, and

Chambers (2007) found that median scores of a dental student cohort for the Tweezer test using slightly different scoring parameters was men = 327 and women = 323, which was significantly better than published norms of men = 360 and women = 342.20. The same study found that the Tweezer test also significantly correlated with the Perceptual Ability Test at r = 0.24 and concluded that the original O'Connor Tweezer Test was a weak predictor of grades in dental school when compared with the modified O'Connor Tweezer Dexterity Test #18 which requires pins to be removed from holes and placed in holes requiring more speed and accuracy than the original.

Advantages

The Tweezer Dexterity Test itself is an original concept and there are few performance measures that assess the same complex fine motor control sought after in the Tweezer Test. Both the Finger and Tweezer Test have been in use since the 1920s and there are a number of studies with age-referenced norms available. The assessments require no special training or certifications and can be administered inn less than 20 minutes.

Disadvantages

Fleishman (1953) argues that relative to other dexterity tests (i.e., Minnesota Rate of Manipulation and Purdue Pegboard), the test takes considerably longer to administer at a typical range of 8 to 15 minutes. Also, the test yields only one score, whereas the Purdue Pegboard Test, for example, can yield five scores (right, left, both hands, total of those, and assembly), and the Minnesota Rate of Manipulation Test yields at least two scores (placing and turning). Additionally, the amount of current research pertaining to the batteries is limited.

Administration

Detailed instructions are included in the examiner's manual as well as standardized norms and percentile ranks of each assessment when purchased. During assessment the clinician uses specific prompts, whereby the subject is asked to take pins from the shallow bowl at the top of each board and place them into specific grooved holes that accept the pins on the board. The Finger Test requires the placement of 3 pins into 1 hole and the tweezer test requires 1 pin in 1 hole using only tweezers. Scoring is based on how fast the person can complete the assigned task of filling the 100 holes on the board. Errors and misplaced pins are accounted for during scoring, which is usually in minutes/seconds. Scoring for each assessment requires unique algorithms. For example, the finger test requires the following computation:

$$\text{Raw score} = \frac{\text{first half time} + (1.1 \times \text{second half time})}{2}$$

Permission

The O'Connor Dexterity Tests can be purchased from various therapy supply companies and cost varies from $125 to $175 each. To use in research or publication contact where purchased or where published. More information about the battery can be found in the following original journal articles:

Hines M., & O'Connor J. (1926). A measure of finger dexterity. *Journal of Personnel Research, 4*, 379-382.
Fleishman, E. A. (1953). A modified administration procedure for the O'Connor Finger Dexterity Test. *Journal of Applied Psychology, 37*(3), 191-194.

Summary

POPULATION	Suspected hand/finger injury; work rehabilitation; general
TYPE OF MEASURE	Activity-based functional performance
WHAT IT ASSESSES	Fine motor; hand dexterity; visual component
TIME	< 20 minutes
COST	$125 to $175

Contact

Lafayette Instrument Company

P.O. Box 5729

Lafayette, IN 47903

Phone: (800) 428-7545

E-mail: info@lafayetteinstrument.com

Web: www.lafayetteevaluation.com/product_detail.asp?itemid=162

Web: www.lafayetteevaluation.com/product_detail.asp?itemid=161

CHAPTER 48: PURDUE PEGBOARD TEST (PPT)

Description

The Purdue Pegboard Test (PPT) by Tiffin and Asher (1948), is a test of upper extremity hand function originally designed to assist in the selection of employees in industrial jobs requiring manipulative dexterity, such as assembly, packing, operation of certain machines, and other routine manual jobs of an exacting nature during the manufacturing boom of the late 1940s in the United States. However, the PPT is now used in many work rehabilitation settings as well as patient populations where hand/finger dexterity is of primary concern. The pegboard itself is constructed of wood/plastic polymer that has 4 recessed cups at the top which hold the washers, pins, and collars to be assembled. The board itself is made of an acrylic polymer and is 23 x 11.5 inches where roughly at the center of the board are 2 vertical rows of 25 holes 1/8 inch in diameter designed to receive the assemblies (Desai, Kene, Doshi, Shubhangi, & Desai, 2006). The test measures dexterity for two types of activities, those involving gross movements of hand, fingers, and arms and the other involving the tips of the fingers. Unlike other pegboard tests the PPT requires more fine motor control as activities are more complex and include the placement of pins into a board as well as the assembly of collars and washers onto the pins (Tiffin & Asher, 1948). The PPT provides separate measurements for the right hand, left hand, and both hands together. Each of the 4 subtests take less than 1 minute to complete and scores are based on the number of placements and assemblies.

Psychometrics

A study of subjects that were administered the 4 subtests of the PPT (n = 25) found that test-retest reliability coefficients ranged from 0.85 to 0.90 (1-trial administration) and 0.92 to 0.96 (for 3 trials) (Gallus & Mathiowetz, 2003). Results from a similar designed study of 47 occupational therapy students found that test-retest reliabilities for 1-test administration were only moderate for the 4 subtests (0.37 to 0.71), whereas the 3-trial administration had coefficients that ranged from 0.81 to 0.89 (Buddenberg & Davis, 2000). Original research found that correlations of subtest scores of 434 college men and women ranged from 0.50 to 0.69 (Tiffin & Asher, 1948). A study of healthy subjects found that as age increased performance generally decreased where results showed that young subjects inserted a mean of 16 pegs with the dominant hand, 15 pegs with the non-dominant hand, 27 pegs with both hands, and assembled 42 pieces; middle-aged subjects inserted a mean of 15 pegs with the dominant hand, 14 pegs with the non-dominant hand, 23 pegs with both hands, and assembled 33 pieces; and healthy elderly subjects had a mean score of 13 pegs with the dominant hand, 12 pegs with the non-dominant hand, 20 with both hands, and assembled 26 pieces (Amirjani, Ashworth, Olson, Morhart, & Chan, 2011). The following are further normative values relating to the PPT from a somewhat different population sample.

TABLE 48-1					
NORMATIVE VALUES					
AGE	SEX	DOMINANT	NON-DOMINANT	BOTH	ASSEMBLY
45 to 55 years old	M	16 (SD: 2)	14 (SD: 1)	12 (SD: 1)	30 (SD: 4)
	F	15 (SD: 1)	14 (SD: 1)	12 (SD: 1)	30 (SD: 4)
55 to 65 years old	M	13 (SD: 2)	13 (SD: 2)	11 (SD: 2)	28 (SD: 7)
	F	14 (SD: 2)	13 (SD: 2)	12 (SD: 2)	29 (SD: 6)
n = 600; age range = 5 to 65 years					
Adapted from Desai, K., Kene, K., Doshi, M., Shubhangi, D. & Desai, S. (2006). Normative data of Purdue Pegboard on Indian population. *The Indian Journal of Occupational Therapy, 37*(3), 72.					

Advantages

There is a considerable amount of research available in support of its use in clinical practice and research. The manual provides detailed directions, scoring, and referenced norms across the lifespan. In addition, there are a number of studies that also provide age-valued norms. No special training is required and the test is portable for use in a variety of settings as well as a number of patient populations where dexterity is of concern. The PPT has been in existence in its present state since the 1940s.

Disadvantages

The assessment requires a relatively higher degree of fine motor skills as well as cognitive ability making it more narrowly focused on smaller patient target populations. Studies have also suggested that group administration may lead to increased competitiveness and knowledge of scores can create a situation where subjects try to beat previous scores (Buddenberg & Davis, 2000).

Administration

The PPT has standardized instructions as well as scoring relative to the 4 types of subtests. For example, in the right hand test the client is instructed to pick up one pin at a time with the right hand from the right hand cup and place these pins in the right hand row, starting with the top hole (Tiffin& Asher, 1948). The person is scored by how many pins can be successfully placed in 30 seconds. The left hand test requires the same procedure described except activities occur on left side of the board with the left hand. The both hands subtest requires the client to use a combination of the right and left hand tests mentioned above. The person is allowed 30 seconds to place as many pairs of pins as possible. The assembly test requires minutiae finger dexterity and consists of assembling the pins, collars, and washers where a complete assembly calls for (1) pin placement, (2) washer on pin, (3) collar on washer, and (4) a second washer placed on top (Tiffin & Asher,1948). As the final washer for the first assembly is being placed with the left hand the second assembly is immediately started by picking up another pin with the right hand placing it in the next hole; dropping a washer over it with the left hand; then a collar with the right hand, and so on, completing another assembly (Tiffin & Asher, 1948). The client is allowed 60 seconds to make as many assemblies as possible. Scores for assembly are based on the number of assemblies made (i.e., if 6 complete assemblies were made and the pin and first washer of the seventh assembly are properly placed at the end of the minute, the score is 24 plus 2 or 26) (Tiffin & Asher, 1948). The examiner's manual has detailed instructions as well as scoring norms (ages 5 to 89 years old) from a number of studies involving large cohorts of people.

Permissions

The PPT is a standardized measure that can be purchased from a number of therapy supply stores. Prices vary from $115 to $170. To use in research or publication contact where it can be purchased or where it has been published at the information that follows. More information can be found in the following articles:

Buddenberg, L., & Davis, C. (1999). Test–retest reliability of the Purdue Pegboard Test. *American Journal of Occupational Therapy, 54*(5), 555-558.

Tiffin, J., & Asher, E. J. (1948). The Purdue Pegboard: Norms and studies of reliability and validity. *Journal of Applied Psychology, 32,* 234–47.

Summary

POPULATION	Suspected hand/finger injury; work rehabilitation; general
TYPE OF MEASURE	Activity-based functional performance
WHAT IT ASSESSES	Fine motor; hand dexterity; cognitive component
TIME	< 10 minutes
COST	$115 to $170

Contact

Lafayette Instrument Company

P.O. Box 5729

Lafayette, IN 47903

Phone: (800) 428-7545

Email: info@lafayetteinstrument.com

Web: www.lafayetteevaluation.com/product_detail.asp?ItemID=159

REFERENCES

Aaron, D. & Stegink-Jansen, C. (2003). Development of the Functional Dexterity Test (FDT): Construction, validity, reliability, and normative data. *Journal of Hand Therapy, 16*(1), 12–21.

Amirjani, N., Ashworth, N., Olson, J., Morhart, M., & Chan, K. (2011). Validity and reliability of the Purdue Pegboard Test in carpal tunnel syndrome. *Muscle and Nerve, 43*(2), 171-177.

Bourassa, G., & Guion, R. (1959). A factorial study of dexterity tests. *Journal of Applied Psychology, 43*(3), 199-204.

Buddenberg, L., & Davis, C. (2000). Test–retest reliability of the Purdue Pegboard Test. *American Journal of Occupational Therapy, 54*(5), 555-558.

Candee, B., & Blum, M. (1937). Report of a study done in a watch factory. *Journal of Applied Psychology, 21*(5), 572-582.

Canny, M., Thompson, J., & Wheeler, M. (2009). Reliability of the Box and Block Test of manual dexterity for use with patients with fibromyalgia. *American Journal of Occupational Therapy, 63*(4), 506-510.

Darley J. G. (1934). The reliability of the tests in the standard battery. In D. G. Paterson (Ed.). *Research Studies in Individual , Vol. 3, No. 4* (pp. 194-199). Minneapolis, MN: University of Minnesota Press.

Desai, K., Kene, K., Doshi, M., Shubhangi, D., & Desai, S. (2006). Normative data of Purdue Pegboard on Indian population. *Indian Journal of Occupational Therapy, 37*(3), 69-72.

Desrosiers, J., Bravo, G., Hébert, R., Dutil, E., & Mercier, L (1994). Validation of the Box and Block Test as a measure of dexterity of elderly people: Reliability, validity, and norms studies. *Archives of Physical Medicine and Rehabilitation, 75*(7), 751–755.

Desrosiers, J., Hébert, R., & Bravo, G. (1997). The Minnesota Manual Dexterity Test: Reliability, validity and reference values studies with healthy elderly people. *Canadian Journal of Occupational Therapy, 64*(5), 270-276.

Earhart, G., Cavanaugh, J., Ellis, T., Ford, M., Foreman, K., & Dibble, L. (2011). The 9-Hole Peg Test of upper extremity function: Average values, test-retest reliability, and factors contributing to performance in people with Parkinson disease. *Journal of Neurological Physical Therapy, 35*(4), 157-163.

Fleishman, E. A. (1953). A modified administration procedure for the O'Connor Finger Dexterity Test. *Journal of Applied Psychology, 37*(3), 191-194.

Fouty, H., McWaters, A., Sanchez, H., Mills, R., Brandon, B., & Weitzner, D. (2015). Effect of left-hand peg placement direction on the Grooved Pegboard Test. *Applied Neuropsychology: Adult, 13*, 1-3.

Gallus, J., & Mathiowetz, V. (2003). Test-retest reliability of the Purdue Pegboard for persons with multiple sclerosis. *American Journal of Occupational Therapy, 57*(1), 108-111.

Gloss, D., & Wardle, M. (1982) Use of the Minnesota Rate off Manipulation Test for disability evaluation. *Perceptual and Motor Skills, 55*(2), 527-532.

Hines, M., & O'Connor, J. (1926). A measure of finger dexterity. *Journal of Personnel Research 4*, 379, 382.

Howell, D., & Yancosek, K. E. (2009). A narrative review of dexterity assessments. *Journal of Hand Therapy, 22*, 258–270.

Jurgensen, C. E. (1943). Extension of the Minnesota Rate of Manipulation Test. *Journal of Applied Psychology, 27*, 164-169.

Kirby, T. (1979). Dexterity testing and residents' surgical performance. *Transactions of the American Ophthalmological Society, 77*, 294-307.

Lafayette Instrument Company. (2002). *Grooved Pegboard Test user instructions.* Lafayette, IN.

Lundergan, W., Soderstrom, E., & Chambers, D. (2007). Tweezer dexterity aptitude of dental students. *Journal of Dental Education, 71*(8), 1090-1097.

Mathiowetz, V., Volland, G., Kashman, N., & Weber, K. (1985). Adult norms for the Box and Block Test of manual dexterity. *American Journal of Occupational Therapy, 39*(6), 386-391.

Mathiowetz, V., Weber, K., Kashman, N., & Volland, G. (1985). Adult norms for the Nine Hole Peg Test of Finger Dexterity. *The Occupational Therapy Journal of Research, 5*, 24-33.

Mitrushina, M. N. (2005). *Handbook of normative data for neuropsychological assessment.* Oxford, United Kingdom: Oxford University Press.

Oxford-Grice, K., Vogel, K. A., Le, V., Mitchell, A., Muniz, S., & Vollmer, M. A. (2003) Brief report: Adult norms for a commercially available Nine Hole Peg Test for finger dexterity. *American Journal of Occupational Therapy, 57*, 570–573.

Ranjan, A., Raj, L., Kumar, D., Sandhya, P., & Danda, D. (2015). Reliability of Box and Block Test for manual dexterity in patients with rheumatoid arthritis: A pilot study. *International Journal of Rheumatic Diseases.* Advance online publication. doi: 10.1111/1756-185X.12655.

Ruff, R. & Parker, S. (1993). Gender- and age-specific changes in motor speed and eye-hand coordination in adults: Normative values for the Finger Tapping and Grooved Pegboard Tests. *Perceptual and Motor Skills, 76*(3c), 1219-1230.

Sage, M., Bryden, P., Roy. E., & Almeida, Q. (2012). The relationship between the grooved pegboard test and clinical motor symptom evaluation across the spectrum of Parkinson's disease severity. *Journal of Parkinson's Disease, 2*(3), 207-213.

Sartorio, F., Bravini, E., Vercelli, S., Ferriero, G., Plebani, G., Foti, C., & Franchignoni, F. (2013). The Functional Dexterity Test: Test-retest reliability analysis and up-to date reference norms. *Journal of Hand Therapy, 26*(1), 62-68

Schubert, C, Cruickshanks, K., Fischer, M., Huang, G. H., Klein, R., Pankratz, N.,…Nondahl, D. (2013). Odor identification and cognitive function in the Beaver Dam Offspring Study. *Journal of Clinical and Experimental Neuropsychology, 35*(7), 669-676.

Sommerfeld, D., Eek, E., Svensson, A. K., Widén Holmqvist, L., & von Arbin, M. (2004). Spasticity after stroke: Its occurrence and association with motor impairments and activity limitation *Stroke, 35*, 134-139.

Strenge, H., Niederberger, U., & Seelhorst, U. (2002) Correlation between tests of attention and performance on Grooved and Purdue Pegboards in normal subjects. *Perceptual and Motor Skills, 95*(2), 507-514.

Surrey, L., Nelson, K., Delelio, C., Mathie-Majors, D., Omel-Edwards, N., Shumaker, J., & Thurber, G. (2003). A comparison of performance outcomes between the Minnesota Rate of Manipulation Test and the Minnesota Manual Dexterity Test. *Work, 20*(2), 97-102.

Tajmir, P., M., & Carnahan, H. (2013). Interactions between cold ambient temperature and older age on haptic acuity and manual performance. *Canadian Journal on Aging, 32*(2), 195-202.

Tiffin, J., & Asher, E. J. (1948). The Purdue Pegboard: Norms and studies of reliability and validity. *Journal of Applied Psychology, 32*(3), 234-247.

Wang, Y-C., Magasi, S., Bohannon, R., Rueben, D., McCreath, H., Bubela, D.,...Rymer, W. (2011). Assessing dexterity function: A comparison of two alternatives for the NIH Toolbox. *Journal of Hand Therapy, 24*(4), 313–321.

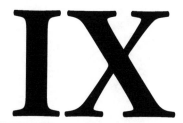

Driving Assessment

Bortnick, K.
*Occupational Therapy Assessments for Older Adults: 100 Instruments for
Measuring Occupational Performance* (pp. 137-145).
© 2017 Taylor & Francis Group.

CHAPTER 49: ADELAIDE DRIVING SELF-EFFICACY SCALE (ADSES)

Description

The Adelaide Driving Self-Efficacy Scale (ADSES) is a self-report questionnaire designed to measure an individual's perceived abilities as they relate to 12 driving-related activities/conditions and is loosely based on self-efficacy theoretical models, such as that postulated by Bandura, that argue that a belief in one's own ability to organize and execute the necessary courses of action are necessary to achieve goal attainment (George, Clark, & Crotty, 2007). The ADSES is composed of 12 driving scenarios, such as driving in heavy traffic or driving at night, in which the subject is asked to rate how confident he or she feels when performing or if asked to perform those scenarios along a scale from 1 to 10 where 1 is not confident and 10 is completely confident. The measure has a maximum score of 120 with higher scores signifying that the subject has more self-perceived driving ability. The ADSES can be completed in less than 10 minutes.

Psychometrics

Developmental research established that the Cronbach's alpha coefficient was $\alpha = 0.98$ and could not be improved by deleting any of the 12 items, indicating a high degree of internal consistency (George et al., 2007). The same study found that overall scores for the control group (n = 79; mean age: 41 years) were 110.3 for men and 109.7 for women while for the intervention/cerebrovascular accident (CVA) group (n = 81; mean age: 67 years) scores were 88.5 for men and 65.9 for women, suggesting that the ADSES is a valid tool able to discriminate levels of driver self-efficacy in both healthy controls and CVA populations (George et al., 2007). Criterion validity of the measure was determined by comparing ADSES scores with on-road driving test scores of 45 healthy controls (mean age: 60 years) where it was determined that of those that passed (n = 22) had a mean score of 108 on the ADSES, while those that failed (n = 23) scored only 96 (George et al., 2007). Similar results were found for a CVA cohort where those that passed (n = 14) scored 107 and those who failed (n = 21) scored 96, suggesting that 96 may be a possible cutoff point when considering a subjects self-perceived driving ability with actual ability (George et al., 2007). A subsequent study of 40 subjects (average age: 65 years), who were 17 months post-CVA, found mean ADSES scores to be 103.50 (McNamara, Walker, Ratcliffe, & George, 2015). The same study found that questions on the assessment exhibiting the least confidence for the group were driving at night (25%), planning

travel to a new destination (12.5%), driving in unfamiliar areas (10%), and parallel parking (10%); whereas those displaying the most confidence were responding to road signs and traffic signals (95%), driving in a local area (90%), and maneuvering through a roundabout (87.5%) (McNamara et al., 2015). Further results explored the Driving Habits Questionnaire and the ADSES and found that how far participants drove and how much they limited their driving to their local area was moderately associated with self-reported confidence levels at 0.35, p = 0.027 (McNamara et al., 2015). Similar results were found for those drivers who avoided or found difficulties driving in the rain, driving on high-traffic roads, and parallel parking, which occurred more often in women, were also associated with lower self-reported confidence at r = 0.63, p = 0.000 (McNamara et al., 2015).

Advantages

The ADSES is a fast and simple measure whose results can be used in a number of ways. For example, it can assist in identifying those who are likely to stop driving due to low self-efficacy scores, which can enable interventions aimed at minimizing the potential negative consequences associated with driving cessation and its effect on quality of life or it can identify those people who are at a heightened risk of reduced safety when driving, thus allowing for the development of intervention strategies to modify those risk-associated driving behaviors (George et al., 2007).

Disadvantages

There is a limited amount of research pertaining to the assessment and that which is available found that both gender and the interactions between diagnosis and gender to be associated with ADSES scores (George et al., 2007). Also, a study of 6 post-CVA subjects (mean age: 64 years) found the presence of a ceiling effect on all items, which could be the product of difficulty of subjects being able to delineate between previous driving ability and the potential impact that stroke has on current driving ability (Stapleton, Connolly, & O'Neill, 2012).

Administration

The ADSES is a self-report questionnaire in which the subject is asked to consider how confident they feel doing 12 driving-related activities. He or she is then asked to quantify that level of confidence along a scale of 1 to 10, where 0 is not confident and 10 is completely confident.

TABLE 49-1
EXAMPLE ITEMS OF THE ADELAIDE DRIVING SELF-EFFICACY SCALE
• Driving at night
• Driving with people in the car
• Responding to road signs/traffic signals
• Attempting to merge with traffic
• Turning right across oncoming traffic
• Parallel parking
Adapted from George, S., Clark, M., & Crotty, M. (2007). Development of the Adelaide Driving Self-Efficacy Scale. *Clinical Rehabilitation, 21*, 61.

George, S., Clark, M., & Crotty, M. (2007). Development of the Adelaide Driving Self-Efficacy Scale. *Clinical Rehabilitation, 21*, 56-61.

Summary

POPULATION	General; driving ability or impairment
TYPE OF MEASURE	Self-report questionnaire
WHAT IT ASSESSES	Self-perceived driving efficacy
TIME	< 10 minutes
COST	Free

Permissions

The ADSES is free to use in private practice and can be downloaded from the Flinders University Department of Rehabilitation Aged and Extended Care website at the information that follows. Use of the measure in research, publication, or for commercial purposes can be obtained by contacting one of its authors also at the information following. More data can be found in the following journal article:

Contact

Dr. Stacey George

Department of Rehabilitation and Aged Care

Flinders University

Bedford Park, Australia

Repatriation General Hospital

Daw Park, Australia

Web: www.flinders.edu.au/sohs/sites/raec/research/adses.cfm

CHAPTER 50: FITNESS TO DRIVE SCREENING MEASURE (FTDS)

Description

The Fitness to Drive Screening Measure (FTDS) is a self-report or informant-based questionnaire of driving ability which has shown to be especially useful for family members, caregivers, or practitioners to help identify potentially at-risk older drivers. Maintained by the University of Florida and accessed remotely via the Internet, the tool enables the rater to quantify performance relative to 54 driving skills over a 90-day time frame. The FTDS is based on three theoretical models:

1. The Precede-Proceed Model of Health Promotion, which is designed to guide the assessment of both the personal and environmental factors that influence health as well as planning targeted interventions.

2. The Haddon's Matrix for Injury Prevention, which provides a framework for crash prevention and injury reduction focusing on interactions among the person, his or her car, and the physical and social environment.

3. Michon's Model of Driving Behavior, which categorizes driving behaviors as operational (on the sub-conscious level), tactical (car handling and maneuvers), and strategic (driving decisions and planning).

The FTDS is also comprised of the following three interrelated constructs relative to driving skill:

1. The Person-Vehicle, which includes behaviors related to use of car controls or features, such as the driver's use of emergency brake.

2. The Person-Environment, which are those behaviors in response to physical factors such as terrain, weather, or social factors such as interactions with passengers.

3. The Person-Vehicle-Environment, which encompasses skills, attitudes, and behaviors in the use of vehicle features or controls and a response to environmental factors such as controlling one's car on an icy road (Classen et al., n.d.).

The FTDS has four sections: (1) demographics and general information about the rater, (2) demographics and general information about the driver, (3) driving history profile, and (4) ratings of driving difficulty pertaining to 54 driving skills. As the FTDS is web-based, upon completion a scoring matrix is generated which classifies the driver into one of three categories: at-risk driver, routine driver, or accomplished driver. Recommendations are also generated relative to the subject's overall score and includes such things as an evaluation by a physician, an occupational therapist, or a certified driver rehabilitation specialist for at-risk or routine drivers, while suggestions for accomplished drivers include guidelines for maintaining their fitness-to-drive such as receiving regular health care check-ups or taking a driving class (Classen et al., n.d.). In addition to recommendations, resources to assist in the transition to driving retirement are given including local transportation options (Classen et al., n.d.). The FTDS requires access to a computer and can be completed in 20 minutes.

Psychometrics

Research into the development of the FTDS with 80 older drivers, 80 caregivers, and 2 raters found that item reliability had a range of $r = 0.93$ to 0.96, while strong Cronbach alphas were demonstrated with a range of $\alpha = 0.96$ to 0.99, suggesting excellent item correlation (Classen et al., 2012). A study to obtain proxy rater input on the clarity, usefulness, understandability, and meaningfulness of the measure of 7 subjects (median age 69 years old) found an overall high level of acceptance (9.13/10) relative to 6 questions pertaining to the usability of the measure (range 8.61 to 9.31) with the lowest rating given for the question "Is the key form meaningful?" (i.e., does it provide helpful recommendations regarding follow-up steps for the driver?) while the highest rating was for the question, "How well was the purpose of the key form explained?" (Winter, Classen, & Shanahan, 2015).

Advantages

Due to self-report bias, which can arise at the possible loss of a valued occupation, such as driving, a screening by way of proxy may be preferable (Classen Winter, Velozo, Hannold, & Rogers, 2013). The FTDS is also able to provide recommendations for follow-up as well as relevant resources. Finally, the FTDS is a free web-based measure developed in conjunction with the University of Florida, which maintains a helpful interactive website devoted to the assessment.

Disadvantages

There is a limited amount of independent research pertaining to the FTDS (i.e., that not indirectly involving its creators). Some have also argued that results of a off-road evaluations, are not necessarily valid predictors of on-road driving performance in subjects with mild traumatic brain injury (TBI) however, they could be considered valid for those with moderate to severe TBI (Classen et al., 2009).

Administration

The person begins the assessment as he or she enters the gateway accessed through the Institute for Mobility, Activity and Participation (I-MAP) website where both instructional text and videos are available to guide the rater through testing. Example directives include the rater being told to use his or her best judgment and use the driver's past experiences to rate level of performance relative to each item on the test, which are organized along a hierarchy of less to more difficult and includes such items as ability to stay in the proper lane to more challenging items such as his or her ability to drive on an icy road (Winter et al., 2015).

TABLE 50-1	
SCORING CHOICES FOR THE FITNESS TO DRIVE SCREENING MEASURE	
Very difficult	The driving skill presents a major challenge.
Somewhat difficult	The driving skill presents a moderate challenge.
A little difficult	The driving skill presents a minor challenge.
Not difficult	The driving skill presents little or no challenge.
Adapted from by Classen, S., Velozo, C., Winter, S., Brumback, B., Bédard, M., Lutz, B.,…Rogers, J. (n.d.). *Fitness-To-Drive Screening Measure (FTDS) user manual.* Gainesville, FL: University of Florida: Institute for Mobility, Activity, and Participation. Retrieved from http://fitnesstodrive.phhp.ufl.edu/pdf/user_manual.pdf	

Permissions

The FTDS is maintained by the University of Florida I-MAP and is free to use in educational or clinical practice. All other uses require permission from the University of Florida. The measure, manual, and other information can be accessed from the FTDS website at the information following. More information can be found in the following publication:

Classen, S., Velozo, C., Winter, S., Brumback, B., Bédard, M., Lutz, B.,…Rogers, J. (n.d.). *Fitness-To-Drive Screening Measure (FTDS) user manual.* Gainesville, FL: University of Florida: Institute for Mobility, Activity, and Participation.

TABLE 50-2	
DEFINITIONS OF TOTAL SCORE CLASSIFICATIONS	
At-risk driver	The driver can perform some basic driving skills; there are safety concerns that need immediate attention.
Routine driver	The driver shows early signs of needing intervention with some skills that are causing concern.
Accomplished driver	Driving is overall good, but difficulty may be experienced with some challenging driving situations.
Adapted from by Classen, S., Velozo, C., Winter, S., Brumback, B., Bédard, M., Lutz, B.,…Rogers, J. (n.d.). *Fitness-To-Drive Screening Measure (FTDS) user manual.* Gainesville, FL: University of Florida: Institute for Mobility, Activity, and Participation. Retrieved from http://fitnesstodrive.phhp.ufl.edu/pdf/user_manual.pdf	

Summary

POPULATION	General; driving ability or impairment
TYPE OF MEASURE	Proxy or self-report questionnaire; web-based
WHAT IT ASSESSES	Driving ability
TIME	20 minutes
COST	Free

Contact

University of Florida

Institute for Mobility, Activity, and Participation

Gainesville, FL 32611

Phone: (352) 273-6817

Email: ftds@phhp.ufl.edu

Web: http://fitnesstodrive.phhp.ufl.edu/

Chapter 51: Performance Analysis of Driving Ability (P-Drive)

Description

The Performance Analysis of Driving Ability (P-Drive) by Patomella (2004), is a comprehensive standardized driving assessment designed to determine an individual's fitness to drive and is based on three theoretical assumptions: The Model of Human Occupation activity analysis as well as psychological theory about a person's decision making while on road. Originally developed for use with a driving simulator, the P-Drive, has been adapted to real life driving situations and is composed of 27 items that form 4 subgroups: (1) maneuvering, (2) orientation, (3) ability to follow regulations, and (4) attending and acting on different stimuli in the traffic context (Patomella & Bundy, 2015). During assessment the subject is graded on his or her ability to safely and effectively engage in task items that, as a whole, lead to safe driving and include such items as steering, using turn signals, wayfinding, trip planning, obeying stop and speed regulations, and problem solving behind the wheel (Patomella & Bundy, 2015). Scoring requires the clinician to grade the safety and quality of observed performance as the subject drives along a predetermined route or simulated program if using a driving simulator. Each item is scored along a 4-point criterion-referenced scale (1 to 4) where a score of (4) suggests that the person is competent and safe, (3) they are questionable, (2) problematic, and a score of (1) denotes an incompetent and unsafe performance. A total score of 108 is possible with higher scores indicting better driving ability. The P-Drive can be completed in 30 to 60 minutes.

Psychometrics

A study of 85 volunteer drivers (mean age: 76 years) determined that the median fail score for 18 subjects was 78 (range: 74 to 81), while for those that passed (n = 67) it was 94 (range: 90 to 96) (Selander, 2012). The most challenging items were observing signs, attending to the left and right, following speed regulations, and giving the right of way, while the most frequent errors were made in obeying the speed limit, changing gears, use of indicators, and attention to the left and right (Selander, 2012). A subsequent study of 99 subjects with neurological impairment referred for driving evaluation determined that the P-Drive was able to separate drivers into 4 different strata with a reliability of r = 0.92, while at a cutoff score of 81 the sensitivity was 93% and specificity was 92% (Patomella & Bundy, 2015). Using the same cutoff score, the positive predictive value was 0.95 and the negative predictive value

was 0.90 (Patomella & Bundy, 2015). A similar study of 101 subjects post-cerebrovascular accident (CVA) determined that the P-Drive was also able separate subject driving ability into different strata at a reliability of only r = 0.84 (Patomella, Tham, & Kottorp, 2006). The same study's investigation of criterion dimensionality found that the first component accounted for 64% of the variance indicating good uni-dimensionality, whereas the second component explained 6% of the variance (Patomella et al., 2006). When researchers analyze components of a scale the first or main one should explain at least 20% of the variance and the second one should not explain more than 5% of the variance.

Advantages

Findings suggest that, overall, the P-Drive is a valid and stable assessment tool with sound psychometric properties that can differentiate people with diverse driving abilities across a number of patient populations including those related to age. Since it was developed by an occupational therapist, it could also be considered specific to that profession.

Disadvantages

Researchers have noted inherent problems with driving tests in general that can effect standardization, and those that affect the P-Drive in particular are variations in the choice of driving routes, as each clinician develops his or her own, the choice of vehicle, as well as individual differences in how testing is conducted. Also, the study by Patomella et al. (2006) of persons post-CVA, discussed earlier, determined that although most items displayed goodness of fit at the 95% confidence interval, controlled speeding did not fit model expectations at only 0.54, suggesting that item may need to be reworked. The same study found that a score of 4 was obtained 56% of the time and a score of 1 only 7% denoting a possible ceiling effect. Finally, P-Drive is still considered a work in progress and although its administration is discussed at length in several articles an examiner's manual is not yet available.

Administration

If using a simulator, the subject is allowed to practice for up to 15 minutes to get used to the controls of the car, such as the pedals, gear, and steering. Similarly, familiarity is allowed in the vehicle prior to actual driving.

Route creation for both simulated and on-road assessment requires the clinician to design one that includes specific challenging traffic situations based on a list from the manual to include such items as yielding and stop regulations, problem solving tasks using unstructured instructions (i.e., find your way back to the gas station where we recently parked), as well as driving in different situations, at different speeds, in rural areas, on highways, and in city traffic (Patomella & Bundy, 2015). Scoring requires the clinician to grade the subject's ability as they relate to the 27 task items of the assessment which may include such observations as the participant collided with a car coming from the right as they had no right-of-way (simulator); the subject was able to pay attention to the right and was able to successfully give the right-of-way when necessary; or the subject was able to control speed by adapting it appropriately up to and through a crossing (Patomella et al., 2006).

TABLE 51-1
EXAMPLE ITEMS OF THE P-DRIVE
• Using pedals
• Controlling speed
• Reversing
• Keeping distance
• Yielding right-of-way
• Attending and acting straight ahead
• Attending and acting to left
• Attending and acting to right
• Attending and acting to mirrors
• Attending and acting to fellow road users

Adapted from Patomella, A. & Bundy, A. (2015). P-Drive: Implementing an assessment of on-road driving in clinical settings and investigating its internal and predictive validity. *American Journal of Occupational Therapy, 69*(4), 4.

Permissions

Use of the P-Drive in practice, research, or publication can be obtained by contacting its author at the information following. When the examiner's manual becomes available there will be a purchase fee, which is as of yet is undetermined. The assessment can be found in its entirety the following journal article:

Selander, H., Lee, H., Johansson, K., & Falkmer, T. (2011). Older drivers: On-road and off-road test results. *Accident Analysis and Prevention, 43*, 1348–1354.

Summary

POPULATION	General; driving ability or impairment
TYPE OF MEASURE	Functional performance; on-road driving test; simulated
WHAT IT ASSESSES	Driving ability
TIME	30 to 60 minutes
COST	n/a

Contact

Ann-Helen Patomella, PhD

Assistant Professor

Division of Occupational Therapy

Department of Neurobiology, Care Science and Society

Karolinska Institutet

Solna, Sweden

Web: http://ki.se/en/people/annpat

REFERENCES

Classen, S., Levy, C., McCarthy, D., Mann, W. C., Lanford, D., & Waid-Ebbs, J. K. (2009). Traumatic brain injury and driving assessment: An evidence-based literature review. *American Journal of Occupational Therapy, 64*, 580–591.

Classen, S., Velozo, C., Winter, S., Brumback, B., Bédard, M., Lutz, B.,...Rogers, J. (n.d.). *Fitness-To-Drive Screening Measure (FTDS) user manual*. Gainesville, FL: University of Florida: Institute for Mobility, Activity, and Participation. Retrieved from http://fitnesstodrive.phhp.ufl.edu/pdf/user_manual.pdf

Classen, S., Wen, P-S., Velozo, C. A., Bédard, M., Winter, S. M., Brumback, B., & Lanford, D. N. (2012). Psychometrics of the self-report Safe Driving Behavior Measure for older adults. *American Journal of Occupational Therapy, 66*, 233–241.

Classen, S., Winter, S. M., Velozo, C., Hannold, E., & Rogers, J. (2013). Stakeholder recommendations to refine the Fitness-to-Drive Screening. *Open Journal of Occupational Therapy, 1*(4), 1-14.

George, S., Clark, M., & Crotty, M. (2007). Development of the Adelaide Driving Self-Efficacy Scale. *Clinical Rehabilitation, 21*, 56-61.

McNamara, A., Walker, R., Ratcliffe, J., & George, S. (2015). Perceived confidence relates to driving habits post-stroke. *Disability and Rehabilitation, 37*(14), 1228–1233

Patomella, A., & Bundy, A. (2015). P-Drive: Implementing an assessment of on-road driving in clinical settings and investigating its internal and predictive validity. *American Journal of Occupational Therapy, 69*(4), 1-8.

Patomella, A., Kottorp, A., & Tham, K. (2008). Awareness of driving disability in people with stroke tested in a simulator. *Scandinavian Journal of Occupational Therapy, 15*(3), 184-192.

Selander, H. (2012). *Driving assessment and driving behavior*. Dissertation Series No. 36, Jönköping University. School of Health Sciences. Jönköping, Sweden.

Stapleton, T., Connolly, D., & O'Neill, D. (2012). Exploring the relationship between self-awareness of driving efficacy and that of a proxy when determining fitness to drive after stroke. *Australian Occupational Therapy Journal, 59*, 63–70.

Winter, S., Classen, S., & Shanahan, M. (2015). User evaluation of the Fitness-to-Drive Screening Measure. *Physical & Occupational Therapy in Geriatrics, 33*(1), 64-71.

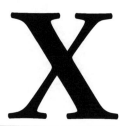

Executive Function

Bortnick, K.
*Occupational Therapy Assessments for Older Adults: 100 Instruments for
Measuring Occupational Performance* (pp. 147-161).
© 2017 Taylor & Francis Group.

Chapter 52: Behavior Rating Inventory of Executive Function—Adult Version (BRIEF-A)

Description

The Behavior Rating Inventory of Executive Function—Adult Version (BRIEF-A) by Gioia et al. (2002) is a self-report/informant-based questionnaire designed to measure a person's self-regulation in his or her everyday environment and is intended for numerous populations where executive impairment is suspected such as developmental disorders, cognitive impairment including neurocognitive disorders of the Alzheimer's and related types, traumatic brain injury (TBI), depression, or psychiatric illnesses (Dean & Dean, 2012). Developed as an extension of the original BRIEF, the BRIEF-A is considered a composite of two indexes: the Behavioral Regulation Index (BRI) and the Metacognitive Index (MI) (Rabin et al., 2006). The BRI index is comprised of four subscales: (1) inhibit, (2) shift, (3) emotional control, and (4) self-monitor, while the MI index comprises five subscales: (1) initiate, (2) working memory, (3) plan/organize, (4) task monitor, and (5) organization of materials (Rabin et al., 2006). The measure contains 75 items that explore such issues as "I have angry outbursts," "I forget my name," and "I make careless errors when completing tasks," which are scored along a scale from often to never. The BRIEF-A takes approximately 20 minutes to complete and yields an overall score called the Global Executive Composite (GEC). Scores are also calculated for each of the subscales which in turn yield three validity scales relative to negativity, infrequency, and inconsistency (Rabin et al., 2006). Higher scores reflect greater executive impairment.

Psychometrics

Author established internal consistency found that for the self-report form coefficients ranged from α=0.73 to 0.90 for the norm sample of 1050 subjects and α=0.80 to 0.94 for a mixed sample of clinical patients with schizophrenia and healthy adults (n=233) (Dean & Dean, 2012). The same study found correlation coefficients for the BRI, MI, and GEC subscales ranged from 0.93 to 0.96 for the norm and 0.96 to 0.98 for the mixed sample, also suggesting strong internal consistency. Similar results were produced for the informant-report-based version where coefficients ranged from 0.80 to 0.93 for the norm (n=1200) and 0.85 to 0.95 for the mixed sample (n=196) (Dean & Dean, 2012). The study also determined that the informant-based

BRI, MI, and GEC subscales had internal consistency scores that ranged from α=0.95 to 0.98 for the norm sample and α=0.96 to 0.98 for the mixed sample (Dean & Dean, 2012). A subsequent study of informant ratings of 89 individuals diagnosed with TBI demonstrated good reliability at r=0.94 and 0.96 and also determined that each index measured a latent trait which separated individuals into five or six ability levels (Waid-Ebbs, Wen, Heaton, Donovan, & Velozo, 2012).

TABLE 52-1		
BEHAVIOR RATING INVENTORY OF EXECUTIVE FUNCTION—ADULT VERSION SELF-REPORT NORMS		
DOMAIN	**NORMAL CONTROLS MEAN ± (SD)**	**SUBJECTS WITH SCHIZOPHRENIA**
Inhibit	10.4 (2.6)	13.4 (2.5)
Shift	8.0 (1.8)	12.3 (2.8)
Emotional control	13.3 (3.3)	19.0 (5.3)
Self-monitor	7.9 (1.9)	10.2 (2.5)
Initiate	10.0 (1.7)	16.4 (3.6)
Working memory	9.9 (1.8)	15.3 (3.5)
Plan/organize	12.6 (2.4)	18.9 (3.9)
Task monitor	7.8 (1.5)	11.2 (2.5)
Organization of materials	10.9 (2.4)	14.8 (3.6)
GEC	90.8 (13.4)	129.2 (23.1)

Schizophrenia: n=31; 40±10 years; healthy controls: n=38; 45.1±12.8 years

Adapted from Bulzacka, E., Vilain, J., Schürhoff, F., Meary, A., Leboyer, M., & Szoke, A (2013). A self-administered executive functions ecological questionnaire (the Behavior Rating Inventory of Executive Function - Adult Version) shows impaired scores in a sample of patients with schizophrenia. *Mental Illness, 5*(e4), 15.

Advantages

The BRIEF-A is a standardized assessment owned by Psychological Assessment Resources (PAR) Inc. that has a significant amount of peer-reviewed literature in support of its use in clinical practice. Several versions are also available, such as the BRIEF, BRIEF-P preschool, and the BRIEF-SR self-report only version. A software portfolio (BRIEF-A SP) is also available that can be used to score and compare referenced norms, and generate interpretive feedback, summary reports, and protocol summary reports (Psychological Assessments Australia, 2014).

Disadvantages

Roth, Lance, Isquith, Fischer, and Giancola (2013) argue that reliance on use of the GEC score as representative of executive function, as measured by the BRIEF-A, might obscure more specific relationships between executive functioning in everyday life which may be reflected in a more detailed examination of subscale scores. A study of young adults found that a three-factor model consisting of metacognition, behavioral regulation, and emotional regulation contributed only 14%, 19%, and 24% of unique variance to the model; however, results may not be applicable to older adults (Roth et al., 2013).

Administration

During testing the subject is asked to consider each of the 75 items and then to indicate whether the behavior described occurred in the past month. Answer choices include never, sometimes, or often. The outcome measure employs a unique scoring algorithm and the manual's interpretation of scores are facilitated by tables showing T-scores and equivalent percentile ranks for the nine clinical subscales as well as the BRI, the MI, and the total score GEC (Dean & Dean, 2012). Reported norms are provided for ages 18 through 90 years old as well as detailed instructions for administration and scoring.

Permission

The BRIEF-A can be purchased from PAR Inc. for $220. PAR Inc. also handles requests for use in research or other purposes. Further inquiries can be directed toward its creator at the information that follows. The original scale is discussed in the following journal article:

Waid-Ebbs, J., Wen, P., Heaton, S. C., Donovan, N., & Velozo, C. (2012). The item level psychometrics of the Behavior Rating Inventory of Executive Function-Adult (BRIEF-A) in a TBI sample. *Brain Injury, 26*(13/14), 1646-1657.

Summary

POPULATION	Suspected executive impairment
TYPE OF MEASURE	Informant or self-report questionnaire.
WHAT IT ASSESSES	Everyday self-regulation
TIME	< 20 minutes
COST	$220

Contact

Robert M. Roth, PhD

Dartmouth College

Hitchcock Medical Center

Department of Psychiatry

Hanover, New Hampshire

Web: https://geiselmed.dartmouth.edu/faculty/facultydb/view.php?uid=2188

PAR, Inc.

16204 North Florida Avenue

Lutz, FL 33549

Phone: (800) 331-8378

Web: www4.parinc.com/Products/Product.aspx?ProductID=BRIEF-A

CHAPTER 53: EXECUTIVE FUNCTION PERFORMANCE TEST (EFPT)

Description

The Executive Function Performance Test (EFPT) is designed to quantify the amount of assistance necessary for an individual to carry out specific daily tasks and is loosely based on the Kitchen Task Assessment described in Chapter 86. However, the EFPT replaces the task of preparing cooked pudding with preparing cooked oatmeal along with three other activities: completing a telephone call, managing medication, and paying a bill (Baum et al., 2008; Baum & Wolf, 2013). The EFPT examines executive functions in the context of performing a task and serves three purposes: (1) to determine which executive function components are deficient during task engagement; (2) to determine an individual's capacity for independent functioning; and (3) the amount and type of assistance necessary for completion of the task (Baum, Morrison, Hahn, & Edwards, 2007; Baum & Wolf, 2013). This is done by assessing client performance relative to five domains: (1) the client's initiation of a task (beginning the task); (2) organization (retrieval and arrangement of tools); (3) sequencing (execution of steps in the correct order); (4) safety and judgment (avoids a dangerous situation); and (5) completion (Baum & Wolf, 2013). The assessment employs a unique standardized system of cueing in order to capture the functional abilities of people during tasks across those domains and is based on the progressive need for assistance associated with varying levels of cognitive impairment thereby giving the clinician a way to record the amount of assistance required to successfully perform the task. (Baum & Wolf, 2013). Amount and type of cues are then factored into scoring descriptors from (0) no cues required to (5) physical assistance or do the task for the participant. Higher scores are reflective of the need for more cueing and is associated with more severe deficits. The EFPT can be completed in 60 minutes or less.

Psychometrics

Inter-rater reliability, as determined by it's the creators in a sample of 10 subjects with 3 trained raters was r = 0.91, with subtest intra-class correlation coefficient scores of 0.94 for the cooking task, 0.89 for paying bills, 0.87 for managing medication, and 0.79 for the using the telephone (Baum et al., 2008). Internal consistency of the sample was also high at α = 0.94 with subtest Cronbach's alpha at 0.86 for the cooking task, 0.78 for paying bills, 0.88 for managing medication, and 0.77 for using the telephone. (Baum et al., 2008). The same study found that the EFPT correlated well among each of the test domains and the total score as follows: initiation 0.91, organization 0.93, sequencing

0.88, safety and judgment 0.78, and completion of all steps 0.89. Significant moderate correlations were also found between the recall score of the Wechsler Memory Scale at r = −0.59, the Short Blessed Scale (r = 0.39), and the Functional Independence Measure (r = −0.40) (Baum et al., 2008). In a study of 30 subjects in acute and chronic stage, 31 schizophrenia researchers found internal consistency reliability to be high at α = 0.88, whereas the correlation coefficients between each executive function component and total scores were initiation 0.71, planning 0.81, transfer between stages 0.87, error detection 0.80, error correction 0.88, safe performance 0.82, and completion 0.53 (Katz, Tadmor, Felzen, & Hartman-Maeir, 2007). The same study found correlations between the individual EFPT tasks and the Behavioural Assessment of the Dysexecutive Syndrome total scores ranged from r = 0.39 to 0.67 within the acute group and 0.33 to 0.63 within the chronic group.

Advantages

The EFPT is located in the public domain, thus it is free to use in clinical practice, research, and publication. No special training is needed and it has been validated in a number of settings. The cueing system can provide helpful insight into the amount of direct supervision needed for successful occupational engagement as well as the ability to test, in a standardized format, populations who otherwise might not be able to be assessed. Washington University—St. Louis maintains a website devoted to the scale where it and supporting information can be downloaded.

Disadvantages

There is a limited amount of direct research in support of its use in clinical practice. The EFPT can take an hour or more to complete and can be involved because it requires an amount of space and material to prepare hot oatmeal such as a stove.

Administration

The EFPT can be used pre- and post-treatment and the examiner's manual has detailed instructions as well as interpretations for the clinician to follow, which includes several pre-test questions. The test delivers three separate scores: (1) an executive function (EF) component score, (2) a task score, and (3) a total score. The EF component score is calculated by summing the numbers-recorded prompts relative to each of the domains of the task and can range from 0 to 5. The task score is calculated by summing the

5 domain scores for each task and ranges from 0 to 25. The total score is the sum of all domain scores of all 4 tasks and can range from 0 to 100 (Baum & Wolf, 2013). Further scoring interpretations quantifies the practitioner's clinical judgment of subject performance.

TABLE 53-1
EXAMPLE DOMAINS AND TYPES OF PROMPTS USED
VERBAL
• Is there anything you need to do first?
• Do you need another item?
GESTURE
• Point in the direction of items needed
• Point to the name of the container
DIRECT VERBAL CUE
• Check that name
• Get the magnifier from the box on table
PHYSICAL ASSISTANCE
• Open the medicine bottle for the subject
• Pour water in glass for the subject

Adapted from Baum, C. M., & Wolf, T. J. (2013). *Executive Function Performance Test (EFPT)* (p. 2-3). St. Louis, MO: Washington University School of Medicine.

Permissions

The EFPT is a public domain instrument that can be used without fee and can be downloaded from the Washington University—St. Louis occupational therapy website. Several materials are included when downloaded such as the training manual, forms, scoring and interpretation, and frequently asked questions. More information can be found in the following journal article:

Baum, C. M., Connor, L., Morrison, T., Hahn, M., Dromerick, A., & Edwards, D. (2008). Reliability, validity, and clinical utility of the executive function performance test: A measure of executive function in a sample of people with stroke. *American Journal of Occupational Therapy, 62*, 446-455.

Summary

POPULATION	Suspected executive impairment
TYPE OF MEASURE	Activity based
WHAT IT ASSESSES	Executive function; level of independence; types of assistance needed
TIME	≥60 minutes
COST	Free

Contact

Carolyn Baum, PhD, OTR, FAOTA

Program in Occupational Therapy

Washington University—St. Louis

St. Louis, Missouri

Web: www.ot.wustl.edu/about/resources/executive-function-performance-test-efpt-308

CHAPTER 54: LOEWENSTEIN OCCUPATIONAL THERAPY COGNITIVE ASSESSMENT (LOTCA) I AND II

Description

The Loewenstein Occupational Therapy Cognitive Assessment (LOTCA), developed by Katz, Itzkovich, Averbuch, and Elazar (1989), is based on Luria's and Piaget's neuropsychological and developmental theories and is designed to measure cognitive abilities such as that which is defined as the intellectual functions thought to be prerequisite for managing everyday encounters with the environment (Najenson, Rahmani, Elasar, & Averbuch, 1984). Originally validated with traumatic brain injury subjects, information from the battery as well as the evaluation of an individual's engagement in activities of daily living can be used to plan occupational therapy treatment (Katz et al., 1989). The LOTCA consists of 20 subtests divided into four domains: (1) orientation, (2) visual and spatial perception, (3) visuomotor organization, and (4) thinking operations and includes such items as object identification, shape identification, overlapping figures, copying geometric forms, reproducing a 2-dimensional model, constructing a pegboard design, constructing a colored block design, constructing a plain block design, reproducing a puzzle, and drawing a clock (Katz et al., 1989). To address inherent shortcomings of the original, the revised LOTCA-II by Itzkovich et al. (2000) was developed which consists of 26 items grouped into 6 subtests: (1) orientation (2 items); (2) visual perception (4 items); (3) spatial perception (3 items); (4) motor praxis (3 items); (5) visuomotor organization (7 items); and (6) thinking operations (7 items). Both tests are similar and take approximately 45 minutes to administer. For the LOTCA-II each item is rated on a scale from (1) low to (4) high, except for the orientation subtest, which is scored on a scale from 1 to 8, as well as 3 items in the thinking operations subtest that are scored on a scale from 1 to 5 (Su, Chen, Tsai, Tsai, & Su, 2007). Scores for both are graded according to criteria based on the degree to which the subject correctly answers questions and performs tasks. A subtest score as well as a total score is achieved that can range from 26 to 115. Higher scores suggest less impairment in basic executive abilities (Su et al., 2007).

Psychometrics

Initial research into the battery found good inter-rater reliability coefficients of r = 0.82 to 0.97 across the 19 subtests with an alpha coefficient of 0.85 and above for the areas of perception, visuomotor organization, and thinking operations (Katz et al., 1989). A subsequent study of people with intellectual disabilities (n = 140) concluded that results showed good internal consistency for the items of orientation (α = 0.82), visual perception (0.74), spatial perception (0.76), visuomotor organization (0.86), and thinking operations (0.80); however, internal consistency of the motor praxis subscale was only α = 0.48 (Yuh, J., Jen-suh, C. & Keh-chung, 2009). A study by Wang et al. (2014) showed that LOTCA scores were strongly and positively correlated (r = 0.93) with Mini-Mental State Exam in patients with cognitive impairment (n = 60). LOTCA-II test-retest reliability from a subsample of 48 persons with schizophrenia was r = 0.95 (total score), for the orientation subtest, the intra-class correlation coefficient was 0.63, visual perception it was 0.77, spatial perception 0.49, motor praxis 0.67, visuomotor organization 0.87, and for the thinking operations subtest it was 0.89. (Su et al., 2007). Weak to moderate correlations were also found between scores on the LOTCA-II and the Wechsler Adult Intelligence Scale—Third Edition subscales with values ranging from 0.37 to 0.69, the Wisconsin Card Sorting two subtests (-0.56 and 0.42), the Allen Cognitive Level Screen (0.55), and the Daily Living Function Scale (0.55).

Advantages

There is a significant amount of research in support of the LOTCA assessments for use in clinical practice and several versions are also available for the adult population such as the LOTCA, LOTCA-II, and the LOTCA-G (geriatric version). Another value of the LOTCA batteries are their ability to measure client strengths and weaknesses across several constructs of orientation, perception, visuomotor organization, thinking operations, and attention where results can then be used to establish starting points for rehabilitation, to formulate specific goals, monitor treatment effects, and serve as a screening for further assessment (Hooper, 2012).

Disadvantages

Both versions are lengthy assessments and the original may be confusing to some as clearly established testing procedures and established norms are limited. Su et al. (2007) found that substantial ceiling effects existed in their LOTCA-II study of subjects with schizophrenia. One possible explanation was that the items studied may have been too easy for that sample. Low internal consistency was also noted for the visual perception, spatial perception, and motor praxis subtests which only had a range of α = 0.20 to 0.45.

Administration

The LOTCA batteries have detailed instructions as well as scoring interpretations and referenced norms outlined in the examiner's manual. When purchased several items are included, such as card decks, colored blocks, pegboard set, and multiple choice questionnaire forms. During administration of both versions the client is asked to complete several standardized activities, which are then graded according to how well the subject answers questions or performs tasks correctly using variable scales from 1 to 8 depending on the particular subtest. A subtest score is generated as well as a total score. Higher scores represent less impairment.

Permissions

The LOTCA battery of assessments can be accessed through various therapy supply outlets where they can be purchased for $205. Permission to use in research or publication can be pursued by contacting the creators of the assessment at the information that follows. More information can be found in the following journal article:

Katz, N., Itzkovich, M., Averbuch, S., & Elazar, B. (1989). Loewenstein Occupational Therapy Cognitive Assessment (LOTCA) battery for brain-injured patients: Reliability and validity. *American Journal of Occupational Therapy, 43*(3), 184-192.

Summary

POPULATION	Suspected executive impairment
TYPE OF MEASURE	Activity based
WHAT IT ASSESSES	Executive abilities; neurological deficits
TIME	≤45 minutes
COST	$205

Contact

Noomi Katz, PhD

Professor Emeritus of Occupational Therapy

Hebrew University of Jerusalem

Jerusalem, Israel

Web: www.huji.ac.il/dataj/controller/ihoker/MOP-STAFF_LINK?sno=8205746&Save_t=

CHAPTER 55: PERCEIVE, RECALL, PLAN, AND PERFORM SYSTEM OF TASK ANALYSIS (PRPP)

Description

The Perceive, Recall, Plan, and Perform System of Task Analysis (PRPP) system is a standardized, two-stage assessment based upon the Australian Occupational Performance Model that uses a task analysis method to examine the effectiveness of executive function relative to information processing that results in the measurement of occupational performance, information processing capacity, as well as other contextual influences (Aubin, Chapparo, Stip, & Rainville. 2012; Chapparo & Ranka, 1997). Clinicians using this system first identify occupational performance errors in stage 1 as a person engages in a task, then determine the cognitive strategy deficits resulting in performance errors during stage 2 (Nott & Chapparo, 2012). Stage 1 uses a behavioral task analysis to determine the steps of the task that need to be assessed through observation and depending on the nature and complexity of the task being performed, the stage 2 cognitive task analysis explores how cognitive strategies are implemented during functional task performance by evaluating the information processing strategies that underpin occupational performance which is divided into 4 areas of cognitive processing identified as central quadrants of performance and include attention and sensory perception (the ability to perceive), memory (ability to recall), response planning and evaluation (ability to plan), and performance monitoring (ability to perform) (Fry & O'Brien, 2002; Nott & Chapparo, 2012). As a client engages in an activity, errors in cognition in each quadrant are identified as those observable behaviors can then be targeted for intervention. The model uses 34 strategies, termed descriptors that are rated on a 3-point scale, indicating how effectively the person applies the 4 outlined cognitive strategies during performance (Fry & O'Brien, 2002; Nott & Chapparo, 2012). The PRPP can be completed in less than 30 minutes.

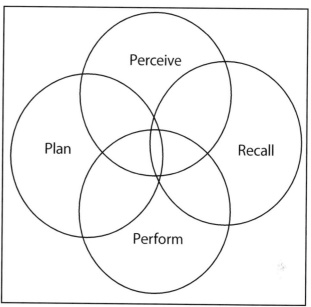

Figure 55-1. A variation of the four-quadrant system of the PRPP showing the interrelated associations of executive functions thought necessary for successful occupational performance.

Psychometrics

Research involving 9 occupational therapists found only a moderate level of inter-rater reliability with an intra-class correlation coefficient (ICC) of r = 0.60, which may be a result of model complexities (Nott, Chapparo, & Heard, 2009). Test-retest reliability was better with an ICC of r = 0.88 with a range from 0.83 to 0.88 for each quadrant (Nott et al., 2009). Intra-rater agreement using a Bland-Altman plot was 62.15% (time 1) and 57.63% (time 2) (Nott et al., 2009). In a schizophrenia sample (n = 10) Aubin et al. (2009) showed inter-rater reliability for the PRPP total score to be r = 0.77, for the perceive quadrant it was 0.65, recall 0.65, plan 0.69, and perform 0.63. A study of 28 community-dwelling persons with neurocognitive disorder dementia along with 25 raters found inter-rater reliability to be r=0.63 for stage 1 and (0.46) for stage 2; however, excellent agreement was found for test reliability for both stages at r=0.94 and 0.90, respectively (Steultjens, Voigt-Radloff, Leonhart, & Graff, 2012).

Advantages

The PRPP evaluation is distinct from other assessments in its use of a conceptual model that behaves more like a flow chart that, for the clinician, relies heavily on the visual presentation of the model where unique synergies takes place. The PRPP also measures both task and information processing performance over time as well as the context in which it occurs, affording the clinician a mechanism to measure intervention outcomes at both the level of body structure and function and at the level of activity and participation (Nott & Chapparo, 2012).

Disadvantages

Several studies have noted only moderate ICC values for various properties of the assessment where values of 0.70 and higher are usually considered acceptable; however, other studies investigating inter-rater reliability suggest that ICC values of 0.80 or more should be obtained in order to recommend a tool for use in confounding situations or for specific interventions (Donohue, 2006; Slagle, Weinger, Dinh, Brumer, & Williams, 2002) Aubin et al. (2009) argue that these limitations should be taken into account for future studies and in clinical settings.

Administration

During the assessment the clinician chooses an activity for the client to perform where their abilities are then rated relative to the four quadrants of the model where close attention is paid to the interplay between them as it is that relationship that determines a person's level of performance. A total of 34 behavioral descriptors of performance can then be used individually or cumulatively to identify client processing strengths or deficits within each of the four overlapping quadrants representing the PRPP and are featured on the outer rings of the conceptual model (Aubin et al., 2009). The 34 descriptors are typically those observable behaviors, such as maintains and monitors in the perceive quadrant; contextualizes to duration and recalls steps in the recall quadrant; and may be targeted as rehabilitation goals or may contribute to the focus of intervention and refining the decision-making process at the clinical level (Fry & O'Brien, 2002; Aubin et al., 2009).

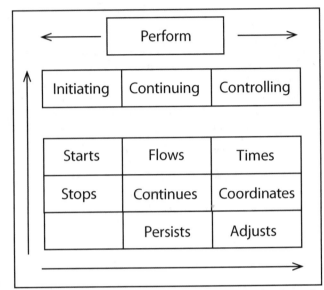

Figure 55-2. An example of the relationship of the 11 descriptors for perform quadrant. (Adapted from Aubin, G., Chapparo, C. I., Stip, E., & Rainville, C. (2009). Use of the Perceive, Recall, Plan, and Perform System of Task Analysis for persons with schizophrenia: A preliminary study. *Australian Occupational Therapy Journal, 56,* 191.)

Permissions

The PRPP is free to use in clinical practice and can be downloaded from several sites as well as being wholly contained in several studies. Use in research or publication can be obtained by contacting its creators or where published. More information can be found in the following publications:

Chapparo, C., & Ranka, J. (2005). *The PRPP System of Task Analysis: User's training manual.* Lidcombe, New South Wales, Australia: University of Sydney.

Nott, M., & Chapparo, C. (2012) Exploring the validity of the Perceive, Recall, Plan and Perform System of Task Analysis: Cognitive strategy use in adults with brain injury. *British Journal of Occupational Therapy, 75*(6), 256-263.

Summary

POPULATION	Suspected executive impairment
TYPE OF MEASURE	Activity based; descriptive rating scale
WHAT IT ASSESSES	Information processing; occupational performance errors
TIME	<30 minutes
COST	Free

Contact

Christine Chapparo, DipOT, MA, PhD

Senior Lecturer, Occupational Therapy

The University of Sydney, Australia

Sydney, New South Wales, Australia

Web: www.occupationalperformance.com/the-perceive-recall-plan-perform-prpp-system-of-task-analysis/

Web: www.prpp.nl/documenten/PRPP_Stage_2_model_%28ENG%29.pdf

CHAPTER 56: TRAIL MAKING TEST (TMT)

Description

The Trail Making Test (TMT) is a neuropsychological assessment that examines speed of cognitive processing and level of executive functioning by requiring an individual to complete two tasks related to connecting objects together in long sequences or *trail making*. Originally part of the Army Individual Test Battery (1944), it was later adopted into the Halstead–Reitan Neuropsychological Test Battery by Reitan (1955). It consists of two parts: Part A is a simple visual scanning and tracking task that requires the subject to connect numbered circles in order from 1 to 25 using a pen or pencil and Part B, which is more complex, requires the subject to connect 25 circles alternating between sequences of numbers and letters (Beckham, Crawford, & Feldman, 1998; Piper et al., 2012). Although, the measure seems quite simple, successful TMT ability comprises complex and multi-factorial cognitive mechanisms, such as visual search, perceptual/ motor speed, speed of processing, working memory, and general intelligence (Sánchez-Cubillo et al., 2009). The TMT takes 5 to 10 minutes to complete and scores are based on the amount of time it takes to complete each task as well as the type and number of errors. Higher scores typically indicate more executive impairment.

Psychometrics

In a study of individuals 18 to 89 years old (n = 680) Tombaugh (2004) examined the relative effects of age, education, and gender on the TMT-A and TMT-B tests in which results showed that age accounted for 34% and 38% of the variance for Trails A and B, while education accounted for only 3% and 6%, and gender accounted for less than 1%. A study by Salthouse, (2011) suggested that performance may be strongly related to speed and fluid cognitive abilities. Ratcliff, Dodge, Birzescu, and Ganguli (2003) found significant longitudinal decline over 2 years for adults 65 to 74 years of age, and Chen et al. (2001) reported similar results where they noted 2-year longitudinal changes of between 0.07 and 0.10 standard deviation units in adults 65 years old and over. A series of exploratory Pearson correlations by Sánchez-Cubillo et al. (2009) confirmed the relationship between TMT-A and TMT-B scores at r = 0.73, supporting the general assumption of common cognitive factors modulating both scores. The same study found that 45% of the variance of TMT-A was explained by speed of visual search (as measured by Wechsler Abbreviated Scale of Intelligence [WAIS-III] Digit Symbol score); whereas the ability to manipulate information in working memory (as measured by WAIS-III Digit Backward score) explained the greater portion of TMT-B variance compared to other variables.

Advantages

The TMT is a simple well-established assessment that has a good amount of peer-reviewed literature in support of its use in clinical practice. Several studies are available pertaining to normative data across the adult life span.

Disadvantages

Once an individual has taken the test he or she may become familiar with it and, due to its simplicity, this can lead to skewed test-retest and intra-rater reliability results at later testing points. Several versions of the assessment are also available along with competing research which may distract from its standardization.

Administration

The TMT is given in two parts: Part A, which requires the rapid connection of sequentially ordered numbers and Part B, which requires the individual to connect alternating letters and numbers (O'Rourke et al., 2011). Performance is typically based on the time required to complete Parts A and B; however, the number and type of errors can also be analyzed to provide additional clinical information (O'Rourke et al., 2011). Normative data examine the relationship between Parts A and B (i.e., time to complete each subtest is available). For example, a common condition thought to influence TMT performance is depression, as it has been shown influence slower test completion times, most likely due to associated bradyphrenia (slowness of thought) and psychomotor slowing (O'Rourke et al., 2011).

TABLE 56-1

TRAIL MAKING TEST-A AND B TEST MEAN SCORES FOR EACH AGE GROUP FROM A CANADIAN SAMPLE

Age	TRAILS—A		TRAILS—B	
	Mean (seconds)	SD	Mean (seconds)	SD
20 to 29 years old	36.10	10.00	85.70	38.70
30 to 39 years old	35.50	9.40	79.60	20.40
40 to 49 years old	40.00	13.30	105.20	42.20
50 to 59 years old	45.30	13.60	103.20	43.30
60 to 72 years old	68.90	21.20	158.80	49.50

n = 122; age range = 20 to 72 years old

Adapted from Fernandez, A. L., & Marcopulos, B. A. (2008). A comparison of normative data for the Trail Making Test from several countries: Equivalence of norms and considerations for interpretation: Cognition and neurosciences. *Scandinavian Journal of Psychology, 49,* 241.

variations of the measure are also available such as the 5-item Comprehensive TMT available through Psychological Assessment Resources Inc. for $67. More information can be found in the following publication:

Reitan, R. (1993). *Halstead-Reitan neuropsychological test battery: Theory and clinical interpretation* (2nd ed.). Tucson, AZ: Neuropsychology Press.

Summary

POPULATION	Suspected executive impairment
TYPE OF MEASURE	Activity based
WHAT IT ASSESSES	Speed of cognitive processing; level of executive functioning
TIME	< 10 minutes
COST	$50 to $67

Contact

Reitan Neuropsychology Laboratory

2517 W Monterey Ave

Mesa, AZ 85202

Phone: (480) 755-7543

Email: reitanlabs@aol.com

Web: www.mcssl.com/store/reitan-neuropsychology-laboratory/catalog/search

Permissions

The original TMT can be purchased from the Reitan Neuropsychology Laboratory for $50 where its use in research or publication can also be obtained. Other

REFERENCES

Aubin, G., Chapparo, C. I., Stip, E., & Rainville, C. (2009). Use of the Perceive, Recall, Plan, and Perform System of Task Analysis for persons with schizophrenia: A preliminary study. *Australian Occupational Therapy Journal, 56*, 189–199.

Baum, C., Connor, L., Morrison, T., Hahn, M., Dromerick, A., & Edwards, D. (2008). Reliability, validity, and clinical utility of the Executive Function Performance Test: A measure of executive function in a sample of people with stroke. *American Journal of Occupational Therapy, 62*(4), 446-455.

Baum, C., Morrison, T., Hahn, M., & Edwards, D. (2007). Executive Function Performance Test: Test protocol booklet. Retrieved from www.practicechangefellows.org/documents/efpt.pdf

Baum, C. M., & Wolf, T. J. (2013). Executive Function Performance Test (EFPT). St. Louis, MO: Washington University School of Medicine.

Beckham, J., Crawford, A., & Feldman, M. (1998). Trail Making Test performance in Vietnam combat veterans with and without post-traumatic stress disorder. *Journal of Traumatic Stress, 11*(4), 811-819.

Bulzacka, E., Vilain, J., Schürhoff, F., Meary, A., Leboyer, M., & Szoke, A. (2013). A self-administered executive functions ecological questionnaire (the Behavior Rating Inventory of Executive Function—Adult Version) shows impaired scores in a sample of patients with schizophrenia. *Mental Illness, 5*(e4), 14-16.

Chapparo, C., & Ranka, J. (1997). The Perceive: Recall: Plan: Perform (PRPP) System of task analysis. In C. Chapparo and J. Ranka (Eds.). *Occupational Performance Model (Australia). Monograph 1* (pp. 189-198). Lidcombe, New South Wales, Australia: University of Sydney.

Chen, P., Ratcliff, G., Belles, S. H., Cauley, J. A., DeKosky, S. T., & Ganguli, M. (2001). Patterns of cognitive decline in presymptomatic Alzheimer disease: a prospective community study. *Archives of General Psychiatry, 58*(9), 856-858.

Dean, G., & Dean, S. (2012). Review of the Behavior Rating Inventory of Executive Function—Adult version. In R. M. Roth, P. K. Isquith, & G. A. Gioia. (Eds.). *Mental measurements yearbook* (17th ed.). Lincoln, NE: Buros Institute of Mental Measurements.

Donohue, M. V. (2006). Interrater reliability of the social profile: Assessment of community and psychiatric group participation. *Australian Occupational Therapy Journal, 53*, 1–10. In G. Aubin, C. I. Chapparo, E. Stip, & C. Rainville. (2009). Use of the Perceive, Recall, Plan, and Perform System of Task Analysis for persons with schizophrenia: A preliminary study. *Australian Occupational Therapy Journal, 56*, 189–199.

Fernandez, A. L., & Marcopulos, B. A. (2008). A comparison of normative data for the Trail Making Test from several countries: Equivalence of norms and considerations for interpretation: Cognition and neurosciences. *Scandinavian Journal of Psychology, 49*, 239–246

Fry, K., & O'Brien, L. (2002). Using the Perceive, Recall, Plan and Perform system to assess cognitive deficits in adults with traumatic brain injury: A case study. *Australian Occupational Therapy Journal, 49*(4), 182-187.

Hooper, S. (2012). Review of the Loewenstein Occupational Therapy Cognitive Assessment. In R. M. Roth, P. K. Isquith, & G. A. Gioia. (Eds.). *Mental measurements yearbook* (18th ed.). Lincoln, NE: Buros Institute of Mental Measurements.

Katz, N., Itzkovich, M., Averbuch, S., & Elazar, B. (1989). Loewenstein Occupational Therapy Cognitive Assessment (LOTCA) battery for brain-injured patients: Reliability and validity. *American Journal of Occupational Therapy, 43*(3), 184-192.

Katz, N., Tadmor, I., Felzen, B., & Hartman-Maeir, A. (2007). Validity of the Executive Function Performance Test in individuals with schizophrenia. *OTJR: Occupation, Participation and Health, 27*(2), 44-51.

Najenson, T., Rahmani, L., Elasar, B., & Averbuch, S. (1984). An elementary cognitive assessment and treatment of the craniocerebrally injured patient. In B. A. Edelstein & E. T. Couture (Eds.). *Behavioral assessment and rehabilitation of the traumatically brain damaged* (pp. 313-338). New York, New York: Plenum Press

Nott, M., & Chapparo, C. (2012). Exploring the validity of the Perceive, Recall, Plan and Perform System of Task Analysis: Cognitive strategy use in adults with brain injury. *British Journal of Occupational Therapy, 75*(6), 256-263.

Nott, M., Chapparo, T., & Heard, R. (2009). Reliability of the Perceive, Recall, Plan and Perform System of Task Analysis: A criterion-referenced assessment. *Australian Occupational Therapy Journal, 56*, 307–314.

O'Rourke, J., Beglinger, L., Smith, M., Mills, J., Moser, D., Rowe, K.,... Paulsen, J. (2011). The Trail Making Test in prodromal Huntington disease: Contributions of disease progression to test performance. *Journal of Clinical and Experimental Neuropsychology, 33*(5), 567–579.

Piper, B., Li, V., Eiwaz, M., Kobel, Y., Benice, T., Chu, A.,...Mueller, S. (2012). Executive function on the Psychology Experiment Building Language tests. *Behavior Research Methods, 44*(1), 110–123.

Psychological Assessments Australia. (2014).Product information. Retrieved from www.psychassessments.com.au/Category. aspx?cID=282.

Rabin, L., Roth, R., Isquith, P., Wishart, H., Nutter-Upham, K., Pare, N., ...Saykin, A. (2006). Self-and informant reports of executive function on the BRIEF-A in MCI and older adults with cognitive complaints. *Archives of Clinical Neuropsychology, 2*, 721–732.

Ratcliff, G., Dodge, H., Birzescu, M., & Ganguli, M. (2003). Tracking cognitive function over time: Ten-year longitudinal data from a community-based study. *Applied Neuropsychology, 10*, 76–88.

Roth, R., Lance, C., Isquith, P., Fischer, A., & Giancola, P. (2013). Confirmatory factor analysis of the Behavior Rating Inventory of Executive Function—Adult Version in healthy adults and application to attention-deficit/hyperactivity disorder. *Archives of Clinical Neuropsychology, 28*(5), 425–434.

Salthouse. T. (2011). Cognitive correlates of cross-sectional differences and longitudinal changes in trail making performance. *Journal of Clinical and Experimental Neuropsychology, 33*(2), 242–248.

Sánchez-Cubillo, I., Periáñez, J., Adrover-Roig, D., Rodríguez-Sánchez, J., Ríos-Lago, M., J. Tirapu, J., & Barceló, F. (2009). Construct validity of the Trail Making Test: Role of task-switching, working memory, inhibition/interference control, and visuomotor abilities. *Journal of the International Neuropsychological Society, 15*, 438–450

Slagle, J., Weinger, M., Dinh, M.-T., Brumer, V., & Williams, K. (2002). Assessment of the intrarater and interrater reliability of an established clinical task analysis methodology. *Anesthesiology, 96*, 1129-1139. In G. Aubin, C. I. Chapparo, E. Stip, & C. Rainville. (2009). Use of the Perceive, Recall, Plan, and Perform System of Task Analysis for persons with schizophrenia: A preliminary study. *Australian Occupational Therapy Journal, 56*, 189-199.

Steultjens, E. J., Voigt-Radloff, S., Leonhart, R., & Graff, M. L. (2012). Reliability of the Perceive, Recall, Plan, and Perform (PRPP) assessment in community-dwelling dementia patients: Test consistency and inter-rater agreement. *International Psychogeriatrics, 24*(4), 659-665.

Su, C-Y., Chen, W-L., Tsai, P-C., Tsai, C-Y., & Su, W-L. (2007). Psychometric properties of the Loewenstein Occupational Therapy Cognitive Assessment–Second Edition in Taiwanese persons with schizophrenia. *American Journal of Occupational Therapy, 61,* 108-118.

Tombaugh, T. (2004). Trail Making Test A and B: Normative data stratified by age and education. *Archives of Clinical Neuropsychology. 19,* 203–214

Waid-Ebbs, J., Wen, P., Heaton, S. C., Donovan, N. J., & Velozo, C. (2012). The item level psychometrics of the Behaviour Rating Inventory of Executive Function-Adult (BRIEF-A) in a TBI sample. *Brain Injury, 26*(13/14), 1646-1657.

Wang, S., Gong, Z., Sen, J., Han, L., Zhang, M., & Chen, W. (2014). The usefulness of the Loewenstein Occupational Therapy Cognition Assessment in evaluating cognitive function in patients with stroke. *European Review for Medical and Pharmacological Sciences, 18*(23), 3665-3672

Yuh, J., Jen-suh, C., & Keh-chung, L. (2009). Validity of the Loewenstein Occupational Therapy Cognitive Assessment in people with intellectual disabilities. *American Journal of Occupational Therapy, 63*(4), 414-422

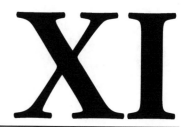

Feeding and Nutritional Status

Bortnick, K.
Occupational Therapy Assessments for Older Adults: 100 Instruments for
Measuring Occupational Performance (pp. 163-173).
© 2017 Taylor & Francis Group.

Chapter 57: Edinburgh Feeding Evaluation Questionnaire (EdFED-Q)

Description

The Edinburgh Feeding Evaluation Questionnaire (EdFED-Q) is an outcome measure designed to quantify the quality of mealtime interactions with caregivers as well as the level of help a client may need while eating typical of that seen in those with late stage neurocognitive disorder (NCD) of the Alzheimer's and related types or other debilitating conditions known to effect mealtime activities of daily living. The EdFED-Q is delivered through observations completed during mealtime performance. The results then allow the clinician to determine an individual's level of impairment as well as the need for possible psychosocial and clinical interventions as well as referrals for more detailed occupational or speech therapy services, environmental modifications, dietary alterations, and other special communication techniques designed to support the nutritional intake of a compromised individual (Amella & Lawrence, 2007). The assessment contains 11 items that form 3 groups of indicators pertaining to patient behavior: obstinacy/aversion and passivity (7 items); clinical interventions (3 items); and feeding difficulties (1 item). The seven behavior items, in particular, form a hierarchy of mealtime behavior such that those behaviors should be predictable in persons with mealtime difficulties (Amella & Lawrence 2007). Items 1 to 10 of the assessment are scored as either (0) never, (1) sometimes, or (2) often, whereas item 11 is a subjective measure of the level of assistance needed as determined by the clinician. The EdFED-Q can be completed during one meal, less than 30 minutes, with higher scores indicating more problematic feeding.

Table 57-1
Items of the Edinburgh Feeding Evaluation Questionnaire
1. Level of supervision while feeding
2. Physical help with feeding
3. Spillage
4. Food on the plate at the end of the meal
5. Refusal to eat
6. Turns head away while eating
7. Refusal to open mouth
8. Spits out food
9. Leaves mouth open allowing food to drop out
10. Refusal to swallow
11. Level of assistance needed

Adapted from Liu, W., Watson, R., & Lou, F. (2014). The Edinburgh Feeding Evaluation in Dementia scale (EdFED): Cross-cultural validation of the simplified Chinese version in mainland China. *Journal of Clinical Nursing, 23*(1/2), 47.

Psychometrics

In a community-based study using 24 pairs of raters the EdFED-Q was found to have an inter-rater reliability of $r = 0.59$ and intra-rater reliability of $r = 0.95$ (Watson,

MacDonald, & McReady, 2001). Personal idiosyncrasies and difficult populations might explain low inter-rater reliability scores. Development of the C-EdFED (Chinese version) revealed only moderate internal consistency, However, when the question, "Does the patient tend to leave food on the plate at the end of the meal?" was omitted, the correlation of item-to-total increased to $\alpha = 0.83$, which may imply the item lacks a substantive relation with other items measuring feeding difficulty in Chinese populations or that cohort in particular (Lin, Watson, Lee, Chou, & Wu, 2008). When scoring of the Chinese version (n = 20) was expanded to include a fourth descriptor (1 = not relevant; 2 = somewhat relevant; 3 = quite relevant; 4 = highly relevant) pre-test internal consistency showed high correlation with the overall scale at 0.87 with item-to-total correlation coefficients ranging from 0.38 to 0.79 (Liu, Watson, & Lou, 2014). Full test internal consistency from a sample of 102 subjects was $\alpha = 0.91$ and results showed moderate inter-rater and intra-rater reliabilities at $r = 0.81$ and 0.89, respectively (Liu et al., 2014). Results also determined that the 3 factor model discussed prior of (1) obstinacy or passivity, (2) nursing intervention, and (3) indicator of feeding difficulty was able to explain 83% of the variance (Liu et al., 2014). A subsequent study of 211 subjects with an average age of 83.3 years found that negative correlations existed between the EdFED-I (Italian version) and the Mini Mental State Exam at –0.27, whereas correlation with the Barthel Index was –0.32 (Bagnasco et al., 2015).

Advantages

The EdFED-Q can be used to determine if further services are needed. It is easy to administer (1 feeding session) and no special training or certifications are needed. Mealtime assessment using the EdFED-Q can also help to identify persons who could benefit from an intervention as research has shown that those individuals who were considered moderately dependent, who typically can feed themselves with appropriate support from staff, are often ignored by staff and not given any feeding assistance resulting in low food intake. Highlighting the importance for the clinician to accurately identify those subjects whose food intake is associated with eating difficulty, feeding assistance, moderate dependence and frequency of family visits (Lin, Watson, & Wu, 2010). The measure has also been adapted to Italian and Chinese versions suggesting cross-cultural validity of the assessment.

Disadvantages

There is a limited amount research pertaining to the EdFED-Q outside of that involving its author.

Administration

During assessment the clinician observes and rates the quality of mealtime interaction across 11 items in which 10 are factored into the final score relative to the presence or absence of adverse feeding behavior. Each item is then scored along a 3-point scale (0 to 2) as either never (0), sometimes (1), or often (2). Scores range from 0 to 20 with higher scores considered more problematic.

Permission

The EdFED-Q is in the public domain and can be used in clinical practice as well as research or publication with no special permissions. More information can be found in the following journal article:

Watson, R., Green, S. M., & Legg, L. (2001) The Edinburgh Feeding Evaluation in Dementia Scale #2 (EdFED-Q #2): Convergent and discriminant validity. *Clinical Effectiveness in Nursing, 5*(1), 44-46.

Summary

POPULATION	Nutritionally compromised; NCD; dysphagia; general
TYPE OF MEASURE	Activity-based rating scale
WHAT IT ASSESSES	Quality of feeding skills
TIME	< 30 minutes
COST	Free

Contact

Roger Watson, PhD

Faculty of Health and Social Science

The University of Hull

Hull, United Kingdom

Web: http://publicationslist.org/roger.watson

CHAPTER 58: McGILL INGESTIVE SKILLS ASSESSMENT (MISA)

Description

The McGill Ingestive Skills Assessment (MISA) outcome measure is an occupational therapy tool designed to quantify a person's ability to safely and independently consume a variety of food and liquid textures and was developed for use with older populations as well as those with neurologic impairment to assess their mealtime routine (Lambert, Gisel, Groher, Abrahamowicz, & Wood-Dauphinee, 2006). The MISA includes 43 items comprising 5 skill domains: (1) positioning, which has 4 items that address the ability to maintain a position that is safe for eating and drinking; (2) self-feeding skills, which has 7 items that examine self-feeding skills, behavior, and judgement; (3) liquid ingestion, which has 7 items that are considered necessary oropharyngeal skills for liquid intake; (4) solid ingestion, which has 12 items that are the oropharyngeal skills for solid intake; and (5) texture management, which has 13 items that explore the ability to manage 8 solid foods and 5 liquid textures (Lambert, Gisel, Groher, & Wood-Dauphinee, 2003). During assessment the clinician notes client abilities or impairments relative to the 5 skill domains during mealtime feeding. The MISA employs a 3-point ordinal scale and, when summed, gives a composite score as well as subscale scores, which can then be used to determine ability across the functional domains as well as areas to address for rehabilitation. The MISA can be completed in 60 minutes or less with higher scores indicative of fewer ingestive problems.

Psychometrics

Initial field testing of the MISA showed that internal consistency of all scales was α = ≥0.86 and inter-rater agreement was r = ≥0.92 (Lambert et al., 2003). A following study determined that the total item inter-rater reliability using 76 subjects with 50 raters was r = 0.85, while for the positioning subscale it was 0.68, self-feeding 0.88, liquid ingestion 0.84, solid ingestion 0.68, and texture management r = 0.74)(Lambert et al., 2006). The same study found total item intra-rater reliability to be r = 0.92, while for the positioning subscale it was 0.69, for self-feeding 0.88, liquid ingestion 0.77, solid ingestion 0.92, and texture management 0.72 (Lambert et al., 2006). Finally, that study also determined that all of the subscales of the MISA were positively correlated with the Functional Independence Measure scale with self-feeding (0.67) being stronger than the others (range; 0.22 to 0.40). An examination of 102 subjects with an average age of 77 years from acute and long-term care facilities found that an increasing total MISA

score had statistically significant associations with reduced risk of death, where a 1-point increase in total MISA score was associated with a 4% decrease in the risk of death, and a 1-point increase in both the self-feeding and solid ingestion scales was associated with an approximately 11% risk reduction (Lambert, Abrahamowicz, Groher, Wood-Dauphinee, & Gisel, 2005).

TABLE 58-1		
PERCENT DIFFICULTIES FOR ACUTELY-HOSPITALIZED SUBJECTS		
DOMAIN	FRAIL	ROBUST
Positioning	41% to 95%	10% to 60%
Self-feeding skills	30% to 86%	5% to 40%
Liquid ingestion	22% to 78%	3% to 48%
Solid ingestion	44% to 77%	10% to 60%
Texture management	38% to 67%	13% to 65%

Frail: n = 64; 82.4 years; SD 7.3
Robust: n = 40; 82.;1 SD 7.3

Adapted from Hansen, T., Lambert, H. C., & Faber, J. (2012). Ingestive skill difficulties are frequent among acutely-hospitalized frail elderly patients, and predict hospital outcomes. *Physical & Occupational Therapy in Geriatrics, 30*(4), 277-279.

Advantages

There is a good amount of research in support of the MISA for use in clinical practice. No special training or certifications are needed and it can be purchased form the Canadian Association of Occupational Therapists (CAOT) website. The assessment has also shown good discriminant ability and one unique aspect of the MISA is its emphasis on ability rather than impairment as defined by the World Health Organization (Lambert et al., 2003).

Disadvantages

Reliability and stability of the positioning and solid ingestion subscales have shown the least stability where in one study, research by MISA creators found the inter-rater reliability inter-class correlation coefficients for those subscales to be only between 0.60 and 0.70 (Lambert et al.,

2006). Although, those values are still considered moderate to good, the lower scores may be influenced by the small number of items in each subscale or possibly by variations in the person's alertness, behavior, or physical vitality during assessment (Lambert et al., 2006).

Administration

The MISA is composed of 43 items across 5 functional domains where during assessment the clinician rates a person's ability as it relates to items on the test. The MISA employs a 3-point-variable ordinal scale depending on the item and has a maximum total score of 129 with higher scores indicating fewer difficulties with feeding, eating, and swallowing (Francis-Bacz, Wood-Dauphinee, & Gisel, 2013).

Permissions

The MISA can be purchased from the CAOT website for $72. Use in research, publication, or for commercial purposes can be obtained by contacting CAOT or its author at the information that follows. More information can be found in the following journal article:

Lambert, H., Gisel, E., Groher, M., & Wood-Dauphinee, S. (2003). McGill Ingestive Skills Assessment (MISA): Development and first field test of an evaluation of functional ingestive skills of elderly persons. *Dysphagia, 18*, 101-113.

Summary

POPULATION	Nutritionally compromised; neurocognitive disorder; dysphagia; general
TYPE OF MEASURE	Activity-based rating scale
WHAT IT ASSESSES	Ability to consume various food/liquid textures
TIME	≤60 minutes
COST	$72

Contact

Heather Lambert, BSc, PhD

McGill University

Montreal, Quebec, Canada

Web: www.mcgill.ca/spot/our-faculty/lambert

Canadian Association of Occupational Therapists Store

100-34 Colonnade Rd

Ottawa, ON K2E 7J6 Canada

Phone: (800) 434-2268

Web: www.caot.ca/store/detail.aspx?id=PUB-ML48

TABLE 58-2

EXAMPLE ITEMS/SCORING OF THE MCGILL INGESTIVE SKILLS ASSESSMENT

ITEM	1 POINT	2 POINTS	3 POINTS
Seals lips on cup	Never/rarely	Sometimes	Always (almost)
Able to sit upright without leaning on arm	Requires constant support of arm	Occasional support	No support needed
Tolerates physical effort of meal	Fatigues throughout the meal	Becomes fatigued part way through meal	No fatigue noted

Adapted from Charmine Francis, C. (2009). *The discriminative validity of the McGill Ingestive Skills Assessment (MISA).* Master's Dissertation. McGill University, Montreal, Quebec.

CHAPTER 59: MINI NUTRITIONAL ASSESSMENT—SHORT FORM (MNA-SF)

Description

The Mini Nutritional Assessment (MNA), by Vellas and Guigoz (1989), is a short nutrition-screening tool designed to help identify geriatric patients (65 years old and over) who are malnourished or at risk of malnutrition. The short form of the MNA (MNA-SF) consists of 6 questions that have shown to have high correlations with the original 18-item long form, which should be used if further investigations into the client's condition are warranted after administration of the MNA-SF. Items on the assessment include an examination of (1) decline of food intake over the past 3 months due to loss of appetite, digestive problems, chewing or swallowing difficulties; (2) weight loss during the last 3 months; (3) mobility; (4) psychological stress or acute disease in the past 3 months; (5) neuropsychological problems; and (6) body mass index (BMI), which is determined by solving weight in kg/height in m^2. The MNA-SF allows for the substitution of BMI, if it cannot be obtained, with calf circumference without losing validity. Each item of the MNA-SF is scored along a variable scale of 0 to 3 with total scores ranging from of 0 to 14. The assessment takes less than 10 minutes to complete with lower scores suggestive of poorer nutritional intake.

Psychometrics

A study of 881 subjects with a mean age of 76.4 years, 73.8% of which were community dwelling, determined that the MNA-SF had a sensitivity of 96%, specificity of 98%, and positive predictive value of 97% when using a score of ≥ 11 as normal cut point (Rubenstein, Harker, Salva, Guigoz, & Vellas, 2001). Using the MNA-SF in a study of nonagenarians (age 90 to 99 years old) found that 66.4% of the screened individuals were at risk of malnutrition (MNA-SF score ≤ 11) and risk of malnutrition was more prevalent in women than in men (68.9% vs 49.5%), while actual malnutrition, based on BMI, was observed in 21.9% of the participants and also tended to be higher in women than in men (22.9% vs 15.0%) (Vandewoude & Gossum, 2013). A study investigating the association between MNA-SF results and frailty status in community-dwelling older adults over 75 years old (n = 206) without cognitive impairment found 15.1% of the participants were at risk of malnutrition with no participant actually malnourished; however, 90% of those at risk of malnutrition were considered either pre-frail (15.5%) or frail (40%) (Bollwein et al., 2013). A population-based study of older adults (average

age: 86 years) found that the mean MNA-SF score was 9.8, which is considered at risk, and that total MNA-SF scores were a significant predictor of mortality according to a Hazard Ratio, which is a measure of survival at any point in time in a group cohort, of 0.83 (Lilamand et al., 2015). Results also found that 198 (25.6%) presented with normal nutritional status (12 to 14 points), 454 (58.7%) were at risk of malnutrition (8 to 11 points), and 121 (15.7%) were malnourished and after 1 year of follow-up 135 (17.5%) had died (Lilamand et al., 2015).

Advantages

The MNA-SF has a significant amount of research in support of its use in clinical practice. The MNA-SF as well as the long version are considered gold standards of nutritional assessment and are utilized across many disciplines. No special training or certifications are needed and research has shown it to be a good predictor of feeding problems in those 65 years old and older. The Nestlé Nutrition Institute hosts an intuitive interactive website devoted to the MNA batteries which can be an excellent resource for the practitioner. Also, the scale has been well-validated in numerous cultural settings.

Disadvantages

The MNA-SF may be limited in its use as a quick screen only to suggest further testing if needed and should not necessarily be used to replace a full assessment if malnourishment is suspected. Finally, the MNA is only validated for patients over the age of 65 years old.

Administration

The MNA-SF is an interactive activity/questionnaire that is comprised of 6 items rated between 0 to 3 relative to aspects of subject's nutritional intake. Scores can range from 0 to 14 with lower scores considered more problematic. A score of 0 to 7 suggests that the person is malnourished, 8 to 11 he or she is considered at risk, and 12 to 14 suggests normal nutritional status.

Permission

The MNA was developed by the Nestlé Nutrition Institute and is freely available to use in clinical practice. The MNA form is protected by copyright laws and is also a registered trademark of Société des Produits Nestlé S.A.

By downloading the MNA form the user agrees to keep the original form unchanged. Permission to use the assessment for research or for commercial purposes can be obtained upon formal request. Further information about the MNA-SF can be found in the following article:

Rubenstein, L. Z., Harker, J. O., Salva, A., Guigoz, Y., & Vellas, B. (2001). Screening for undernutrition in geriatric practice: Developing the short-form mini-nutritional assessment (MNA-SF). *The Journals of Gerontology. Series A, Biological Sciences and Medical Sciences, 56*(6), M366-M372.

Summary

POPULATION	≥65 years; suspected malnutrition; general
TYPE OF MEASURE	Questionnaire/rating scale
WHAT IT ASSESSES	Malnutrition risk
TIME	< 10 minutes
COST	Free

Contact

Nestlé Nutrition Institute

Email: info@mna-elderly.com

Web: www.mna-elderly.com/

Chapter 60: Minimal-Eating Observation Form—Version II (MEOF-II)

Description

The Minimal-Eating Observation Form—Version II (MEOF-II) is an outcome measure developed to provide the clinician with a description of subject mealtime problems and to assess the need for possible interventions (Westergren, Norberg, Vallen, & Hagell, 2011). The assessment is an interactive observation tool composed of three domains: ingestion, deglutition, and energy and appetite, and has six subscales relating to (1) the presence of unintentional weight loss; (2) body mass index (BMI) or calf circumference (CC); (3) eating problems; (4) swallowing and mouth problems; (5) energy and appetite; and (6) the indication of clinical signs. Designed as a modification to the original MEOF by Axelsson (1996), changes included the replacement of opening/closing the mouth and aberrant eating time with chewing ability and appetite (Westergren, Lindholm, Mattsson, & Ulander, 2009). During assessment the clinician notes the presence or absence of particular adverse mealtime behaviors as well as the measurement of a person's BMI or CC if BMI is unattainable. Items on the MEOF-II may include several observations that are scored as either 0 or 2 or 0 or 1. The measure can be completed in less than 10 minutes where a higher score is suggestive of more risk.

Psychometrics

A study of 24 inpatients, median age 69 years, found MEOF-II total score inter-rater and intra-rater reliabilities to be r=0.92 and r=0.84, respectively (Westergren, Torfadóttir, & Hagell. 2014). Another study found inter-rater agreement between a trained observer and less trained observers (n=20) to be r=0.89 when testing 50 subjects post-cerebrovascular accident where agreement ranged from 0.82 for manipulation of food on the plate and mouth to 0.94 for ability to chew and swallow (Westergren et al., 2009). The same study determined that internal consistency for the trained observer was α=0.76 and for the less-trained observers it was 0.71 (Westergren et al., 2009). Another study found that total values were above r=0.80 for both inter- and intra-rater reliabilities using 8 raters with no prior experience among 24 subjects (Westergren et al., 2014). A study by Vallen, Hagell, & Westergren (2011) of various patient populations (n=33 each) found that the number of those found to be at risk were 38.2% for orthopedic, 28.1% for cardiology, and 45.4% for stroke populations. When using the BMI version its results had exact agreement of 82% with the full Mini Nutritional Assessment—Long Form (MNA), which is much longer, and when CC was used agreement was 81%. A similar examination involving 87 persons receiving inpatient care found that out of 18 undernourished patients, according to gold standard (MNA), only 13 were considered to be at high risk according to MEOF-II resulting in a sensitivity (i.e., the proportion of people correctly identified according to the 18-item MNA) of 0.61, whereas the specificity and accuracy were 79% and 68%, (Westergren, Norberg, & Hagell, 2011). Furthermore, a positive MEOF-II result for undernutrition, was associated with an 82% probability that the individual really was undernourished according to the MNA and a negative result was associated with a 57% probability that the individual really was not undernourished (Westergren, Norberg, & Hagell, 2011).

Advantages

The MEOF-II is an easy to use, relatively quick assessment that has shown both acceptable sensitivity and specificity in detecting undernutrition if used in the same manner as the MNA-SF (short form). For example, Vallen et al. (2011) found that it took, on average, only 8.8 minutes to complete the assessment. Administration also allows for substituting BMI with CC in situations where measures of patient height and weight cannot be easily obtained. Another advantage of using the MEOF-II compared to other quick screening tools is that it has the ability to identify actual problems for immediate intervention (Westergren, Norberg, Vallen, et al., 2011). Finally, the MEOF-II is not limited to only patient populations ≥65 years of age like the MNA-SF.

Disadvantages

Differing inter- and intra-rater agreement between trained and untrained observers as well as the presence of outlier scores have been observed suggesting that instruction in performing eating observations may be required; however, the authors argue that only minimal training is needed (Westergren et al., 2009). Also, the amount of independent research (i.e., work that does not indirectly involve one of the original authors) is limited.

Administration

The MEOF-II is an interactive observational tool in which the practitioner notes the presence or absence of aberrant eating, feeding, or swallowing behaviors as well as defining a person's BMI or CC. Each item is scored along a variable scale of 0 or 1 and yields a total score ranging from 0 to 8. A final score of 0 to 2 is considered low risk for under-nutrition, a score of 3 or 4 is a moderate risk, and a score ≥ 5 is considered a high risk for undernutrition (Valle et al., 2011).

Permissions

The MEOF-II can be downloaded and used free of charge from the website listed in Contact however, the author asks that a simple form be filled out when downloading the material. Use of the MEOF-II for research or other purposes can be obtained by contacting its creators. The assessment can also found in its entirety in the following journal article:

Vallen, C., Hagell, P., & Westergren, A. (2011). Validity and user-friendliness of the Minimal Eating Observation and Nutrition Form—Version II (MEONF-II) for under-nutrition risk screening. *Food and Nutrition Research, 55*, 5801. doi: 10.3402/fnr.v55i0.5801

Summary

POPULATION	Suspected malnutrition; general
TYPE OF MEASURE	Questionnaire/rating scale
WHAT IT ASSESSES	Malnutrition risk
TIME	< 10 minutes
COST	Free

Contact

Albert Westergren, PhD

Kristianstad University School of Health and Society

Kristianstad, Sweden

Web: www.hkr.se/meof

REFERENCES

Amella, E. J., & Lawrence, J. F. (2007). *Eating and feeding issues in older adults with dementia: Part I: Assessment*. New York, New York: Hartford Institute of Geriatric Nursing, New York University and the Alzheimer's Association.

Bagnasco, A., Watson, R., Zanini, M., Rosa, F., Rocco, G., & Sasso, L. (2015). Preliminary testing using Mokken scaling of an Italian translation of the Edinburgh Feeding Evaluation in Dementia (EdFED-I) scale. *Applied Nursing Research, 28*(4), 391-396.

Bollwein, J., Volkert, D. D., Diekmann, R. R., Kaiser, M. M., Uter, W. W., Vidal, K. K.,…Bauer, J. J. (2013). Nutritional status according to the Mini Nutritional Assessment (MNA) and frailty in community dwelling older persons: a close relationship. *Journal of Nutrition, Health & Aging, 17*(4), 351-356.

Charmine Francis, C. (2009). *The discriminative validity of the McGill Ingestive Skills Assessment (MISA)*. Master's dissertation. McGill University. Montreal, Quebec.

Francis-Bacz, C., Wood-Dauphinee, S., & Gisel, E. (2013). The discriminative validity of the McGill Ingestive Skills Assessment. *Physical and Occupational Therapy in Geriatrics, 31*(2), 148–158.

Hansen, T., Lambert, H. C., & Faber, J. (2012). Ingestive skill difficulties are frequent among acutely-hospitalized frail elderly patients, and predict hospital outcomes. *Physical & Occupational Therapy in Geriatrics, 30*(4), 271-287.

Lambert, H., Abrahamowicz, M., Groher, M., Wood-Dauphinee, S., & Gisel, E. G. (2005). The McGill Ingestive Skills Assessment predicts time to death in an elderly population with neurogenic dysphagia: Preliminary evidence. *Dysphagia, 20*(2), 123-132.

Lambert, H., Gisel, E., Groher, M., Abrahamowicz, M., & Wood-Dauphinee, S. (2006). Psychometric testing of the McGill Ingestive Skills Assessment. *American Journal of Occupational Therapy, 60*(4), 409-419.

Lambert, H., Gisel, E., Groher, M., & Wood-Dauphinee, S. (2003). McGill Ingestive Skills Assessment (MISA): Development and first field test of an evaluation of functional ingestive skills of elderly persons. *Dysphagia, 18*, 101-113.

Lilamand, M., Kelaiditi, E., Demougeot, L., Rolland, Y., Vellas, B., & Cesari, M. (2015). The Mini Nutritional Assessment-Short Form and mortality in nursing home residents—Results from the INCUR study. *Journal of Nutrition, Health and Aging, 19*(4), 383-388.

Lin, L. C., Watson, R., Lee, Y. C., Chou, Y. C., & Wu, S. C. (2008). Edinburgh Feeding Evaluation in Dementia (EdFED) scale: Cross-cultural validation of the Chinese version. *Journal of Advanced Nursing, 62*(1), 116-123.

Lin, L. C. Watson, R., & Wu, S. C. (2010). What is associated with low food intake in older people with dementia? *Journal of Clinical Nursing, 19*(12), 53-59.

Liu, W., Watson, R., & Lou, F. (2014). The Edinburgh Feeding Evaluation in Dementia scale (EdFED): Cross-cultural validation of the simplified Chinese version in mainland China. *Journal of Clinical Nursing, 23*(1/2), 45-53.

Rubenstein, L., Harker, J., Salva, A., Guigoz, Y., & Vellas, B. (2001). Screening for undernutrition in geriatric practice: Developing the short-form Mini-Nutritional Assessment (MNA-SF). *The Journals of Gerontology. Series A, Biological Sciences and Medical Sciences, 56*(6), M366-M372.

Vallen, C., Hagell, P., & Westergren, A. (2011). Validity and user-friendliness of The Minimal Eating Observation and Nutrition Form— Version II (MEONF-II) for undernutrition risk screening. *Food and Nutrition Research, 55,* 5801. doi: 10.3402/fnr.v55i0.5801

Vandewoude, M. M., & Gossum, A. A. (2013). Nutritional screening strategy in nonagenarians: the value of the MNA-SF (Mini Nutritional Assessment Short Form) in NutriAction. *Journal of Nutrition, Health & Aging, 17*(4), 310-314.

Watson, R., MacDonald, J., & McReady, T. (2001). The Edinburgh Feeding Evaluation in Dementia scale #2 (EdFED #2): Inter- and intra-rater reliability. *Clinical Effectiveness in Nursing, 5*(4), 184–186.

Westergren, A., Lindholm, C., Mattsson, A., & Ulander, K. (2009). Minimal Eating Observation Form: Reliability and validity. *Journal of Nutrition, Health & Aging, 13*(1), 6-12.

Westergren, A., Norberg, E., & Hagell, P. (2011). Diagnostic performance of the Minimal Eating Observation and Nutrition Form— Version II (MEONF-II) and Nutritional Risk Screening 2002 (NRS 2002) among hospital inpatients—A crosssectional study. *BMC Nursing, 10*(24). doi:10.1186/1472-6955-10-24

Westergren, A., Norberg, E., Vallen, C., & Hagell, P. (2011). Cut-off scores for the Minimal Eating Observation and Nutrition Form— Version II (MEONF-II) among hospital inpatients. *Food and Nutrition Research, 55.* doi:10.3402/fnr.v55i0.7289

Westergren, A., Torfadóttir, O., & Hagell, P. (2014). Inter- and intra-rater reliability of Minimal Eating Observation and Nutrition Form–version II (MEONF-II) nurse assessments among hospital inpatients. *BMC Nursing, 13*(18). doi:10.1186/1472-6955-13-18

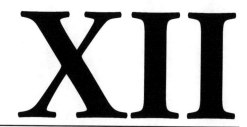

XII

Memory Assessment

Bortnick, K.
Occupational Therapy Assessments for Older Adults: 100 Instruments for
Measuring Occupational Performance (pp. 175-181).
© 2017 Taylor & Francis Group.

Chapter 61: Rivermead Behavioural Memory Test (RBMT)

Description

The Rivermead Behavioural Memory Test (RBMT) outcome measures are standardized assessments of memory designed to quantify problems associated with episodic and prospective memory and orientation difficulties, as well to monitor change following therapeutic interventions (Quemada et al., 2003). The RBMT was originally composed of 12 subtests that represent typical everyday activities, such as remembering an appointment, a name, or a short route as well as picture or face recognition. During assessment the client receives a stimuli and must recall that stimuli or perform certain activities based on recall when asked by the examiner. The original RBMT uses a dichotomous scoring system in which the person either receives a pass or fail, thus more items passed indicates better memory performance. Although the RBMT has shown to be ecologically valid at detecting impairment, especially in low-functioning individuals, the simplified pass/fail scoring system is considered less sensitive to a spectrum of possible scores, which lead to the development of the RBMT-E (extended version) as well as the RBMT second and third editions, whose scoring is more perceptive of the subtler decrements of memory performance (Wills, Clare, Shiel, & Wilson, 2000). The latest version, RBMT-3 is a 10 item restructured edition that includes updated stimuli from the original, improved data and norms, as well as a new novel task subtest, which is a puzzle that has to be solved in a fixed order. It comprises six domains relative to verbal and nonverbal episodic memory, spatial memory, aspects of prospective memory, and procedural memory (Wester, Leenders, Egger, & Kessels, 2013; Wester, van Herten, Egger, & Kessels, et al. 2013). Administration time is less than 30 minutes and in addition to the raw scores on subtests, a Global Memory Index (GMI) can be computed for overall performance (Wester, van Herten, et al., 2013).

Psychometrics

Original research by Quemada et al. (2003) found test-retest reliability of the original RBMT to be high at r = 0.96. Reliability was also good for the four parallel forms (the assessment when purchased comes with four separate but similar types) with a range of r = 0.65 to 0.85. With respect to discriminant ability, when comparing mild cognitive impairment and mild neurocognitive disorders of the Alzheimer's type, it was determined that the profile score correctly classified 90.9% of subjects, while the screening score of the RBMT alone was able to correctly classify 81.8% of subjects (Adachi et al., 2013). Using the revised RBMT-3 in a comparison of healthy controls of those with alcoholism and Korsakoff's syndrome (KS), which is a type of alcohol related cognitive impairment, showed through ROC analysis that the RBMT-3 GMI (total score GMI) was able to distinguish KS from those with alcoholism at AUC = 0.85 (at the 95% confidence interval [CI]), where AUC is considered the area under the curve (Wester, van Herten, et al., 2013). While at a cutoff score of < 67.5 the RBMT-3 had a sensitivity of 0.80 and a specificity of 0.69 in differentiating the 2 types of alcohol syndromes (Wester, van Herten, et al. 2013). The same study determined that the GMI score could also distinguish those with alcoholism from healthy controls as well at AUC = 0.83 (at the 95% CI) and a GMI cutoff score of 87.5 for this group had a sensitivity of 0.80 and a specificity of 0.62 (Wester, van Herten, et al. 2013). A similar study of 25 subjects with alcohol-related memory impairment and 25 healthy controls found that RBMT-3 scores resulted in less ceiling and floor effects in both groups when compared to the original RBMT (Wester, Leenders, et al. 2013).

Table 61-1		
Comparison Ceiling Effects Shown in Percentages		
	RBMT	RBMT-3
Sub-Test	Total Percent	Total Percent
Names	46%	26%
Belonging	66%	56%
Appointment	54%	32%
Pictures	68%	54%
Faces	76%	18%
Route (immediate)	68%	46%
Orientation	64%	26%

Adapted from Wester, A. J., Leenders, P., Egger, J. M., & Kessels, R. C. (2013). Ceiling and floor effects on the Rivermead Behavioural Memory Test in patients with alcohol-related memory disorders and healthy participants. *International Journal of Psychiatry in Clinical Practice, 17*(4), 286-291.

Advantages

The RBMT batteries are relatively easy to administer and each has a fair amount of research in support of their use in clinical practice. The several versions are available from Pearson Clinical where each has established norms and scoring algorithms clearly defined in their respective manual. Although, the original RBMT, when compared to the other versions, has shown to have both floor and ceiling effects this suggests that it may be a more suitable measure for those with more severe memory impairment.

Disadvantages

The RBMT measures have been criticized by some for being atheoretical (i.e., developed on the basis of clinical experience with memory and not on any particular theory). Others have noted sensitivity and specificity issues at high- and low-end memory functioning (Pereira, 2007).

Administration

All forms of the measure use a standardized format where detailed instructions as well as score interpretations are outlined in the examiner's manual. Example RBMT-3 items include (1) two possessions belonging to the examinee are borrowed and hidden, and the subject is required to remember where the items have been hidden at a later point; (2) the subject is shown two photographic portraits and asked to remember the first and second names of both people in the photographs at a later point; and (3) the subject is shown a set of faces and then is asked to recognize them from a further set of faces at a later time (Wilson, 2011). A person receives a subtest score based on their ability to complete the task correctly. These scores are then converted to scaled scores where percentile ranks are provided in the manual that contains stratified data across the lifespan from 16 to 89 years of age (Wilson, 2011). In addition to scaled scores, a GMI score is calculated by summing the scaled scores and then converting its sum using the appropriate conversion table provided in the manual, which also provides CIs and percentile ranks (Wilson, 2011). The GMI, which represents overall memory performance, has a standardized mean of 100 with a standard deviation of 15 (Wilson, 2011).

Permissions

The RBMT battery of assessments can be accessed through the Pearson Clinical Psychology website where the RBMT-3, in particular, can be purchased for $70. Authorization to use in research or publication can be obtained by Pearson Clinical as well. More information can be found in the following original journal article:

Wilson, B., Cockburn, J., Baddeley, A., & Hiorns, R. (1989). The development and validation of a test battery for detecting and monitoring everyday memory problems. *Journal of Clinical and Experimental Neuropsychology.* 11(6), 855-70.

Summary

POPULATION	Suspected memory impairment; general
TYPE OF MEASURE	Activity-based rating scale
WHAT IT ASSESSES	Working memory
TIME	<30 minutes
COST	$70

Contact

Pearson Education, Inc.

Attn: Inbound Sales and Customer Support

P.O. Box 599700

San Antonio, TX 78259

Phone: (800) 627-7271

Email: clinicalcustomersupport@pearson.com

Web: www.pearsonclinical.com/psychology/products/100000644/rivermead-behavioural-memory-test-third-edition-rbmt-3.html

Chapter 62: Wechsler Memory Scale—Fourth Edition (WMS-IV)

Description

The Wechsler Memory Scale—Fourth Edition (WMS-IV), first introduced by Wechsler (1945), is a standardized measure of visual, auditory, and working memory in adults ages 16 to 69 years old and older adults ages 65 to 90 years old, and is designed to assess memory deficits in a variety of patient populations, such as those with neurological and psychiatric disorders (Chittooran, 2012). Theoretical underpinnings of the battery include visual memory encompassing the Designs II and Visual Reproduction II subtests, visual working memory covering the Symbol Span and Spatial Addition subtests, and auditory memory, which includes Logical Memory II and Verbal Paired Associates II subtests, as well as a two-factor model consisting of visual (Designs II, Visual Reproduction II, Spatial Addition, and Symbol Span subtests) and auditory (Logical Memory II and Verbal Paired Associates II subtests) (Hoelzle, Nelson, & Smith, 2011). The Adult Battery includes six primary subtests and an optional Brief Cognitive Status Exam, whereas the Older Adult Battery only includes four primary subtests as well as the optional Brief Cognitive Status Exam. The WMS-IV could be considered a complex assessment where each individual subtest can take up to 30 minutes to complete with total administration times ranging from 130 to 190 minutes. Although time consuming, its results can generate unique insights into client ability (Chittooran, 2012). The WMS-IV generates 5 individual index scores, 12 primary subtest scores, 9 secondary subtest scores, and 13 contrast scores where raw scores as well as age-adjusted scaled scores can be evaluated for use as predictor variables in primary logistic regressions (Miller, 2010).

Psychometrics

Data from normative samples across several age groups for Spatial Addition (n = 900) and Symbol Span (n=1400) subtests established robust internal consistency where Spatial Addition scores ranged from $\alpha = 0.89$ to 0.93 and Symbol Span ranged from 0.76 to 0.92 (Holdnack & Drozdick, n.d). Test-retest reliabilities were r = 0.77 for Spatial Addition and 0.72 for Symbol Span, whereas concurrent validity found that Spatial Addition and Symbol Span correlated at 0.58 and 0.52 with WMS-III Spatial Span, respectively suggesting that the newer fourth edition is indeed different (Holdnack & Drozdick n.d). Data from clinical samples also collected as part of standardization of the WMS-IV included traumatic brain injury (n = 30), right temporal lobectomy (n = 15), math disorder (n = 22), schizophrenia (n = 55), and autism (n = 22); obtained measures of internal consistency for the subtests of Immediate Total at $\alpha = 0.83$ to 0.90), Immediate Content (0.66 to 0.88), Immediate Spatial (0.70 to 83), Delayed Total (0.80 to 0.90), Delayed Content (0.70 to 0.84), and Delayed Spatial (0.67 to 0.82); whereas test-retest reliabilities were Immediate Total (r = 0.73), Immediate Content (0.64), Immediate Spatial (0.50), Delayed Total (0.72), Delayed Content (0.64), and Delayed Spatial (.50) (Holdnack & Drozdick, n.d). The study also found that the Designs Total Immediate section correlated at 0.38 with the Immediate Memory section of the Repeatable Battery for the Assessment of Neuropsychological Status (RBANS) and Designs Delayed correlated at (0.44) with RBANS Delayed Memory (Holdnack & Drozdick, n.d). Finally, a factor analysis by Hoelzle et al. (2011) found that a robust two-dimensional WMS–IV structure was supported across age-based normative samples that emphasized moderately correlated dimensions of (a) auditory learning/memory and (b) visual attention/memory. The auditory learning/memory dimension reflected Logical Memory and Verbal Paired Associates subtests, whereas the Designs subtests were primarily reflected on visual attention/memory dimensions.

Advantages

There is a significant amount of research in support of previous editions on which the WSM-IV is based. The battery is available from Pearson Clinical, where further information regarding the most recent and previous versions can be found. Finally, established norms for the WMS-IV are based on large clinical samples.

Disadvantages

The amount of direct evidence pertaining to the latest WMS-IV is limited. It is also a complex assessment to administer and score and training may be required. The basic kit is roughly $800, making it rather expensive to use in private practice, and as administration time can be long as well, in certain settings that demand the delivery of expedient occupational therapy services, the WMS-IV may not be practical.

Administration

The examination manual includes complete standardized instructions as well as scoring procedures where during assessment, the quality of responses and the patterns of success and failures, along with the individual scores are considered during the evaluation process (Sattler & Ryan, 2009).

Permissions

The WMS-IV can be accessed through the Pearson Clinical Psychology website where a paper-based version can be purchased for $779. Web-based administration, scoring and the generation of reports are also available. Authorization to use in research or publication can be obtained by contacting Pearson or where it has been published. More information can be found in the following article:

Carlozzi, N. E., Grech, J., & Tulsky, D. S. (2013). Memory functioning in individuals with traumatic brain injury: An examination of the Wechsler Memory Scale–Fourth Edition (WMS–IV). *Journal of Clinical and Experimental Neuropsychology, 35*(9), 906-914.

Summary

POPULATION	Suspected memory impairment; general
TYPE OF MEASURE	Activity-based rating scale
WHAT IT ASSESSES	Working memory
TIME	130 to 190 minutes
COST	$779

Contact

Pearson Education, Inc.

Attn: Inbound Sales and Customer Support

P.O. Box 599700

San Antonio, TX 78259

Phone: (800) 627-7271

Email: clinicalcustomersupport@pearson.com

Web: www.pearsonclinical.com/psychology.html

REFERENCES

Adachi, H., Shinagawa, S., Komori, K., Toyota, Y., Takaaki Mori, T.,… Ikeda, M. (2013). Comparison of the utility of everyday memory test and the Alzheimer's Disease Assessment Scale-Cognitive part for evaluation of mild cognitive impairment and very mild Alzheimer's disease. *Psychiatry and Clinical Neurosciences, 67*, 148–153.

Chittooran, M. (2010). Wechsler Memory Scale—Fourth Edition. In P. M. Roth, P. K. Isquith, & G. A. Gioia. (Eds.). *Mental measurements yearbook* (18th ed.). Lincoln, NE: Buros Institute of Mental Measurements.

Hoelzle, J. B., Nelson, N. W., & Smith, C. A. (2011). Comparison of Wechsler Memory Scale—Fourth Edition (WMS–IV) and Third Edition (WMS–III) dimensional structures: Improved ability to evaluate auditory and visual constructs. *Journal of Clinical and Experimental Neuropsychology, 33*(3), 283-291.

Holdnack, J., & Drozdick, L. (n.d). Clinical and Psychometric Properties of the new WMS-IV Design Memory Subtest. Pearson Clinical. Retrieved from http://images.pearsonclinical.com/images/products/wms-iv/WMS-IV_Ins_Posters.pdf

Miller, J. (2010). *Assessment of memory function and effort using the Wechsler Memory Scale—4th Edition.* Wayne State University Dissertations. Paper 201: DigitalCommons@WayneState

Pereira, A. (2007). Assessment of memory in rehabilitation counseling. *Journal of Rehabilitation, 73*(2), 15-25.

Quemada, J., Munoz Cespedes, J., Ezkerra, J., Ballesteros, J., Ibarra, N., & Urruticoechea, I. (2003). Outcome of memory rehabilitation in traumatic brain injury assessed by neuropsychological tests and questionnaires. *Journal of Head Trauma Rehabilitation, 18*(6), 532-540.

Sattler, J., & Ryan, J. (2009). *Assessment with the WAIS-IV.* La Mesa, CA: Jerome M. Sattler Publisher, Inc.

Wester, A. J., Leenders, P., Egger, J. M., & Kessels, R. C. (2013). Ceiling and floor effects on the Rivermead Behavioural Memory Test in patients with alcohol-related memory disorders and healthy participants. *International Journal of Psychiatry in Clinical Practice, 17*(4), 286-291.

Wester, A. J., van Herten, J. C., Egger, J. I., & Kessels, R. P. (2013). Applicability of the Rivermead Behavioural Memory Test—Third Edition (RBMT-3) in Korsakoff's syndrome and chronic alcoholics. *Neuropsychiatric Disease and Treatment, 9*, 875–881.

Wills, P., Clare, L., Shiel, A., & Wilson, B. (2000). Assessing subtle memory impairments in the everyday memory performance of brain injured people: Exploring the potential of the Extended Rivermead Behavioural Memory Test. *Brain Injury, 14*(8), 693-704.

Wilson, B. (2011). *Rivermead Behavioural Memory Test—Third Edition (RBMT-3).* Retrieved from http://images.pearsonclinical.com/images/assets/RBMT-3/RBMT3MrktCollateral.pdf

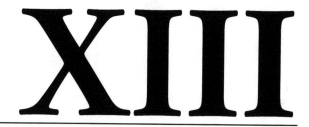

Mental Health Assessment

CHAPTER 63: BECK ANXIETY INVENTORY (BAI)

Description

The Beck Anxiety Inventory (BAI), by Beck, Epstein, Brown, and Steer (1988), is a 21-item self-report/interview questionnaire designed to quantify the symptoms of anxiety a person may be experiencing over the past week and has proved to be a valid indicator of conditions associated with anxiety across a number of patient populations. The theoretical basis of the measure is reflective of a somatic factor composed of 14 physical symptoms, such as numbness, feeling hot, and having difficulty breathing, and a subjective factor composed of 7 psychological symptoms, such as being unable to relax or being nervous. The BAI was originally developed out of a need to consolidate other anxiety inventories for use in psychiatric populations and to have a scale that could reliably discriminate anxiety from depression as well as to differentiate the various types of anxiety diagnostic groups, like those with panic or generalized anxiety disorder (Beck et al., 1988; Leentjens et al., 2008; Steer, 1993). Each of the BAI's 21 items are scored along a 4-point Likert scale with answer choices ranging from 0 to 3. Total scores range from 0 to 63 with higher scores suggestive of more anxiety. The BAI can be completed in less than 10 minutes.

Psychometrics

A study of 75 older adults diagnosed with generalized anxiety disorder (GAD) found internal consistency to be $\alpha = 0.90$, while for the normal control group it was 0.81 (Loebach-Wetherell & Gatz, 2005). Further results of the study determined that 2 items, fearing the worst and nervousness, were able to correctly distinguish 86.5% of patients with GAD and 93.8% of normal controls (Loebach-Wetherell & Gatz, 2005). The BAI was also found to have good internal consistency at $\alpha = 0.91$ in an outpatient population (n=137, median age 41 years old) (Enns, Cox, Parker, & Guertin, 1998). The same study determined that a four-factor model proposed by Steer (1993) was best able to explain results when compared with other models and encompassed the subjective, neurophysiological, autonomic, and panic; while the mean BAI score of the study was 24.0 (SD = 12.7) (Enns et al., 1998). A study by Steer (2009) determined that the mean BAI total score was 21.42 (SD = 13.06) for an outpatient sample of 525 adults (M = 41, SD = 15) indicating that the sample was moderately anxious. An examination of 117 community-dwelling older adults, mean age 75 years, found that the correlation between the Geriatric Anxiety Scale and the BAI was 0.61 while the correlation between the BAI and the Geriatric Anxiety Inventory was only 0.36 (Yochim, Mueller, June, & Segal, 2011). A sample of 281 older adults who were either community-dwelling (82.6%) or living in a residential care facility (17.4%) determined the mean score to be 6.5 (SD = 7.2), indicating a minimal amount of anxiety; however, there was a trend for older subjects to score higher as well as females and those living in residential facilities vs those in the community.

Advantages

The BAI is a simple assessment both to administer and score and has a significant amount of research in support of its use in clinical practice. It is also a widely accepted measure of anxiety that has been translated into numerous languages signifying its cross-cultural relevance. Its use can also foster a common language throughout the health professions because it is considered by many to be a gold standard of its respective measurement properties.

Disadvantages

A study by Morin et al. (1999), comprising subjects > 75 years old, found that results were not easily explained using either the common two-factor model of cognitive or somatic or the four-factor model already discussed as a more complex six-factor solution, in which multiple subjective, motoric, and physiological dimensions of anxiety emerged in this sample. This suggests that clinicians and researchers need to be careful when interpreting scores of the BAI, which is not designed specifically for use with the elderly (the BAI is validated for persons 17 to 80 years old) because it contains several somatic items and it is known that somatic symptoms typically increase with age often reflecting underlying medical illnesses. The authors went on to suggest that it may be necessary to consider a differential weight system when computing a severity index of anxiety symptomatology for older adults.

Administration

During assessment the person reads a list of 21 common symptoms of anxiety and is asked to consider each and indicate whether he or she has been bothered by any of them during the past week and, if so, how much by numerically choosing the best answer from 4 possible choices (0 to 3). Items are then summed with score interpretation as follows: 0 to 21, very low anxiety; 22 to 35, moderate anxiety; and > 36 is a potential cause for concern.

TABLE 63-1
SCORING CHOICES FOR THE BECK ANXIETY INVENTORY
0. Not at all
1. Mildly— but it didn't bother me much
2. Moderately— it wasn't pleasant at times
3. Severely—it bothered me a lot

Adapted from Beck, A. Epstein, N., Brown, G., & Steer, R. (1988). An inventory for measuring clinical anxiety: Psychometric properties. *Journal of Consulting and Clinical Psychology, 56*(6), 895.

TABLE 63-2
EXAMPLE ITEMS OF THE BECK ANXIETY INVENTORY
• Heart pounding/racing
• Feeling of choking
• Hands trembling
• Difficulty breathing
• Indigestion
• Faint/lightheaded

Adapted from Beck, A. Epstein, N., Brown, G., & Steer, R. (1988). An inventory for measuring clinical anxiety: Psychometric properties. *Journal of Consulting and Clinical Psychology, 56*(6), 895.

Permissions

The BAI is available as paper-, software-, or web-based versions that can be purchased from Pearson Inc. Price for the full kit is $131, whereas price for the manual is $83. Progress and interpretive reports can also be procured.

Permission to use for commercial purposes, publication, or research can also be obtained by contacting Pearson. More information can be found in the following journal article:

Beck, A., Epstein, N., Brown, G., & Steer, R. (1988). An inventory for measuring clinical anxiety: Psychometric properties. *Journal of Consulting and Clinical Psychology, 56*(6), 893-897.

Summary

POPULATION	Suspected anxiety; general ages 17 to 80 years old
TYPE OF MEASURE	Self-report or interview questionnaire
WHAT IT ASSESSES	Anxiety level
TIME	< 10 minutes
COST	$131

Contact

Pearson Inc.

Attn: Inbound Sales and Customer Support

P.O. Box 599700

San Antonio, TX 78259

Phone: (800) 627-7271

Email: clinicalcustomersupport@pearson.com

Web: www.pearsonclinical.com/psychology/products/100000251/beck-anxiety-inventory-bai.html

Chapter 64: Beck Depression Inventory-II (BDI-II)

Description

The Beck Depression Inventory-II (BDI–II), by Beck, Steer, Ball, and Ranieri (1996), is a self-report/interview questionnaire designed to quantify the amount of depression a person may be experiencing and its use is considered appropriate for a number of general client populations. Composed of 21 items, it assesses a wide range of depressive symptoms over a 2-week period. The original BDI instrument has gone through multiple revisions and today the BDI-II is arguably a gold standard of depression measurement. First mentioned in the literature in 1961, the most recent revision includes (1) the removal and replacement of 4 items that assess agitation, worthlessness, concentration difficulty, and loss of energy; (2) the time frame for responses was lengthened from 1 to 2 weeks; and (3) 2 items were changed to assess changes in appetite and sleep (Hall et al., 2013). Each item of the BDI-II is rated along a 4-point Likert scale from 0 to 3 where the descriptors for each item vary and include such answers as self-dislike, which is scored as (0) I feel the same about myself as ever, (1) I have lost confidence in myself, (2) I am disappointed in myself, and (3) I dislike myself. Items are summed to produce a total score with higher scores representing more depressive symptoms. Administration time can be less than 10 minutes.

Psychometrics

Beck et al. (1996) provided evidence that the BDI-II possesses adequate reliability and validity for clinical purposes where they found that for 26 subject in an outpatient setting the 1-week test-retest reliability was high (r = 0.93). With respect to its convergent and discriminant validities, they also reported that the BDI-II was more positively correlated with the revised Hamilton Psychiatric Rating Scale for Depression (0.71) than it was with the revised Hamilton Rating Scale for Anxiety (0.47). Measurement of depression among bariatric subjects established that total BDI-II scores demonstrated excellent internal consistency at α = 0.90, whereas factor analysis produced 3 items that explained a large percent of the variance: affective (0.72), cognitive (0.82), and somatic (0.80) (Hall et al., 2013). Osman et al. (1997) found that reliability estimates for the total BDI-II score resulted in a coefficient of r = 0.90, similar to that reported in the manual, whereas indices of a factor analysis produced 3 items that explained variance: negative attitude (0.84), performance difficulty (0.77), and somatic elements (0.68). An analysis of healthy college students showed that the mean score of women was 11.8, (SD = 8.65), which was significantly higher than men's scores of 9.41 (SD = 6.44) (Osman et al., 1997). A study by Steer, Rissmillera, and Beck (2000) concurred with those results in which the mean BDI-II total scores of 80 geriatric women and 50 men were 25.42 (SD = 12.68) and 23.18 (SD = 12.86), respectively.

Advantages

There is a significant amount of evidenced-based research in support of the BDI in it various forms for use in clinical practice and no special training or certifications are needed. Web-based and local software administration, scoring, and reporting are available through Pearson Clinical where the assessment can be purchased.

Disadvantages

Factor analysis of the BDI–II has shown that scores typically break down into two or three latent symptom sets such as the somatic or cognitive, raising questions about its utility and meaningfulness (Quilty, Zhang, & Bagby, 2010). The issue is highlighted in a normative sample (n = 500) with various psychiatric disorders where scores were found to reflect two positively correlated dimensions: (1) a non-cognitive (somatic-affective) factor represented by somatic symptoms, such as loss of energy and affective symptoms, such as irritability and (2) cognitive factors composed of psychological symptoms, such as self-dislike and worthlessness (Steer et al., 2000).

Administration

The BDI-II examiner's manual includes detailed instructions as well as standardized norms across a wide range of age groups. The recommended cutoff for minimal depression is 13, a score of 14 to 19 indicates mild depression, 20 to 28 indicates moderate depression, and 29 to 63 indicates serious depression (Skule et al., 2014). During assessment the subject is asked to consider each question and how it relates to his or her own personal experience over the preceding 2 weeks.

TABLE 64-1
EXAMPLE ITEMS OF THE BECK DEPRESSION INVENTORY-II
• Sadness
• Pessimism
• Past failure
• Loss of pleasure
• Guilty feelings
• Punishment feelings
• Self-dislike
• Self-criticalness
• Suicidal thoughts
• Crying
• Agitation
Adapted from Whisman, M., Perez, J. E., & Ramel, W. (2000). Factor structure of the Beck Depression Inventory-Second Edition (BDI-II) in a student sample. *Journal of Clinical Psychology, 56*(4), 548.

Permissions

The BDI can be accessed through the Pearson Clinical Psychology website where it can be purchased. A number of options are available such as pen-and-paper and software-or web-based scoring. Prices vary from $56 to $81. Authorization to use in research or publication can be obtained by contacting the creators of the measure, its publishers, or Pearson directly. More information can be found in the following journal articles:

Beck, A. (1996). Comparison of Beck Depression–IA and –II in psychiatric patients. *Journal of Personality Assessment, 67*(3), 588-597.

Beck. A., Steer, R. A., & Brown, G. (1996). *Manual for the Beck Depression Inventory-II.* San Antonio, TX: Psychological Corporation.

Summary

POPULATION	Suspected depression; general; ages 13 to 80 years old
TYPE OF MEASURE	Self-report or interview questionnaire
WHAT IT ASSESSES	Level of depression
TIME	< 10 minutes
COST	$56 to $81

Contact

Pearson Education, Inc.

Attn: Inbound Sales and Customer Support

P.O. Box 599700

San Antonio, TX 78259

Phone: (800) 627-7271

Email: clinicalcustomersupport@pearson.com

Web: www.pearsonclinical.com/psychology/
    products/100000159/beck-depression-inventoryii-
    bdi-ii.html

Aaron T. Beck, MD

Beck Institute for Cognitive Behavior Therapy

Bala Cynwynd, Pennsylvania

Web: www.beckinstitute.org/aaron-beck/

CHAPTER 65: CORNELL SCALE FOR DEPRESSION IN DEMENTIA (CSDD)

Description

The Cornell Scale for Depression in Dementia (CSDD) is a 19-item, clinician-administered scale specifically developed to assess signs and symptoms of major depression in persons with neurocognitive disorders (NCD) of the Alzheimer's and related types of cognitive impairment (Alexopoulos, 2002). The CSDD uses a comprehensive interview approach that derives information from both the patient and an informant, thus information is elicited through two semi-structured interviews (Alexopoulos, 2002). The interviews focus on depressive symptoms during the previous week where many of the items can be filled in through direct observation of the patient (Alexopoulos, 2002). The signs and symptoms of depression are measured by the CSDD scale and categorized into five general content areas: (1) mood-related signs (anxiety, sadness, lack of reactivity to pleasant events, irritability); (2) behavioral disturbances (agitation, multiple physical complaints, loss of interest); (3) physical signs (loss of appetite, weight loss, lack of energy); (4) cyclic functioning (diurnal variation of mood, difficulty falling asleep, multiple awakenings during sleep, early morning awakenings); and (5) ideational disturbances (suicide, poor self-esteem, pessimism, mood-congruent delusions) (Harwood, Ownby, Barker, & Duara, 1998). The CSDD has 38 items total (19 each for patient and informant) and all items are rated for severity on a scale of 0 to 2 where (0) suggests the symptom is absent, (1) mild or intermittent, and (2) severe. Scores above 10 indicate a probable major depression and scores above 18 indicate a definite major depression, while scores below 6 are typically associated with absence of significant depressive symptoms (Alexopoulos, 2002). The CSDD can be completed in less than 15 minutes.

Psychometrics

Using 2 studies of 103 and 32 subjects the correlation between 2 raters for the total score was r = 0.81 and 0.97, respectively (Lage-Barca, Engedal, & Selbaek, 2010). The same study found that for nursing home patients a cutoff score of 6/7 produced a sensitivity of 0.79 and a specificity of 0.68; a score of 7/8 the sensitivity was 0.76 and specificity was 0.75; and at 8/9 the sensitivity was 0.69 and the specificity was 0.81 (Lage-Barca et al., 2010) A subsequent study of 63 subjects with early onset neurocognitive disorder (NCD) found that at an optimal cutoff score of 5/6 results yielded a sensitivity of 0.83 and a specificity of 0.57 (Leontjevas, van Hooren, & Mulders, 2009). Their research also suggested

that the following 3 of the 19 items were able to discriminate depressed patients from non-depressed patients: (1) sadness, (2) loss of interest, and (3) lack of energy (Leontjevas et al., 2009). The same study also established congruent validity between the Montgomery-Asberg Depression Rating Scale and the CSDD, which was significant at 0.79 (Leontjevas et al., 2009). Snowdon, Rosengren, Daniel, and Suyasa (2011) found that of 223 residents of a nursing home in Australia, 23% scored > 12 which indicated probable depression, 21% were possibly depressed, and 29% were not depressed; however, clinicians also found themselves unable to make CSDD ratings in 14% of cases because of severe dementia and rating proved impossible in another 10%, thus meaningful scores were not available for a substantial proportion of the residents suggesting that its usefulness may be limited to only specific populations, such as those with mild to moderate symptomology. Finally, a factor analysis by Kurlowicz, Evans, Strumpf, and Maislin (2002) concluded that the CSDD has a psychobiological orientation, with a broad spectrum of depressive symptoms in the affective, cognitive, somatic, and behavioral realms and that somatic items comprised 37% (7/19) of items on the test.

Advantages

There is a significant amount of research in support of the CSDD for use in clinical practice and no special training or certifications are needed. The assessment is unique from other interview/self-report scales in that scores are based on information collected from both the subject and informant giving the clinician unique insight into depressed subjects.

Disadvantages

The assessment is specific to those with NCD relative to Alzheimer's and related types and accurate assessment may be difficult for certain sub-populations as noted in the study by Kurlowicz et al. (2002), thus scores may be weighted more heavily toward informant responses in those patient groups.

Administration

The 38 items of the CSDD are delivered according to a standardized format that is done through the use of two structured interviews, with the client and with an informant, where each interview has clearly outlined instructions as well as scoring interpretations contained in the examiner's manual. Items are scored as either 0 = absent, 1 = mild to intermittent, 2 = severe, or A = unable to evaluate. The total score range for both forms is 0 to 38, with higher values representing greater severity of depressive symptoms.

TABLE 65-1
EXAMPLE ITEMS ON THE CORNELL SCALE FOR DEPRESSION IN DEMENTIA
PHYSICAL SIGNS
• Appetite loss
• Weight loss
• Lack of energy
MOOD-RELATED SIGNS
• Anxiety
• Sadness
• Lack of reactivity to pleasant events
BEHAVIORAL DISTURBANCE
• Agitation
• Multiple physical complaints
• Loss of interest
IDEATIONAL DISTURBANCE
• Suicide
• Self-depreciation
• Pessimism
• Mood congruent delusions
Adapted from Alexopoulos, G. (2002). *The Cornell Scale for Depression in Dementia administration & scoring guidelines* (pp. 2-5). New York, New York: Cornell Institute of Geriatric Psychiatry: Cornell University.

Permissions

The CSDD is readily available on the web and if requested it is free to use in clinical practice. To use in research or publication contact the author of the assessment at the information that follows or where it has been published. It is wholly contained in the following journal article:

Alexopoulos, G., Abrams, R., Young, R., & Shamoian, C. (1988). Cornell Scale for Depression in Dementia. *Biological Psychiatry, 23*(3), 271-284.

Summary

POPULATION	Suspected depression; NCD and cognitive impairment specific
TYPE OF MEASURE	Interview questionnaire
WHAT IT ASSESSES	Presence and level of depression
TIME	< 15 minutes
COST	Free

Contact

George S. Alexopoulos, MD

Cornell Institute of Geriatric Psychiatry

Weill Medical College of Cornell University

New York, New York

Web: http://vivo.med.cornell.edu/display/cwid-gsalexop

Access to the instrument: www.caltcm.org/assets/documents/forms/cornell%20scale%20for%20depression%20in%20dementia.pdf

CHAPTER 66: GENERAL HEALTH QUESTIONNAIRE (GHQ-12)

Description

The General Health Questionnaire (GHQ-12) by Goldberg (1976) is a self-administered questionnaire designed to detect persons that are symptomatic or at risk of developing the common, non-psychotic mental health problems associated with depression, anxiety, somatic symptoms, and social dysfunction (Jackson, 2007). Designed for the general population, available versions include the 60-, 30-, 28-, and the 12-item (GHQ-12) versions. The GHQ-12 was introduced in 1988 and is now considered one of the most extensively used outcome measures across a number of health professions (del Pilar Sánchez-López & Dresch, 2008). The GHQ-12 covers several domains associated with a person's psychological well-being and is worded in such a way as to comprise six positive and six negative items concerning the past few weeks of a person's life and includes such items as "Have you recently felt capable of making decisions about things?" while, negative items include "Have you recently felt constantly under strain?" (Hu, Stewart-Brown, Twigg, & Weich, 2007). Positively worded items have responses of "better than usual," "same as usual," "less than usual," and "much less than usual," while responses to negatively worded items are "not at all," "no more than usual," "rather more than usual," and "much more than usual." Scoring is along a 4-point ordinal scale (0 to 3) with higher scores suggestive of more distress. The GHQ-12 can be completed in less than 10 minutes.

Psychometrics

A study of 897 men and 911 women (59% ≥ 50 years old) determined that Cronbach's alpha coefficients (estimates of reliability) were 0.83 for men and 0.85 for women (Doi & Minowa, 2003). Whereas Kihc et al. (1997) determined that the internal consistency of the GHQ-12 was α = 0.76, which compared to results of the GHQ-30 at 0.92 in their study of a stratified sample of 400 cases (15 to 65 years old). Although the GHQ-12 is often regarded as measuring only a single dimension of psychological health, a confirmatory factory analysis using a cohort of 9000 (mean age: 41 years; n = 2077 ≥ 56 years of age), suggested that 2 factors best described as *symptoms of mental disorder* (encompassing negative affect, anxiety, and impaired mental functioning) and *positive mental health* (covering positive mental functioning and positive affect) (Hu et al., 2007). A similar study by Gao et al. (2004) that compared six factor models relative to the measure, found that the one proposed by Graetz (1991) to be the best fit, as strong correlations between the 3 factors of anxiety and depression (4 items),

social dysfunction (6 items), and loss of confidence (2 items) were found (range = 0.83-0.90), suggesting that even if there were 3 different factors, it would be difficult to differentiate them. Examples of other factor models compared in the study were general dysphoria, social, and the cope, stress, and depress model. A study comparing the level of agreement between the GHQ-12 and the Geriatric Depression Scale (GDS-30) using 1172 subjects (≥ 60 years old) found median scores to be 2.7 for the GHQ-12 and 11.7 for the GDS-30 with the prevalence of depressive symptoms based on the GHQ-12 at 40% and 33% using cutoff points of 2/3 and 3/4, whereas 50% and 38% were classified as depressed at cutoff points of 10/11 and 13/14 according to the GDS-30 (Costa, Barreto, Uchoa, & Lima-Costa, 2003). Agreement between the scales ranged from 0.50 to 0.60 with depressive symptoms significantly higher for woman and those individuals ≥ 75 years of age (Costa et al., 2003). A study by del Pilar Sánchez-López and Dresch (2008) of 1001 subjects (50% between 45 and 65 years old) generally concurred with those findings where they too established statistically significant differences between women and men's scores at 7.34 and 9.30, respectively. The study by Hu et al. (2007) discussed previously, however, found that positive mental health was most strongly associated with younger age, being in work, being single, not having any financial strain, and having no or few physical health problems.

Advantages

There is a significant amount of research in support of the GHQ-12 as well as its other versions for use in clinical practice and it is arguably a gold standard measure of the symptoms of psychological distress in the general population. Several alternative scoring methodologies have also been proposed expanding its usefulness, and since its introduction in 1976, the GHQ has been translated into 38 different languages, highlighting its relevance as a cross-cultural assessment (Jackson, 2007). Finally, in certain populations the 28-item version may be considered as it is a more multidimensional outcome measure comprising 4 distinct subscales (somatic symptoms, anxiety and insomnia, social dysfunction, and severe depression) of 7 items each (Gao et al., 2004).

Disadvantages

Some have argued that aspects of the negative and positive wording used by the measure has a latent effect on answer selection and thus on scoring. Also, the GHQ-12 is designed to only give a general indication of psychological distress and should not be considered a replacement for more thorough and accepted psychological assessments.

Administration

The GHQ-12 measure has standardized instructions as well as scoring interpretations for the clinician to follow and is administered as a self-report in which the subject is asked to consider 12 questions and how they relate to his or her personal life over the past few weeks. Total scores range from 0 to 36 with a score of 11 or 12 considered typical, scores >15 suggesting evidence of distress, and scores >20 are considered severe problems with psychological distress.

TABLE 66-1
EXAMPLE ITEMS OF THE GENERAL HEALTH QUESTIONNAIRE-12
• Have you recently lost much sleep over worry?
• Have you recently felt you couldn't overcome your difficulties?
• Have you recently been losing confidence in yourself?
Adapted from Delivering for Mental Health. (2007). Mental Health and Substance Misuse: Consultation Draft The Scottish Government. Retrieved from www.gov.scot/Publications/2007/06/29120532/26

Permissions

The GHQ-12 can be purchased from the GL Education Group at the information that follows for a cost of $150 (pack of 100). To use in research or publication contact the GL group or where published. More information can be found in the following articles:

Goldberg, D. & Hillier, V. F. (1979). A scaled version of the General Health Questionnaire. *Psychological Medicine, 9*, 139-145.

Goldberg, D., & Williams, P. (1988). *A user's guide to the General Health Questionnaire.* Windsor, United Kingdom: NFER-Nelson.

Summary

POPULATION	General; suspected psychological distress
TYPE OF MEASURE	Self-report questionnaire
WHAT IT ASSESSES	Non-psychotic symptomology
TIME	< 10 minutes
COST	$150

Contact

Sir David Goldberg

Professor Emeritus

Institute of Psychiatry

King's College London

London, United Kingdom

The GL Education Group

Customer Services

Freepost London 16517 Swindon SN2 8BR

Phone: +44 (0) 330-123-5375

Email: info@gl-assessment.co.uk

Web: www.gl-assessment.co.uk/products/general-health-questionnaire-0

CHAPTER 67: GERIATRIC DEPRESSION SCALE—SHORT FORM (sfGDS)

Description

The Geriatric Depression Scale—Short Form (sfGDS) by Yesavage et al. (1986) is a 15-item rating scale developed to screen for depression in older populations but may also be appropriate for people who have mild cognitive impairment because it is known that significant depressive symptoms are often observed in 30% to 50% of that population (Debruyne et al., 2009). The sfGDS is a self-report/interview questionnaire based on validation studies of the original 30-item assessment where 15 items were selected that had the highest correlation with depressive symptoms for the revised short form (Lesher & Berryhill, 1994). Sample test items include the following:

- Are you afraid that something bad is going to happen to you?
- Do you feel happy most of the time?
- Do you often feel helpless?
- Do you prefer to stay at home rather than going out and doing new things?
- Do you feel you have more problems with memory than most?

Items are rated as either yes or no, and depending on the question, either response may indicate depressive symptoms. The sfGDS can be completed in less than 10 minutes with higher scores indicative of more depressive symptoms.

Psychometrics

The original GDS and the GDS-15 were found to be highly correlated at $r = 0.84$ (Sheikh & Yesavage, 1986). Results of a study by Lesher & Berryhill (1994) concurred with those results where they too established correlates between the 2 outcome measures at $r = 0.89$. A study of functionally impaired yet cognitively intact community-dwelling persons aged 65 years and older ($n = 960$) found that the internal consistency reliability for the total scale was $\alpha = 0.75$ (Friedman, Heisel, & Delavan, 2005). A study by Incalzi, Pedone, and Carbonin (2003) found that 3 factors were able to explain 47.7% of variance of the sfGDS comprising the following dimensions: positive attitude toward life, distressing thoughts/negative judgment about one's own condition, and inactivity/reduced self-esteem. Research by Lyness et al. (1997) showed that the GDS-15 had 92% sensitivity and 81% specificity when using a cutoff score of 5. Lesher and Berryhill (1994) argued to the contrary and suggested that one area of weakness of the sfGDS was its low specificity rates, where they found that at a score ≥ 5 the sensitivity was 0.91 and specificity was 0.54; however, at a score of ≥ 6 sensitivity was 0.83 and specificity was 0.69, at ≥ 7 sensitivity was 0.83 and specificity was 0.73, and at ≥ 10 sensitivity was 0.72 with a specificity of 0.92. Finally, a study of 198 elderly subjects who completed the sfGDS (34%) scored above a cutoff score of 4/5 for probable depression (D'ath, Katona, Mullan, Evans, & Katona, 1994).

Advantages

The sfGDS is a relatively quick measure to determine if further services are needed. It is easy to administer and can be used by both client and caregiver to determine levels of depression. No training or certifications are needed and there is a significant amount of research pertaining to both the original and short versions. The assessment is located in the public domain, thus no special permissions are required for its use in research or publication. Finally, D'ath et al. (1994) found the questionnaire to be acceptable to older adults as only 3.6% found it difficult or stressful to complete ($n = 198$).

Disadvantages

One study has noted inconsistencies associated with the scale's sensitivity and specificity and another found that the question, "Do you feel that your life is empty?" was able to identify 84% of cases. Continuing with that information, further research found that ad hoc generated 10-, 4-, and 1-item versions displayed significant agreement with the sfGDS at 0.95, 0.91, and 0.79, respectively suggesting possible problems with uni-dimensionality (D'ath et al. 1994).

Administration

The sfGDS is completed as either self-report or interview and consists of 15 items scored yes or no, where specific answers are indicative of depressive symptoms as follows: for *no* answers they are items 1, 5, 7, 11, and 13 and for *yes* answers they are items 2 to 4, 6, 8 to 10, 12, 14, and 15. A score > 5 points is suggestive of depression and should warrant a more thorough investigation. A score ≥ 10 points is indicative of depression.

TABLE 67-1

ITEMS ON THE GERIATRIC DEPRESSION SCALE—SHORT FORM

- Are you basically satisfied with your life?
- Have you dropped many of your activities and interests?
- Do you feel that your life is empty?
- Do you often get bored?
- Are you in good spirits most of the time?
- Are you afraid that something bad is going to happen to you?
- Do you feel happy most of the time?
- Do you often feel helpless?
- Do you prefer to stay at home rather than going out and doing new things?
- Do you feel you have more problems with memory than most?
- Do you think it is wonderful to be alive now?
- Do you feel pretty worthless the way you are now?
- Do you feel full of energy?
- Do you feel that your situation is hopeless?
- Do you think that most people are better off than you are?

Adapted from Crawford, G. B., & Robinson, J. A. (2008). The Geriatric Depression Scale in palliative care. *Palliative & Supportive Care, 6*(3), 216.

Permissions

The sfGDS is located in the public domain and is free to use in clinical practice, research, and publication, in part because of federal funding at the time of its creation. Thus no special permissions are required and it can be downloaded at the website that follows. More information can be found in the following journal article:

Sheikh, J., & Yesavage, J. (1986). Geriatric Depression Scale (GDS): Recent evidence and development of a shorter version. *Clinical Gerontologist, 5*(1-2), 165-173.

Summary

POPULATION	Suspected depression; general
TYPE OF MEASURE	Self-report or interview questionnaire
WHAT IT ASSESSES	Presence and level of depression
TIME	< 10 minutes
COST	Free

Contact

Jerome Yesavage, MD

Stanford University School of Medicine

Stanford, California

Web: www.stanford.edu/~yesavage

Web: www.stanford.edu/~yesavage/GDS.html

REFERENCES

Alexopoulos, G. (2002). *The Cornell Scale for Depression in Dementia Administration & Scoring Guidelines.* New York, New York: Cornell Institute of Geriatric Psychiatry: Cornell University.

Beck, A., Epstein, N., Brown, G., & Steer, R. (1988). An inventory for measuring clinical anxiety: Psychometric properties. *Journal of Consulting and Clinical Psychology, 56*(6), 893-897.

Beck, A., Steer, R., Ball, R., & Ranieri, W. (1996). Comparison of Beck Depression Inventories–IA and –II in psychiatric patients. *Journal of Personality Assessment, 67*(3) 588-597.

Costa, E., Barreto, S., Uchoa, E., & Lima-Costa, M. (2003). Agreement between the Geriatric Depression Scale and the General Health Questionnaire in a population-based elderly cohort: The Bambuí Health & Ageing Study (BHAS). *Clinical Gerontologist, 26*(3/4), 69-82.

Crawford, G. B., & Robinson, J. A. (2008). The Geriatric Depression Scale in palliative care. *Palliative & Supportive Care, 6*(3), 213-223.

D'ath, P., Katona, P., Mullan, E., Evans, S., & Katona, C. (1994). Screening, detection and management of depression in elderly primary care attenders. I: The acceptability and performance of the 15 item Geriatric Depression Scale (GDS15) and the development of short versions. *Family Practice, 11*(3), 260-266.

Debruyne, H., Van Buggenhout, M., Le Bastard, N., Aries, M., Audenaers, K., De Deyn, P., & Engelborghs, S. (2009). Is the geriatric depression scale a reliable screening tool for depressive symptoms in elderly patients with cognitive impairment? *International Journal of Geriatric Psychiatry, 24*, 556–562.

del Pilar Sánchez-López, M., & Dresch, V. (2008). The 12-Item General Health Questionnaire (GHQ-12): Reliability, external validity and factor structure in the Spanish population. *Psicothema, 20*(4), 839-843.

Doi, Y., & Minowa, M. (2003). Factor structure of the 12-Item General Health Questionnaire in the Japanese general adult population. *Psychiatry and Clinical Neurosciences, 57*, 379–383.

Enns, M., Cox, B., Parker, J., & Guertin, J. (1998). Confirmatory factor analysis of the Beck Anxiety and Depression Inventories in patients with major depression. *Journal of Affective Disorders, 47*, 195–200.

Friedman, B., Heisel, M., & Delavan, R. (2005). Psychometric properties of the 15-item geriatric depression scale in functionally impaired, cognitively intact, community-dwelling elderly primary care patients. *Journal of the American Geriatric Society, 53*(9), 1570-1576.

Gao, F., Luo, N., Thumboo, J., Fones, C., Li, S. C., & Cheung, Y. B. (2004). Does the 12-Item General Health Questionnaire contain multiple factors and do we need them? *Health and Quality of Life Outcomes, 2*(63), 1-7.

Graetz, B. (1991). Multidimensional properties of the general health questionnaire. *Social Psychiatry and Psychiatric Epidemiology, 26*(3), 132-138.

Hall, B., Hood, M., Nackers, L., Azarbad, L., Ivan, I., & Corsica, J. (2013). Confirmatory factor analysis of the Beck Depression Inventory-II. Bariatric surgery candidates. *Psychological Assessment, 25*(1), 294-299.

Harwood, D., Ownby, R., Barker, W., & Duara, R. (1998). The factor structure of the Cornell Scale for Depression in Dementia among probable Alzheimer's disease patients. *American Journal of Geriatric Psychiatry, 6*(3), 212-220.

Hu, Y., Stewart-Brown, S., Twigg, L., & Weich, S. (2007). Can the 12-Item General Health Questionnaire be used to measure positive mental health? *Psychological Medicine, 37*, 1005-1013.

Incalzi, R. A., Pedone, C., & Carbonin, P. (2003). Construct validity of the 15-Item Geriatric Depression Scale in older medical inpatients. *Journal of Geriatric Psychiatry and Neurology, 16*(1), 23-28.

Jackson, C. (2007). The General Health Questionnaire. *Occupational Medicine, 57*, 79.

Kihc, C., Rezaki, M., Rezaki, B., Kaplan, I., Ozgen, G., Sagduyu, A.,... Ozturk, M. O. (1997). General Health Questionnaire (GHQ12 & GHQ28): Psychometric properties and factor structure of the scales in a Turkish primary care sample. *Social Psychiatry and Psychiatric Epidemiology, 32*(6), 327-331.

Kurlowicz, L., Evans, L., Strumpf, N., & Maislin, G. (2002). A psychometric evaluation of the Cornell Scale for Depression in Dementia in a frail nursing home population. *American Journal of Geriatric Psychiatry, 10*(5), 600-608.

Lage-Barca, M., Engedal, K., & Selbaek, G. (2010). A reliability and validity study of the Cornell Scale among elderly inpatients, using various clinical criteria. *Dementia and Geriatric Cognitive Disorders, 29*, 438–447.

Leentjens, A., Dujardin, K., Marsh, L., Martínez-Martín, P., Richard, I., Starkstein, S.,...Goetz, C. (2008). Anxiety rating scales in Parkinson's disease: Critique and recommendations. *Movement Disorders, 23*(14), 2015–2025.

Leontjevas, R., van Hooren, S., & Mulders, A. (2009). The Montgomery-Asberg Depression Rating Scale and the Cornell Scale for Depression in Dementia: A validation study with patients exhibiting early-onset dementia. *American Journal of Geriatric Psychiatry, 17*(1), 56-64.

Lesher, E., & Berryhill, J. (1994). Validation of the Geriatric Depression Scale—Short Form among inpatients. *Journal of Clinical Psychology. 50*(2), 256-260.

Loebach-Wetherell, J., & Gatz, M. (2005). The Beck Anxiety Inventory in older adults with generalized anxiety disorder. *Journal of Psychopathology and Behavioral Assessment, 27*(1), 17-24.

Lyness J., Noel, T., Cox, C., King, D., Cornwell, Y., & Caine, E. (1997). Screening for depression in elderly primary care patients. A comparison of the Center for Epidemiologic Studies-Depression Scale and the Geriatric Depression Scale. *Archives of Internal Medicine, 157*(4), 449-454.

Morin, C., Landreville, P., Colecchi, C., McDonald, K., Stone, J., & Ling, W. (1999). The Beck Anxiety Inventory: Psychometric properties with older adults. *Journal of Clinical Geropsychology, 5*(1), 19-29.

Osman, A., Downs, W., Barrios, F., Kopper, B. A., Gutierrez, P., & Chiros, C. (1997). Factor structure and psychometric characteristics of the Beck Depression Inventory-II. *Journal of Psychopathology and Behavioral Assessment, 19*(4), 359-376.

Quilty, L., Zhang, K., & Bagby, R. (2010). The latent symptom structure of the Beck Depression Inventory-II. *Psychological Assessment, 22*(3), 603–608.

Sheikh, J., & Yesavage, J. (1986). Geriatric Depression Scale (GDS): Recent evidence and development of a shorter version. *Clinical Gerontologist, 5*(1-2), 165-173.

Skule, C., Ulleberg, P., Lending, H. D., Berge, T., Egeland, J., Brennen, T.,...Landro, N. (2014). Depressive symptoms in people with and without alcohol abuse: Factor structure and measurement invariance of the Beck Depression Inventory (BDI-II) across groups. *PLusOne, 9*(2) e88321.

Snowdon, J., Rosengren, D., Daniel, F., & Suyasa, M. (2011). Brief Report Australia's use of the Cornell Scale to screen for depression in nursing homes. *Australasian Journal on Ageing, 30*(1), 33–36

Steer, R. A. (2009). Amount of general factor saturation in the Beck Anxiety Inventory responses of outpatients with anxiety disorders. *Journal of Psychopathology and Behavioral Assessment, 31*(2), 112-118.

Steer, R., Rissmillera, D., & Beck, A. (2000). Use of the Beck Depression Inventory-II with depressed geriatric inpatients. *Behaviour Research and Therapy, 38*, 311-318.

Whisman, M., Perez, J. E., & Ramel, W. (2000). Factor structure of the Beck Depression Inventory-Second Edition (BDI-II) in a student sample. *Journal of Clinical Psychology, 56*(4), 545–551

Yochim, B., Mueller, A., June, A., & Segal, D. (2011). Psychometric properties of the Geriatric Anxiety Scale: Comparison to the Beck Anxiety Inventory and Geriatric Anxiety Inventory. *Clinical Gerontologist, 34*(1), 21-33.

XIV

Motor Function—Global

Bortnick, K.
*Occupational Therapy Assessments for Older Adults: 100 Instruments for
Measuring Occupational Performance* (pp. 197-209).
© 2017 Taylor & Francis Group.

Chapter 68: Assessment of Motor and Process Skills (AMPS)

Description

The Assessment of Motor and Process Skills (AMPS) developed by Fisher (1999), is an outcome measure used to evaluate the quality of motor and process skills necessary for effective engagement in activity of daily living (ADL) tasks (Sellers, Fisher, & Duran, 2001). AMPS is comprised of 16 motor and 20 process ADL skills and is considered to be client centered because it is the client who chooses which tasks are to be completed from a list of over 100 standardized activities (Fioravanti, Bordignon, Pettit, Woodhouse, & Ansley, 2012). During assessment, two or more tasks, that are both familiar and relevant, are chosen through negotiation with the clinician and as the client completes those tasks, the occupational therapy practitioner assesses effort, efficiency, safety, and independence with motor and process skills needed for successful performance (Fioravanti et al., 2012). Chosen activities include but are not limited to meal preparation, home maintenance, and laundry and are conceptualized such that each activity entails the use of certain motor and process skills which may include walks, reaches, bends, and transports or initiates, chooses, and accommodates, all of which are thought to be those observable, goal-directed actions that a person uses to organize logically and adapt his or her behavior over time to complete a specified task (Sellers et al., 2001). During the assessment the clinician examines and grades the unique performance attributes of the selected activity that may also include the client's ability to attend, choose, manipulate, or inquire (Fisher, Liu, Velozo, & Pan, 1992). Each task is then rated on a 4-point scale from severe deficit (1) to competent (4) relative to the motor and process skills needed for the activity. Scoring employs a unique algorithm whose results allow the clinician to identify skill deficits to target for intervention. AMPS software can also be used to generate a faceted Rasch analysis of the person's ordinal scores as well as other types of observations to build an occupational profile or plan therapeutic interventions. The time to complete the assessment is 30 to 40 minutes.

Psychometrics

Marom, Jarus, and Josman (2006) have reported high test-retest reliabilities of $r = 0.91$ and 0.90 among certified raters for the motor and process scales and another study also obtained good to excellent results for inter-rater reliability ($r = 0.74$) and test-retest reliability ($r = 0.91$) among a sample of adults with psychiatric disabilities performing the same chosen task; however, test-retest reliability was much lower (0.70) when subjects performed different tasks (Fisher et al., 1992). An early study of the AMPS reported that global internal consistency applied to older persons to be $\alpha = 0.9$ for the process skill items (Fisher et al., 1992). Kizony and Katz (2002) found that women performed significantly higher on the process scale than men and results of their study showed that gender, visual contextual memory, and visual attention was able to explain 59% of the variance of process scale scores. Using data from 118 persons with a cognitive disorder, Bouwens et al. (2007) found that the Mini Mental State Exam and Global Deterioration Scale scores were able to explain 27% and 44% of the variance of AMPS process scores. The same study found a significant relationship between AMPS process scores and total Cambridge Cognition scores at 0.58.

Advantages

There is a significant amount of research in support of AMPS for use in clinical practice and the measure has been validated among various patient populations as well. Several language variants also exist suggesting cross-cultural relevance of the measure. The AMPS International Center for Innovative OT Solutions maintains a website devoted to the measure where, along with general information, training and certification information can also be found. Also, special software is available from the website that streamlines scoring and gives the clinician the ability to generate various types of detailed scoring reports, and professional analysis, as well as the ability to chart client performance over time.

Disadvantages

Some researchers have noted difficulties with the use of AMPS in practice due to rigid time schedules and workplace routines as the assessment can take up to 40 minutes to complete (Chard, 2006). McCluskey and Cusick (2002) found that the introduction of AMPS into the workplace required managerial and administrative support as well as the introduction and adoption of new skills by occupational therapy departments and concluded that a lack of staffing and high workloads can make the AMPS assessment challenging to implement. Also, use of AMPS necessitates the clinician to be certified which entails attendance of a 5-day training course (in person) at a current cost of $1000. The assessment must then be performed on 10 clients in the practitioner's workplace to become certified; however, once certified the candidate will receive verification of 45 contact hours of participation that can be used for documentation of continuing education credits (Center for Innovative OT Solutions, 2013).

Administration

The clinician begins the process by conducting an occupational interview to obtain information about what daily task performances are of most concern to the individual, as well to understand the circumstances and context in which the client is presently operating. Specific ADL tasks are then identified and prioritized into a subset of approximately five from which the person chooses at least two tasks to perform. The AMPS assessment contains 110 unique standardized tasks along with descriptions, instructions, and specific guidelines for scoring. The manual also provides for flexibility if there is no exact match to the client's chosen tasks as activities can be adapted or new ones generated. Scoring is based on the quality of performance relative to the motor and process skills needed to engage in the agreed upon tasks which are scored along a 4-point ordinal scale where (1) suggests a deficit, (2) ineffective, (3) questionable, and (4) competent. Each motor and process score has unique and particular cutoff points, also outlined in the manual, where total scores are then expressed in digits that range from –3 (less able) to +4 (more able). Scores above a certain point indicate an independent level and scores below suggest the need for assistance (Marom et al., 2006).

TABLE 68-1
EXAMPLE MOTOR AND PROCESS SKILLS OF THE ASSESSMENT OF MOTOR AND PROCESS SKILLS
BODY POSITION (MOTOR)
• Stabilizes
• Aligns
• Positions
SUSTAINING PERFORMANCE (MOTOR)
• Endures
• Paces
ADAPTING PERFORMANCE (PROCESS)
• Notices/responds
• Adjusts
TEMPORAL ORGANIZATION (PROCESS)
• Initiates
• Sequences
• Terminates
Adapted from Fisher, A. G., & Jones, K. B. (2010). *Assessment of Motor and Process Skills. Vol. 1: Development, standardization, and administration manual.* (7th ed., pp. 1-5). Fort Collins, CO: Three Star Press.

Permissions

The AMPS battery and its associated products can be purchased form AMPS International: Center for Innovative OT Solutions where price for the software ranges from $69 to $239, whereas an examiner's manual is $95, certification is $995, and a professional score analysis is $250. To use in research and publication contact the original author of the scale or the copyright holders at the information that follows. More information can be found in the following publications:

Fisher, A. G., & Jones, K. B. (2012). *Assessment of Motor and Process Skills. Vol. 1: Development, standardization, and administration manual* (7th ed.) Fort Collins, CO: Three Star Press.

Fisher, A. G., & Jones, K. B. (2014). *Assessment of Motor and Process Skills. Vol. II: User manual* (8th ed.). Fort Collins, CO: Three Star Press.

Summary

POPULATION	General
TYPE OF MEASURE	Activity-based rating scale
WHAT IT ASSESSES	Quality of motor and process skills during task performance
TIME	30 to 40 minutes
COST	$69 to $239

Contact

Anne Fisher, ScD, OT

Division of Occupational Therapy

Umeå University

Umeå, Sweden

Web: www.ot.chhs.colostate.edu/faculty-staff/anne_fisher.aspx

AMPS International: Center for Innovative OT Solutions

P.O. Box 42

Hampton Falls, NH 03844

Phone: (603) 778-2965

Email: info@innovativeOTsolutions.com

Web: www.innovativeotsolutions.com/content/

CHAPTER 69: CHEDOKE-MCMASTER STROKE ASSESSMENT (CMSA)

Description

The Chedoke-McMaster Stroke Assessment (CMSA) is a comprehensive standardized assessment of global motor function that was developed by Gowland et al. (1993) in conjunction with the Chedoke Rehabilitation Centre in Hamilton, Ontario, Canada. Originally validated for use with stroke clients, its application has been widely demonstrated in other populations as well where motor impairment is of primary concern (Miller et al., 2008). The CMSA comprises two components: an Impairment Inventory (II), which is used to assess motor control across six dimensions, including the arm, hand, leg, and foot, postural control, and shoulder pain where performance is quantified using a seven-point staging system based on Brunnstrom's stages of recovery, and Activity Inventory (AI), that assesses functional mobility across such items as gross motor function and walking (Dang et al., 2014; McMaster University, 2015). During assessment the II section requires the subject to perform various motor movements such as shoulder flexion or abduction which are then graded in relation to normal motor movement criteria, whereas the AI section is scored using a method that is analogous to the Functional Independence Measure (FIM; i.e., the amount of assistance needed by the client to complete the functional activity) (McMaster University, 2015). The AI section is further represented by two indices: the Gross Motor Function Index, which measures functional mobility across 10 items and includes such items as moving in bed, transferring in and out of bed, and getting on and off the floor and the Walking Index which assesses a person's ability to walk on various surfaces as well as climb stairs (Dang et al., 2014). The CMSA can take up to an hour to complete across several therapy days where higher scores represent more impairment

Psychometrics

Original research by the authors of 32 subjects in a stroke rehabilitation unit showed that the II section had excellent intra-rater and inter-rater reliability (r=0.98 and 0.97) as well as excellent test-retest and intra-rater reliability for the AI section (r=0.98 and 0.99) (Gowland et al., 1993). The same study found significant positive correlations between the CMSA and the Fugl-Meyer assessment (r=0.95, p<0.001) as well as with the disability inventory of the FIM (r=0.79, p<0.05) (Gowland et al., 1993). A separate study found that correlation values between the CMSA (AI section) and the Clinical Outcome Variables Scale ranged from r=0.59 to 0.93 across subscales and total scales with a confidence level of p<0.01 (Sacks et al., 2010). Poole, et al. (2001) explored the utility of eleven assessments, which included the Fugl-Meyer Assessment Scale (FMA), the Motor Assessment Scale, the Rivermead Motor Assessment, the Frenchay Arm Test, and the Action Research Arm Test among others and determined that the FMA and CMSA had the most sound psychometric evidence compared to the other tests reviewed.

Advantages

There is a good amount of research in support of the use of the CMSA in clinical practice and research. The assessment manual is inexpensive, only $25 dollars, and when purchased it provides a thorough descriptive analysis of all testing parameters. McMaster University also supports a unique interactive website devoted to the scale. Training for use of the CMSA is also available via a 1-day training workshop, videoconferencing, and a bilingual (French) CD-ROM for self-directed learning (Dang et al., 2014).

Disadvantages

The CMSA is a somewhat complex assessment to administer and score, thus it may be beneficial for the clinician to consider training in one form or another. Also, depending on client endurance more than one session may be needed to complete the battery. Finally, the CMSA measure has not been validated for use with clients who are less than 1-week post-stroke.

Administration

The CMSA manual has detailed instructions for testing as well as for scoring and score interpretations. The use of therapy equipment is necessary and includes such things as a foot stool, pillows, stop watch, floor mat, chair with armrests, ball, adjustable table, and a 1-liter plastic pitcher with water (Miller et al., 2008). Scores of the II are determined by the quality of movement (rated 1 to 7) with a score of 1 indicating severe motor impairment and a score of 7 suggesting normal movement. The AI scoring uses a similar 7-point scale with a range of (1) needs maximal assistance to (7) completely independent. The 2-minute walk test is scored according to a paradigm related to age-specific walking speed outlined in the manual. The maximum total score of the AI section is 100 with higher scores indicating better occupational performance. The CMSA scoring manual also includes an index of predictive discharge scores.

Table 69-1

Example Item of the Impairment Inventory

KNEE FLEXION BEYOND 100°

Position	Sitting, hips and knees flexed to 90° and feet supported
Instruction	Bend knee back as far as possible
Required	Knee flexion greater than 100°
Acceptable	Part of the foot can remain in contact with the floor
Not acceptable	Excessive trunk movement

Adapted from Miller, P., Huijbregts, M., Gowland C., Barreca S., Torresin W., Moreland J.,...Barclay-Goddard. R. (2008). *Chedoke-McMaster Stroke Assessment. Development, validation, and administration manual* (pp. 7-24). Hamilton, Ontario, Canada: McMaster University and Hamilton Health Sciences.

Permissions

The CMSA is produced by McMaster University in Hamilton, Ontario, Canada where the administration manual can be purchased for a cost of $15.00 (plus $10.00 shipping). A bilingual (French-English) CD-ROM is also available ($250) that includes administration and scoring guidelines as well as video demonstrations available from the Canadian Physiotherapy Association e-Store website. To use in publication or research, contact McMaster University or associated persons. Further information can be found in the following journal article:

Gowland, C., Stratford, P., Ward, M., Moreland, J., Torresin, W., Van Hullenaar, S.,...Plews, N. (1993). Measuring physical impairment and disability with the Chedoke-McMaster Stroke Assessment. *Stroke, 24*, 58-63.

Summary

POPULATION	General
TYPE OF MEASURE	Activity-based rating scale
WHAT IT ASSESSES	Global motor performance
TIME	≤60 minutes
COST	$25

Contact

Donna Johnston

McMaster University

Hamilton, Ontario, Canada

Web: www.chedokeassessment.ca/

Web: www.chedokeassessment.ca/Default.aspx?tabid=528

Canadian Physiotherapy Association

955 Green Valley Crescent, Suite 270

Ottawa, Ontario K2C 3V4

Phone: (613) 564-5454 or (800) 387-8679

Web: www.physiotherapy.ca/mrm/webstore/ProductDetail.aspx?cwit_itemid=1118

Chapter 70: Fugl-Meyer Motor Assessment (FMA)

Description

The Fugl-Meyer Motor Assessment (FMA), originally described by Fugl-Meyer, Jaasko, Leyman, Olson, and Steglind (1975) as a system for the evaluation of motor function, balance, sensation qualities, and joint function, is now one of the most widely used clinical assessments of motor impairment and recovery such as that found in individuals post-stroke or with hemiplegia. The assessment, as described by Fugl-Meyer et al. (1975), is based on the theoretical hypothesis that the restoration of motor function follows a definable stepwise course such that for persons with hemiparalysis the recurrence of reflexes always precedes volitional motor action, and after initial dependence on those synergies, active motion becomes successively less dependent upon the primitive reflexes and reactions, and finally complete voluntary motor function with normal muscle reflexes may be regained. This is in many ways similar to Brunnstrom's description of the stages of motor recovery; however, the FMA uses only 5 of the 6 stages defined by Brunnstrom, considering the recovery of wrist and hand function as independent of shoulder-arm recovery (Crow & Harmeling-van der Wel, 2008). The hierarchical stages of recovery according to the FMA include (1) reflex activity, (2) voluntary movement in flexor and extensor synergies, (3) voluntary movement partially independent of synergies, (4) voluntary movement independent of synergies, and finally (5) normal reflex activity. The FMA is composed of several domains that measure motor performance, sensory function, balance, joint range of motion, and joint pain where during assessment the person is asked to complete certain movements in order to elicit motor response synergies associated with the levels of recovery described above where they are then scored relative to the presence or absence those synergies using a 3-point ordinal scale as follows: (0) cannot perform, (1) performs partially, or (2) performs fully. The complete test comprises 155 items and can take up to 60 minutes or more to complete depending on subject stamina.

TABLE 70-1	
EXAMPLE MUSCLE/REFLEX SYNERGIES TESTED BY THE FUGL-MEYER MOTOR ASSESSMENT	
UPPER EXTREMITY—SHOULDER, ELBOW, AND FOREARM	
Reflex-activity	Flexors
	Extensors
Shoulder	Retraction
	Elevation
	Abduction
	Outward rotation
	Adduction/inward rotation
Elbow	Flexion
	Extension
Forearm	Supination
	Pronation
LOWER EXTREMITY—HIP, KNEE, AND ANKLE	
Reflex-activity	Flexors
	Extensors
Hip	Flexion
	Extension
	Adduction
Knee	Flexion
	Extension
Ankle	Dorsiflexion
	Plantar flexion

Adapted from Fugl-Meyer, A. R., Jaasko, L., Leyman, I., Olsson, S., & Steglind, S. (1975). The post-stroke hemiplegic patient: A method for evaluation of physical performance. *Scandinavian Journal of Rehabilitation Medicine, 7*(1), 15,17.

Psychometrics

Early research into the validity of the FMA by Duncan, Propst, and Nelson (1983) reported the inter-rater reliability scores using 4 physical therapists as evaluators and 19 persons more than 1-year post-stroke showed that intra-rater correlations for each subscore and the total score varied from r = 0.86 to 0.99. Later research by Platz et al. (2005) found that the FMA upper limb section correlated significantly with the Action Research Arm Test and Box and Block Test (0.92) and moderately with the Hemispheric Stroke Scale (0.66 to 0.69). Sanford, Moreland, Swanson, Stratford, and Gowland (1993) established data for the FMA in which 3 therapists assessed 12 clients 6 days to 6 months post-stroke and found that inter-rater reliability for the total score was r = 0.96, whereas the reliability coefficients for the subsections varied from 0.61 for pain measurements to 0.97 for the upper extremity items. The same study, using guidelines developed by Fugl-Meyer for characterizing the various levels of motor performance, found that 92% of the patients in the study placed in the first 3 categories (n = 3, severe impairment; n = 4, marked impairment; and n = 4, moderate impairment) (Sanford et al., 1993). A final study of 15 persons with hemiparetic stroke involving 17 trained physical therapists and 1 expert rater showed inter-rater agreement between expert and therapist raters to be high for the total motor score at r = 0.98 and within the moderate to high range for the lower extremity motor subscore at 0.91 (Sullivan, Tilson, Cen, & Duncan, 2011). This suggests that the FMA battery is both intuitive and uncomplicated for those therapists not highly trained.

Advantages

The FMA is a well-established outcome measure of motor function across several therapy disciplines that has a significant amount of sustaining research in support of its use in clinical practice making it arguably a gold standard for its respective assessment of motor function. The upper extremity subsection has been widely validated and has shown to be particularly useful when employed among stroke populations. The FMA also requires no special training and a short version is available as well.

Disadvantages

The FMA, in its entirety, can be a time consuming test at greater than 60 minutes and due to the technical nature of prescribed movements it can also be difficult if one is not familiar with the physical or occupational therapeutic process relative to motor control or cerebrovascular accident (CVA). Administration also requires a certain amount of space as well as the following equipment: a chair, bedside table, reflex hammer, cotton ball, pencil, small piece of cardboard or paper, small can, tennis ball, stop watch, and blindfold.

Administration

Detailed instructions as well as scoring interpretations are outlined in the original article as well as in other places. The FMA has a maximum score of 226 which is the sum of all subscales. A subscale score is also generated relative to level of impairment. For example, the motor performance subscale has a range from (0) hemiplegia to (100) normal and is further delineated between the upper extremity, worth 66 points and lower extremity, worth 34 points. An overall FMA score less than 50 is suggestive of severe motor impairment, 50 to 84 is considered marked motor impairment, 85 to 95 is moderate motor impairment, and 96 to 99 indicates slight motor impairment. Example items relative to hand assessment are mass flexion and mass extension where the subject is tested from full active or passive extension/flexion and graded as (0) cannot perform, (1) performs partially, or (2) performs fully.

Permissions

The assessment is free to use in practice. To use in research or publication, contact its creators or where published. The original article by Fugl-Meyer, et al. wholly contains the measure. Several researchers have also created a rough guide manual to the upper extremity subsection geared toward stroke populations that delivers standardized content, procedures, and scoring.

Fugl-Meyer, A. R., Jaasko, L., Leyman, I., Olsson, S., & Steglind, S. (1975). The post-stroke hemiplegic patient: A method for evaluation of physical performance. *Scandinavian Journal of Rehabilitation Medicine, 7*(1), 13-31.

Deakin, A., Hill, H., & Pomeroy, V. (2003). Rough guide to the Fugl-Meyer Assessment. *Physiotherapy, 89*(12), 751–763.

Summary

POPULATION	CVA; suspected motor impairment; hemiplegia; general
TYPE OF MEASURE	Activity-based rating scale of performance
WHAT IT ASSESSES	Global motor and other
TIME	Up to 60 minutes or more
COST	Free

Contact

Copyright Clearance Center

222 Rosewood Drive

Danvers, MA 01923

Phone: (855) 239-3415

E-mail: info@copyright.com

Web Address: www.copyright.com

FMA—Upper Extremity Motor Scale web:

www.gu.se/digitalAssets/1328/1328946_fma-ue-english.pdf

FMA—Lower Extremity Motor Scale web:

http://neurophys.gu.se/digitalAssets/1520/1520595_fma-le-protocol-english-updated-20150311.pdf

Examiner's Manual web:

https://toneurologiaufpr.files.wordpress.com/2013/02/leaps-fugl-meyer-manual-de-utilizac3a7c3a3o.pdf

CHAPTER 71: MOTOR ASSESSMENT SCALE (MAS)

Description

The Motor Assessment Scale (MAS) is a standardized criterion-based measure that assesses functional motor activity from basic gross motor upper and lower extremity to fine hand motor function. Developed by Carr and Shepherd (1985), it includes eight items representing eight areas of motor function and one item related to muscle tone on the affected side. The motor functions tested include (1) supine to side lying, (2) supine to sitting over the side of the bed, (3) balanced sitting, (4) sitting to standing, (5) walking, (6) upper-arm function, (7) hand movements, and (8) advanced hand activities. The items of the MAS are scored on a 7-point scale ranging from (0) no motor function to (6) optimal task performance completed within a set time frame. The assessment is based on a person's ability to perform and sequentially complete specific tasks, thus in each category the assessment is intended to be hierarchical; that is to say, the ability to accomplish task 6 implies the ability to accomplish tasks 1 through 5 (Sabari, Woodbury, & Velozo, 2014). Therefore, not all items need to be tested for each item/category and the clinician can choose the most appropriate starting point which can reduce administration time (Sabari et al., 2014). Each question uses specific scoring descriptors (0 to 6) relevant to the activity and, as a whole, takes less than 20 minutes to complete with higher scores indicative of better performance.

TABLE 71-1
EXAMPLE ITEMS/SCORING OF THE MOTOR ASSESSMENT SCALE
SUPINE TO SITTING OVER SIDE OF BED
1. Side lying, lifts head sideways but cannot sit up
2. Clinician assists patient with movement, patient controls head position throughout
3. Clinician gives stand-by help by assisting legs over side of bed
4. Side lying to sitting over side of bed with no stand-by help
5. Supine to sitting over side of bed with no stand-by help
6. Supine to sitting over side of bed within 10 seconds with no stand-by help
WALKING
1. Stands on affected leg and steps forward with other leg (i.e., weight bearing with stand-by help)
2. Walks with stand-by help from one person
3. Walks 3 meters alone or uses an aid but no stand-by help
4. Walks 5 meters with no aid in 15 seconds
5. Walks 10 meters with no aid, picks up a small sandbag from floor, turns around and walks back in 25 seconds
6. Walks up and down 4 steps with or without an aid but without holding on to the rail 3 times in 35 seconds
*0 = no activity
Adapted from Carr, J., Shepherd, R., Nordholm, L., & Lynne, D. (1985). Investigation of a new motor assessment scale for stroke patients. *Physical Therapy, 65*(2), 175.

Psychometrics

Original research of 15 persons post-cerebrovascular accident (CVA) showed that the test-retest correlations ranged between $r = 0.87$ and 1.00, with an average correlation of 0.98, whereas inter-rater agreement was also high with a range of $r = 0.89$ to 0.99 (Carr, Shepherd, Nordholm, & Lynne, 1985). A study by Poole & Whitney (1988) established concurrent validity of the MAS with the Fugl-Meyer Motor Assessment (FMA) when they compared motor function in stroke patients and found high correlations between the total scores on the MAS and the FMA ($r = 0.88$), while between specific item scores (except sitting balance) correlations ranged from 0.28 to 0.92. A subsequent study by Malouin, Pichard, Bonneau, Durand, and Corriveau (1994) also compared the MAS and the FMA and found that the correlation coefficient for total FMA and total MAS scores was 0.96 and for selected items, correlations ranged from 0.65 to 0.93, except for sitting balance (-0.10), suggesting that the FMA sitting balance test may not be a valid measure and is responsible for the low correlation. Miller, Slade, Pallant, and Galea (2010) found that a floor effect existed upon admission to stroke rehabilitation for item 5 (walking) with participants often scoring the lowest score. Similarly, a ceiling effect on discharge existed for item 4 (sitting to standing) with persons scoring the highest. A ceiling effect on admission to and discharge from stroke rehabilitation was also noted for item 3 (balanced sitting).

Advantages

Due to its hierarchical scale and ease of administration as a clinical evaluation tool, the MAS may be preferable to other assessments such as the Wolf Motor Function Test, Action Research Arm Test, or Arm Motor Ability Test, which require extensive setup and time to complete (Sabari et al., 2014). The MAS also has the ability to test and grade gross motor abilities of low-functioning individuals as well as the ability to document meaningful change in motor ability from gross to refine during the recovery process.

Disadvantages

Sabari et al. (2014) found that problems in the scoring criteria for hand items were a negative factor that decreased the tool's effectiveness and recommended improving the 2-hand items by clearly differentiating between movements and activities, adding criteria that would be appropriate for stroke survivors with lower levels of hand function, and providing a more valid difficulty hierarchy for behavioral criteria. Based on those findings they presented 2 amended items for assessing hand function: hand movements, consisting of 10 behavioral criteria and hand activities, consisting of 8 behavioral criteria. In addition to providing a clear differentiation between motor execution and motor control, they added easier behavioral criteria, thus allowing the items to be used with patients that demonstrate more severe impairment (Sabari et al., 2014).

Administration

The MAS is scored on the person's ability to complete 8 specific motor tasks of increasing difficulty. A score of 0 indicates inability to achieve any of the criteria and a score of 6 indicates ability to perform all the criteria for that specific item. When administering the MAS, the clinician assigns a score (0 to 6) for each item based upon the most difficult criterion the patient was able to achieve for each task. Total MAS scores represent the sum of scores for each of the 8 task items and range from 0 to 48. The assessment requires some set up as well as several items for administration such as a low wide plinth (a sort of base), a stopwatch, polystyrene cup, a pen and pen top, a prepared sheet of paper for drawing lines with one vertical line on the right of the sheet, and a cylindrical object such as a jar.

Permissions

The MAS is located in the public domain and is an instrument that can be used in practice, research, or publication without fee. A template and instructions for administration can be downloaded from numerous websites and is wholly contained in the following journal article:

Carr, J., Shepherd, R., Nordholm, L., & Lynne, D. (1985). Investigation of a new Motor Assessment Scale for stroke patients. *Physical Therapy, 65*(2), 175-180.

Summary

POPULATION	General; CVA
TYPE OF MEASURE	Activity-based hierarchical rating scale
WHAT IT ASSESSES	Global motor performance
TIME	< 20 minutes
COST	Free

Contact

Roberta Shepherd, DipPhty, DHlthSc (honoris causa)

Honorary Professor

Department of Physiotherapy

University of Sydney—Cumberland Campus

Lidcombe, New South Wales, Australia

REFERENCES

Bouwens, S., Van Heugten, C., Aalten, P., Wolfs, C., Baarends, E., Van Menxel, D., & Verhey, F. (2007). Relationship between measures of dementia severity and observation of daily life functioning as measured with the Assessment of Motor and Process Skills (AMPS). *Dementia and Geriatric Cognitive Disorders, 25*(1), 81-87.

Carr, J., Shepherd, R., Nordholm, L., & Lynne, D. (1985). Investigation of a new Motor Assessment Scale for stroke patients. *Physical Therapy, 65*(2), 175-180.

Center for Innovative OT Solutions. (2013). AMPS: Assessment of Motor and Process Skills. Retrieved from www.innovativeotsolutions.com/content/amps/

Chard, G. (2006). Adopting the Assessment of Motor and Process Skills into practice: Therapists' voices. *British Journal of Occupational Therapy, 69*, 50–57.

Crow, J. L., & Harmeling-van der Wel, B. C. (2008). Hierarchical properties of the motor function sections of the Fugl-Meyer Assessment scale for people after stroke: A retrospective study. *Physical Therapy, 88*(12), 1554-1567.

Dang, M., Ramsaran, K., Street, M., Syed, S., Barclay-Goddard, R., Stratford, P., & Miller, P. (2011). Estimating the accuracy of the Chedoke–McMaster Stroke Assessment predictive equations for stroke rehabilitation. *Physiotherapy Canada, 63*(3), 334–341.

Duncan, P., Propst, M., & Nelson, S. G. (1983). Reliability of the Fugl-Meyer Assessment of the sensorimotor recovery following cerebrovascular accident. *Physical Therapy, 63*, 1606-1610.

Fioravanti, A., Bordignon, C., Pettit, S., Woodhouse, L., & Ansley, B. (2012). Comparing the responsiveness of the Assessment of Motor and Process Skills and the Functional Independence Measure. *Canadian Journal of Occupational Therapy, 79*, 167-174.

Fisher, A. G., & Jones, K. B. (2010). *Assessment of Motor and Process Skills. Vol. 1: Development, standardization, and administration manual* (7th ed.). Fort Collins, CO: Three Star Press.

Fisher, A., Liu, Y., Velozo, C., & Pan, A. (1992). Crosscultural assessment of process skills. *American Journal of Occupational Therapy, 46*, 876–885.

Fugl-Meyer, A. R., Jaasko, L., Leyman, I., Olsson, S., & Steglind, S. (1975). The post-stroke hemiplegic patient: A method for evaluation of physical performance. *Scandinavian Journal of Rehabilitation Medicine, 7*(1), 13-31.

Gowland, C., Stratford, P., Ward, M., Moreland, J., Torresin, W., Van Hullenaar, S.,... Plews, N. (1993). Measuring physical impairment and disability with the Chedoke-McMaster Stroke Assessment. *Stroke, 24*, 58-63.

Kizony, R., & Katz, N. (2002). Relationships between cognitive abilities and the process scale and skills of the Assessment of Motor and Process Skills (AMPS) in patients with stroke. *OTJR: Occupation, Participation, and Health, 22*(2), 82-92.

Malouin, F., Pichard, L., Bonneau, C., Durand, A., & Corriveau D. (1994). Evaluating motor recovery early after stroke: Comparison of the Fugl-Meyer Assessment and the Motor Assessment Scale. *Archives of Physical Medicine and Rehabilitation, 75*(11), 1206-1212.

Marom, B., Jarus, T., & Josman, N. (2006). The relationship between the Assessment of Motor and Process Skills (AMPS) and the Large Allen Cognitive Level (LACL) test in clients with stroke. *Physical and Occupational Therapy in Geriatrics, 24*(4), 33-50.

McCluskey, A., & Cusick, A. (2002) Strategies for introducing evidence-based practice and changing clinical behaviour: A manager's toolbox. *Australian Occupational Therapy Journal, 49*, 53-70.

McMaster University. (2015). Chedoke-McMaster Stroke Assessment. Hamilton, ON, Canada. Retrieved from http://www.chedokeassessment.ca/Default.aspx?tabid=510

Miller, P., Huijbregts, M., Gowland, C., Barreca, S., Torresin, W., Moreland, J.,...Stratford, P. (2008). *Chedoke–McMaster Stroke Assessment: Development, validation, and administration manual.* Hamilton, Ontario, Canada: McMaster University and Hamilton Health Sciences.

Miller, K., Slade, A., Pallant, J., & Galea, M. (2010). Evaluation of the psychometric properties of the upper limb subscales of the Motor Assessment Scale using a Rasch analysis model. *Journal of Rehabilitative Medicine, 42*, 315–322.

Platz, T., Pinkowski, C., van Wijck, F., Kim, I., di Bella, P., & Johnson, G. (2005). Reliability and validity of arm function assessment with standardized guidelines for the Fugl-Meyer Test, Action Research Arm Test and Box and Block Test: A multicentre study. *Clinical Rehabilitation, 19*(4), 404-411.

Poole, J., & Whitney, S. (1988). Motor assessment scale for stroke patients: Concurrent validity and inter-rater reliability. *Archives of Physical Medicine and Rehabilitation, 69*(3 Pt 1), 195-197.

Poole, J., & Whitney, S. (2001). Assessment of motor function post stroke: a review. *Physical and Occupational Therapy in Geriatrics, 19*(2), 1-22.

Sabari, J., Woodbury, M., & Velozo, C. (2014). Rasch analysis of a new hierarchical scoring system for evaluating hand function on the Motor Assessment Scale for stroke. *Stroke Research and Treatment, 2014*, 1-10.

Sacks, L., Yee, K., Huijbregts, M., Miller, P., Aggett, T., & Salbach, N. (2010). Validation of the activity inventory of the Chedoke-McMaster Stroke Assessment and the clinical outcome variables scale to evaluate mobility in geriatric clients. *Journal of Rehabilitation Medicine, 42*, 90–92.

Sanford, J., Moreland, J., Swanson, L., Stratford, P., & Gowland. C. (1993). Reliability of the Fugl-Meyer Assessment for testing motor performance in patients following stroke. *Physical Therapy, 73*, 447-454.

Sellers, S., Fisher, A., & Duran, L. (2001). Validity of the Assessment of Motor and Process Skills with students who are visually impaired. *Journal of Visual Impairment and Blindness, 95*(3), 164-167.

Sullivan, J., Tilson, J. Cen, S., & Duncan, P. (2011). Fugl-Meyer Assessment of sensorimotor function after stroke: Standardized training procedure for clinical practice and clinical trials. *Stroke, 42*(2), 427-432.

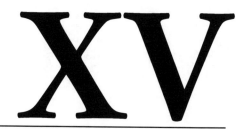

Motor Function—
Upper Extremity Limb

Bortnick, K.
Occupational Therapy Assessments for Older Adults: 100 Instruments for
Measuring Occupational Performance (pp. 211-228).
© 2017 Taylor & Francis Group.

CHAPTER 72: ACTION RESEARCH ARM TEST (ARAT)

Description

The Action Research Arm Test (ARAT) is an observational activity-based measure used to determine the quality of upper limb function that was developed by Lyle (1981) as a modification of the Upper Extremity Function Test. The test consists of 19 items encompassing 4 subtests (grasp, grip, pinch, and gross arm movement) where the subject's performance on each item is rated along a 4-point scale (0 to 3) where (0) equates cannot perform any part of the test, (1) can partially perform the test, (2) can complete the test but took abnormally long or had great difficulty, and (3) can perform the test normally. A maximum score of 57 is considered for each extremity tested and indicates the absence of any dysfunction (Koh et al., 2006). The test has a hierarchical design in which the subject attempts the most difficult item of each subtest first. If subjects correctly complete the first, most difficult item, they are positively credited for all items of the subtest without having to be tested any further (McDonnell, 2008). Thus not all items need to be tested. If the patient fails the first most difficult item the second item tested is the easiest, if he or she receives a score of 0 for the easiest item (i.e., fails) the assessor moves onto the next subtest and so on until all subtests have been attempted (McDonnell, 2008). While the test requires substantial set up as well as a fair amount of equipment, once set up it can be completed in about 10 minutes.

Psychometrics

A study by Nordin, Alt-Murphy, and Danielsson (2014) using 2 raters with 35 subjects ≤22 months post-stroke found that the median ARAT total score for raters A and B was 37 (range; 3 to 54) and 38 (range; 3 to 56). Intra-rater reliability for total score was r = 0.94 for each of the raters. At the subtest level, a satisfactory level of agreement was also found within each rater for all 4 subtests, ranging from 0.91 to 0.94 for the subtests grasp and pinch, and 0.83 to 1.0 for the subtests grip and gross movement. Inter-rater reliability for the ARAT total score was r = 0.91 and 0.99, respectively while inter-rater agreement at the subtest level ranged from 0.81 to 0.91 for grasp and pinch, and from 0.86 to 1.0 for grip and gross movement. An earlier study by Platz et al. (2005) found a significant correlation (0.92) between the ARAT, the Fugl-Meyer Motor Assessment upper limb section, and the Box and Block Test. The same study also showed that the ARAT had moderate to significant correlations with the Hemispheric Stroke Scale (0.66), suggesting that it too is measuring the same phenomenon as other established assessments.

Advantages

No special training is required for administration and once set up the assessment can be completed in < 10 minutes for most patient populations. The ARAT has also been shown to have good responsiveness evidenced by its ability to detect clinically relevant changes in motor function during the acute phase following stroke as well as in patients with chronic conditions (McDonnell, 2008). Another advantage of the ARAT is its unique hierarchical format and scoring design where once an item is completed successfully it is assumed that all easier items can also be completed, which can shorten testing time without sacrificing a valid score. Conversely, if the easiest item is failed it can be assumed that any attempt at a harder item will also result in failure (McDonnell, 2008).

Disadvantages

Koh et al. (2006) examined the construct validity of the current 19-item ARAT and found that although it closely resembled the original design and displayed a consistent hierarchical order relative to continuum of motor function the *pinch ball bearing with 3rd finger and thumb* item was inconsistent with other items in its subtest and its removal should be considered. The poor fit of this item as well as others were also discussed in a study by van der Lee, Roorda, Beckerman, Lankhorst, and Bouter (2002) in which they argued that although overall the assessment displayed a good uni-dimensional hierarchy with a scalability coefficient of 0.79 (range = 0.69 to 0.86) the removal of four items would allow even higher values of the scalability coefficient *H*.

Administration

Testing procedures, scoring, and materials have been standardized and outlined in an article by Yozbatiran, Der-Yeghiaian, and Cramer (2008), where the full notation is under permissions. Conversely, a testing kit can be purchased from a number of therapy supply retailers. The complete list of items needed are a chair without armrests, a table, various-sized wooden blocks, a cricket-type ball, a sharpening stone, alloy tubes, a washer and bolt, 2 glasses, marbles, ball bearings, 2 planks for placing the alloy tubes, 1 plank to place the washer, 2 tobacco tin lids, and 1 37-cm high shelf (Yozbatiran et al., 2008). During assessment, the subject is seated upright and each of the 19 tasks are performed unilaterally until completion of the task or until reaching a time limit defined as 60 seconds (Yozbatiran et al., 2008) The subject starts with the least affected arm first where quality of movement is scrutinized.

TABLE 72-1
EXAMPLE ITEMS OF THE ACTION RESEARCH ARM TEST
• Pinch ball bearing with 3rd finger and thumb
• Pinch marble with 3rd finger and thumb
• Pinch ball bearing with 2nd finger and thumb
• Pour water glass to glass
• Grasp block (10 cm^3)
• Pinch ball bearing with 1st finger and thumb
• Pinch marble with 2nd finger and thumb
• Pinch marble with 1st finger and thumb
• Grasp block
• Grip washer over bolt
Adapted from Koh, C. L., Hsueh, I. P., Wang, W. C., Sheu, C. F., Yu, T. Y., Wang, C. H., & Hsieh, C. L. (2006). Validation of the Action Research Arm Test using item response theory in patients after stroke. *Journal of Rehabilitation Medicine, 38,* 378.

Permissions

The ARAT can be created by the clinician according to instructions outlined by Yozbatiran et al. (2008) or purchased at a price of $600 from Salia Rehab LLC. To use the ARAT in research or publication contact the creator of the measure or where purchased at the information that follows. More information can be found in the following journal articles:

Lyle, R. C. (1981). A performance test for assessment of upper limb function in physical rehabilitation treatment and research. *International Journal of Rehabilitation Research, 4*(4), 483-492.

Yozbatiran, N., Der-Yeghiaian, L., & Cramer, S. C. (2008). A standardized approach to performing the Action Research Arm Test. *Neurorehabilitation and Neural Repair, 22*(1), 78-90.

Summary

POPULATION	General; cerebrovascular accident
TYPE OF MEASURE	Activity-based hierarchical rating scale
WHAT IT ASSESSES	Upper extremity limb motor; hand performance
TIME	< 10 minutes; after some set up
COST	Free to $600

Contact

Johanna H. van der Lee, MD, PhD

Department of Pediatrics, Clinical Epidemiology

The Academic Medical Center—Netherlands

Amsterdam-Zuidoost, Netherlands

Web: www.amc.nl/web/Research/Who-is-Who-in-Research/Who-is-Who-in-Research.htm?p=1935

Salia Rehab LLC

P.O. Box 1192

Traverse City, MI 49685

Phone: (888) 604-0966

Email: info@saliarehab.com

Web: http://saliarehab.com/

CHAPTER 73: ARM MOTOR ABILITY TEST (AMAT-9)

Description

The Arm Motor Ability Test (AMAT), developed by McCulloch, Cook, Fleming, Novack, and Taub (1988), is a standardized assessment of select activities of daily living (ADLs) that quantify a person's unilateral or bilateral performance of their upper extremity and, in particular, arm movement. The original AMAT consisted of 16 compound tasks, broken down into categories of 3 movements each that comprise differential contributions from the 2 arms or of the distal and proximal musculature of the affected arm (Kopp et al., 1997) The assessment is generally stroke-specific and has gone through several revisions with the nine item AMAT-9 being the most recent. ADLs on the scale include such items as cutting meat, eating with a spoon, combing hair, opening a jar, tying shoelaces, and using a telephone where some items have multiple components. During assessment the person is scored according to his or her functional performance and the quality of each movement as well as the time to complete each task. The AMAT-9 uses a 6-point ordinal scale (0 to 5) for each item with higher scores indicating better performance. The test takes approximately 40 minutes to complete.

Psychometrics

An initial reliability assessment of the AMAT with 30 subjects at varying periods after a cerebrovascular accident (CVA) and 10 age-matched unaffected controls indicated high inter-rater reliability (range = 0.96 to 0.99, median = 0.97) (McCulloch et al., 1988). A study of 32 community-dwelling stroke survivors found the AMAT-9 to be a reliable measure with a Cronbach's alpha of $\alpha = 0.93$, significant correlation with the Action Research Arm Test at 0.79, Fugl-Meyer Assessment (FMA) at 0.79, and the Wolf Motor Function Test at 0.78, suggesting that they have similar constructs as well as testing equivalent phenomenon. The same study found a moderate correlation with the Stroke Impact Scale (hand subscore) at 0.40 as well as a significant negative correlation with the Stroke Impact scale (communication subscore) at −0.16 (O'Dell et al., 2013). A study

by Chae, Labatia, and Yang (2003) also found a significant correlation with the FMA (0.94); however, AMAT-9 time of performance exhibited significant ceiling and floor effects and the same study found that it had a negative impact correlation with FMA time at -0.92.

Advantages

The AMAT-9 is unique in that it uses ADLs to test arm motor ability making it specific to occupational therapy practice. There is also a fair amount of research in support of its use in clinical practice. It has also shown to significantly correlate with other more well-known assessments such as the FMA and the Wolf Motor Function test. No special training is required for administration.

Disadvantages

Research by Chae et al. (2003) has suggested that the AMAT quality of movement section is redundant and somewhat based on qualitative observation of the clinician. They also found that the clinical utility of time of performance remains uncertain. The administration of the AMAT can also be longer than other assessments and for more-impaired subjects the test can be tiresome and/or frustrating to complete. A study by Chae et al. (2003) found that the FMA upper extremity arm subtest took less than 5 minutes to complete, whereas the average time to administer the AMAT was approximately 40 minutes.

Administration

The AMAT is composed of 9 bilateral and unilateral ADL-specific tasks. The unilateral activities are performed with the affected arm and the bilateral tasks are performed using (or attempting to use) the dominant or affected limb in the same roles as before onset of the stroke (i.e., tying shoe laces) (Chae et al., 2003). Each task is rated along a 6-point ordinal scale (0 to 5) with respect to functional ability and quality of movement. Each task is also timed, and subjects are given a maximum time limit of 60 or 120 seconds depending on the task (Chae et al., 2003).

TABLE 73-1
ACTIVITIES ON THE ARM MOTOR ABILITY TEST
CUT MEAT
A. Pick up knife and fork
B. Cut meat (Play-Doh [Hasbro])
C. Fork to mouth
EAT WITH SPOON
A. Pick up spoon
B. Pick up bean with spoon
C. Spoon to mouth
PUT ON T-SHIRT
A. Arms in T-shirt sleeve
B. Head through hole
C. Pull down and straighten shirt

Adapted from O'Dell, M. W., Kim, G., Rivera, L., Fieo, R., Christos, P., Polistena, C.,...Gorga, D. (2013). A psychometric evaluation of the Arm Motor Ability Test. *Journal of Rehabilitation Medicine, 45*(6), 520.

TABLE 73-2
RATING SCALES USED ON THE ARM MOTOR ABILITY TEST
FUNCTIONAL ABILITY
0. No use
1. Very slight use
2. Slight use
3. Moderate use
4. Almost normal use
5. Normal use
QUALITY OF MOVEMENT
0. No use
1. Very poor use
2. Poor use
3. Fair use
4. Almost normal use
5. Normal use

Adapted from Chae, J., Labatia, I., & Yang, G. (2003). Upper limb motor function in hemiparesis: Concurrent validity of the Arm Motor Ability test. *American Journal of Physical Medicine and Rehabilitation, 82*(1), 3.

Permissions

The AMAT is free to use in clinical practice and is outlined in several articles. Use of the AMAT in research or publication can be obtained by contacting the journal in which it was published or the developers of the assessment at the information following. More information about the AMAT can be found in the following publication:

Kopp, B., Kunkel, A., Flor, H., Platz, T., Rose, U., Mauritz, K.,...Taub, E. (1997). The Arm Motor Ability Test: Reliability, validity, and sensitivity to change of an instrument for assessing disabilities in activities of daily living. *Archives of Physical Medicine and Rehabilitation, 78*(6), 615-620.

Summary

POPULATION	CVA
TYPE OF MEASURE	Activity-based rating scale using ADLs
WHAT IT ASSESSES	Upper extremity limb motor; hand performance
TIME	< 10 minutes after some set up
COST	Free

Contact

Karen McCulloch, PT, PhD, NCS

The University of North Carolina at Chapel Hill

Division of Physical Therapy

Chapel Hill, North Carolina

Web: www.med.unc.edu/ahs/physical/faculty/karen-mcculloch-pt-phd-ncs

Edward Taub, PhD

Professor/Director C.I. Therapy

University of Alabama—Birmingham

Birmingham, Alabama

Web: www.uab.edu/cas/psychology/psy-fac/33-primary-faculty/63-dr-edward-taub

CHAPTER 74: DASH (DISABILITY OF THE ARM, SHOULDER AND HAND) OUTCOME MEASURE

Description

The DASH (Disability of the Arm, Shoulder and Hand) Outcome Measure, by Hudak et al. (1996), is a 30-item self-report questionnaire designed to measure physical function and symptoms in persons with musculoskeletal disorders of the upper limbs. The assessment examines the degree of difficulty a person has performing various physical activities related to the arm, shoulder, or hand (21 items) as well as the severity of symptoms associated with pain including such things as tingling, weakness, and stiffness (5 items), and the psychological impact the person is experiencing relative to social activities, work, and sleep (4 items). Two optional modules pertaining to sports/performing arts (4 items) and work (4 items) can also be completed. DASH uses several 5-point rating scales from no difficulty to unable, not limited at all to unable, none to extreme, etc. The scale includes items such as (1) place an object on a shelf above your head; (2) rate arm, shoulder, or hand pain while performing a specific activity; and (3) level of agreement with a statement (i.e., less capable, less confident, or less useful because of arm, shoulder, or hand problem). The responses to the 30 items are summed to form a raw score that is then converted to a 0 to 100 scale where a higher score reflects greater disability. DASH can be completed in less than 10 minutes.

Psychometrics

A study by Franchignoni et al. (2010) of 238 subjects with upper extremity muscle disorders revealed that all items showed item-to-total correlations between 0.53 and 0.76, except item 26, tingling, at 0.31. Further analysis revealed 3 factors that were able to explain 67% of the variance: (1) shoulder range of motion at 54%, which included items 1 to 5, 7 to 11, 16 to 18, 20, and 21; (2) symptoms at 8%, which included items 6, 12 to 15, and 19; and (3) consequences at 5%, which included items 22 to 30. A cross-cultural adaptation of the DASH to Swedish using 176 subjects with upper extremity conditions found internal consistency to be high at $\alpha = 0.96$, while test-retest reliability, which was evaluated in a subgroup of 67 subjects who completed the DASH within 7-day intervals, was excellent with an intra-class correlation coefficient of $r = 0.92$ (Atroshi, Gummesson, Andersson, Dahlgreen, & Johansson, 2000). A later study by Franchignoni et al. (2014) also found test-retest reliability of the DASH to be high at $r = 0.93$. A study by Beaton et al. (2001) showed that test-retest reliability exceeded manual guide lines at $r = 0.96$ with mean scores of shoulder patients to be 48.4, whereas wrist/hand patients it was only 34.4. Correlation with the Shoulder Pain and Disability Index pain and function scales were also strong (0.82 and 0.87). A study by Whalley & Adams (2009) found that when used in an outpatient occupational therapy clinic among 22 subjects, the DASH showed responsiveness to change where baseline mean was 50.20 and discharge mean was 30.77. Finally, a study by van Kampen et al. (2013) found the minimal detectable change of the DASH to be 16.3, whereas Franchignoni et al. (2014) found it to be 10.81 points at the 90% confidence level.

Advantages

There is a significant amount of research in support of the DASH for use in clinical practice. The assessment is free to use in certain settings and administration time is less than 10 minutes. The Institute for Work & Health maintains a website devoted to the DASH measures (QuickDASH) where information can be found and downloaded. Access to a free online form and score calculation service is available as well.

Disadvantages

Analysis of the DASH noted that question number 26, tingling along with question number 22, interference with social activities, failed to load meaningfully into a three-factor model that fit for other items, suggesting its inter-item correlation could be improved by reworking these items.

Administration

During assessment the subject is asked to consider each item as it relates to function and feeling relative to issues of the arm, shoulder, and hand and then to choose the most appropriate self-perceived rating descriptor (1 to 5). The assessment has 2 scored components: the disability/symptom section (30 items) and the optional high performance sport/music or work section (4 items each). Scoring employs a unique algorithm in which assigned values for each response are added, divided by 4, and then 1 is subtracted from the sum. That sum is then multiplied by 25 to give a total score.

TABLE 74-1
EXAMPLE ACTIVITIES OF THE DASH MEASURE
• Writing
• Turning a key
• Preparing a meal
• Pushing open a heavy door
• Doing heavy household chores
• Carrying a shopping bag or briefcase
• Carrying a heavy object (over 5 kg)
• Putting on a pullover sweater
• Managing transportation needs
• Pain when performing activities
• Difficulty in sleeping
• Impact on self-image
Adapted from Atroshi, I., Gummesson, C., Andersson, B., Dahlgren, E., & Johansson, A. (2000). The Disabilities of the Arm, Shoulder and Hand (DASH) outcome questionnaire: Reliability and validity of the Swedish version evaluated in 176 patients. *Acta Orthopaedica Scandinavica, 71*(6), 614.

Permission

The DASH Outcome Measure is free to use in clinical practice, not for profit use, and in non-commercial research. Any other use requires permission from the Institute for Work & Health who holds the copyright to the assessment and can be contacted at the information that follows. More information can be found in the following journal article:

Hudak, P. L., Amadio, P. C., Bombardier, C., Beaton, D., Cole, D., Davis, A.,...Marx, R. G. (1996). Development of an upper extremity outcome measure: the DASH (Disabilities of the Arm, Shoulder, and Hand). *American Journal of Industrial Medicine, 29*(6), 602-608.

Summary

POPULATION	Suspected upper extremity-limb/hand; general
TYPE OF MEASURE	Self-report questionnaire
WHAT IT ASSESSES	Perceived level of impairment
TIME	< 10 minutes
COST	Free

Contact

DASH Outcome Measures

Institute for Work & Health

481 University Avenue, Suite 800

Toronto, Ontario

Canada M5G 2E9

Phone: (416) 927-2027 ext. 2173

Email: dash@iwh.on.ca

Web: www.dash.iwh.on.ca/

CHAPTER 75: MICHIGAN HAND OUTCOMES QUESTIONNAIRE (MHQ)

Description

The Michigan Hand Outcomes Questionnaire (MHQ) is a self-report questionnaire designed to assess a person's general hand function as well as change over time and when used by the clinician, it can help to portray an overall sense of what the client feels their strengths and weaknesses are as it relates to their injured extremity. The MHQ has 72 items comprising 6 categories: (1) overall hand function, (2) activities of daily living (ADLs), (3) pain, (4) work performance, (5) aesthetics, and (6) patient satisfaction with hand function. There is also a demographic section that purveys information relating to age, background, and education. The battery uses several numerical value scoring systems that range from (1) not difficult to (5) very difficult, (1) always to (5) never, and (1) strongly disagree to (5) strongly agree. A Brief MHQ (bMHQ) is also available that contains 12 items scored 1 to 5 along a Likert scale and is designed for clinical, rather than research, functions and includes such items as "In the past week, how satisfied are you with the motion of your fingers?" and "How was the sensation (feeling) in your hand(s) during the past week?" The MHQ can be completed in 15 minutes and the bMHQ in less than 5 minutes. Both assessments employ unique scoring algorithms giving the clinician several ways to assess results.

Psychometrics

An early study of the MHQ using 200 consecutive patients at a university-based hand surgery clinic found that test-retest reliabilities of the subscales demonstrated substantial agreement, ranging from r = 0.81 for the aesthetics scale to 0.97 for the ADL scale (Chung, Pillsbury, Walters, & Hayward, 1998). Among a diabetic population Poole, Gonzales, and Tedesco (2010) found that test–retest reliability ranged from r = 0.58 to 0.94, whereas a study by Impens et al. (n.d.) showed overall test-retest reliability to be r = 0.84) with subscales ranging from 0.61 (aesthetic) to 0.86 (ADLs) among subjects with systemic sclerosis. The same study found the internal consistency results of each subscale were greater than α = > 0.80, except for aesthetics, which was 0.62. Another study of 116 and 77 using 2 administrations of the MHQ found that reliabilities ranged from r = 0.84 to 0.95 for the MHQ subscales and correlation coefficients ranged from 0.71 to 0.84 (Chung & Morris, 2014). Horng et al. (2010) found that strong associations existed between the MHQ and the DASH (Disabilities of the Arm, Shoulder and Hand) scale at r = 0.89 and further results confirmed the MHQ to be more sensitive to functional changes, whereas the DASH was more sensitive to disability days. When comparing the MHQ, DASH, and the Patient-Rated Wrist/Hand Evaluation (PRWHE), 45% considered the PRWHE as easiest to complete, followed by the DASH (28%), and the MHQ (27%). However, 49% selected the MHQ as best reflecting current ability to use their hand, followed by the DASH (36%), and the PRWHE (15%) (Weinstock-Zlotnick, Page, Wolff, & Ghomwari, 2012)

Advantages

There is a good amount of research evidence in support of its use in clinical practice and no special training or certifications are needed to administer the assessment. It has also shown to be relatively sensitive in detecting the client's perceived changes in hand function over time, highlighting its usefulness in developing an occupational profile of a client's self-perceived strengths and weaknesses as well as determine client-centered treatment goals. The MHQ is free to use in clinical practice and can be completed in 15 minutes. Finally, the University of Michigan maintains a website devoted to the measure where it can be downloaded along with support material.

Disadvantages

The MHQ has separate questions for the right and left hand in 4 of 6 domains, excluding pain and work, therefore, scores in these domains could potentially be affected by latent symptoms in the unoperated hand of carpal tunnel syndrome, for example (Chatterjee & Price, 2009).

Administration

The MHQ, when downloaded, includes both versions where each has detailed instructions as well as scoring interpretations. Administered as a self-report questionnaire, the subject is asked to consider each question relative to the function of his or her hand(s)/wrist(s) during the past week by selecting the appropriate descriptive scoring choice (1 to 5). A raw scale score for each of the six scales is generated, as is the sum of responses of each scale item. The raw score can then be converted to an overall score ranging from 0 to 100 using a unique algorithm that requires some items to be reversed and recoded. A higher score on the pain scale is suggestive of more pain, whereas on the other five scales, higher scores indicate better hand performance. The end result is typically a score for the affected hand; however, if both hands are affected (i.e., rheumatoid arthritis), the right and left hand scores are averaged (Ames, 2014).

Permission

Both the MHQ and the bMHQ are free to use in private practice or in non-profit, however, they do require the completion of a licensing form. To use in unique for-profit or other patient populations (1 to 1000 people) the cost is $7500, in populations over 1000 the cost is $15,000. To use in research or publication, contact its creator at the information following. More information can be found in the following journal article:

Chung, K. Pillsbury, M., Walters, M., & Hayward, R. (1998). Reliability and validity testing of the Michigan Hand Outcomes Questionnaire. *Journal of Hand Surgery-American, 23*(4), 575-87.

Summary

POPULATION	Suspected hand impairment
TYPE OF MEASURE	Self-report questionnaire
WHAT IT ASSESSES	Perceived level/effect of impairment
TIME	< 15 minutes
COST	Free for private practice (varies)

Contact

Melissa Shauver, MPH

Clinical Research Coordinator

Department of Surgery

University of Michigan Medical School

Ann Arbor, Michigan

Web: http://mhq.lab.medicine.umich.edu/home

CHAPTER 76: MOTOR ACTIVITY LOG (MAL)

Description

The Motor Activity Log (MAL) is a standardized assessment designed to assess the use of a person's affected arm and hand during activities of daily living (ADLs) following a stroke. The MAL is composed of two subtests, one pertaining to the amount of use (AOU) and the other pertaining to the quality of movement (QOM) of the affected extremity, where each is delivered in a structured interview format with either the client or caregiver. The MAL consists of 30 ADL items where the subject is asked to rate his or her level of performance over the past week and explores such capabilities as turning on a light switch, wiping off a kitchen counter or other surface, getting up from a chair with armrests, putting on makeup base, lotion, or shaving cream on face, as well as the ability to write on paper or button a shirt (Taub, McCulloch, Uswatte, & Morris, 2011). The MAL uses an 11-point Likert scale (0 to 5), which includes half points. Scores for the AOU subtest range from (0) never use the affected arm for this activity to (5) always use the affected arm for this activity. Scores for the QOM portion range from (0) inability to use the affected arm for this activity to (5) ability to use the affected arm for this activity just as well as before the stroke (van der Lee, Beckerman, Knol, de Vet, & Bouter,2004). Individual item scores are summed with higher scores indicating better performance. Time to administer the exam is approximately 20 minutes.

Psychometrics

Test-retest reliabilities have been reported to be high at r = 0.91 in stable populations, whereas subacute patient reliabilities have ranged from r = 0.79 to 0.82 (Uswatte, Taub, Morris, Vignolo, & McCulloch, 2005). Using the 14-item version, internal consistency data from 29 patients who had performed all 14 activities was α = 0.88 and 0.91 for the AOU and QOM subscales; however, when data that included missing values of activities that were not performed during the past week of 56 subject's Cronbach's alpha were similar at α = 0.87 and 0.90 (van der Lee et al., 2004). Another study found the correlation coefficient between the 2 subscales to be 0.95, whereas the internal consistency was α = 0.82 for the AOU and α = 0.87 for the QOM (van der Lee et al., 2004). A study of 59 patients post-cerebrovascular accident established the concurrent validity of MAL-AOU scores at both pre- and post-treatment with the Box and Block Test (BBT) as correlations were found to be 0.37 and 0.49, while with the Nine-Hole Peg Test (NHPT) they were stronger at 0.16 and −0.23, and with the Action Research Arm Test (ARAT) they were 0.31 and 0.32 (Lin, Hsieh, & Chang,

2010). The same study found that the MAL-QOM section had pre- and post-treatment correlations of 0.52 and 0.52 with the BBT, −0.26 and −0.33 with the NHPT, and 0.39 and 0.35 with the ARAT (Lin et al., 2010). A later study found the MAL to correlate somewhat better with the Hand Function subscale of the Stroke Impact Scale at 0.68 to 0.72, as well as mildly with accelerometry, which is motor recovery monitoring, at 0.47 to 0.52 (Uswatte, Taub, Morris, Light, & Thompson, 2006).

Advantages

There is a good amount of research in support of its use in clinical practice and requires no special training or certifications to administer. The MAL also uses ADL-specific activities to gauge motor performance making it a relevant assessment to the profession of occupational therapy. Several versions of the MAL are also available including the 14-, 26-, and 30-item versions.

Disadvantages

Some studies have questioned the stability of its published properties with regard to variations in the way interviews have been or can be performed as well as for the number of activities completed. For example, during assessment the person may not have performed all ADLs in the past week, such as eating half a sandwich or finger foods, leading to varying calculations of total scores and psychometric results (van der Lee Knol et al., 2004). Administration of the MAL also requires participants to watch a video that may be inconsistent with some clinical practices.

Administration

The MAL is standardized and has clearly defined testing techniques as well as scoring guidelines outlined in the examiner's manual. During assessment the client is asked to consider his or her ADL engagement during the past week, and how well his or her weaker arm functioned as it relates to each item/activity on the test. It is composed of the following 2 subtests delivered in a structured interview format with the client or caregiver: (1) the AOU section and (2) the QOM section, where each is scored along a 5-point rating scale (0 to 5) with half points being assigned as well by the subject. A mean MAL score is calculated for both scales by adding the rating scores for each scale and dividing by the number of items asked. Higher scores indicate better ADL engagement. Participants may also be asked to watch a brief video.

TABLE 76-1
GENERAL SCORING DESCRIPTORS OF THE TWO MOTOR ACTIVITY LOG SUBSCALES
AMOUNT OF USE SUBTEST
0. Did not use weaker arm (not used).
1. Occasionally used weaker arm but very rarely (very rarely).
2. Sometimes used weaker arm but did the activity most of the time with my stronger arm (rarely).
3. Used weaker arm about half as much as before the stroke (half pre-stroke).
4. Used weaker arm almost as much as before the stroke (3/4 pre-stroke).
5. Used weaker arm as often as before the stroke (same as pre-stroke).
QUALITY OF MOVEMENT SUBTEST
0. Weaker arm was not used at all for the activity (not used).
1. Weaker arm was moved during that activity but was not helpful (very poor).
2. Weaker arm was of some use during that activity but needed some help from the stronger arm; moved very slowly or with difficulty (poor).
3. Weaker arm was used for that activity but the movements were slow or were made only with some effort (fair).
4. The movements made by my weaker arm for that activity were almost normal but not quite as fast or accurate as normal (almost normal).
5. The ability to use weaker arm for that activity was as good as before the stroke (normal).

Adapted from Taub, E., McCulloch, K., Uswatte, .G., & Morris, D. (2011). *Motor Activity Log (MAL) manual* (pp. 2-3). Birmingham, AL: UAB CI Therapy Research Group.

Permissions

The MAL is free to us in clinical practice and can be downloaded at the information that follows. To use in research or publication contact the authors of the measure. More information can be found in the following publication:

Taub, E., McCulloch, K., Uswatte, G., & Morris, D. (2011). *Motor Activity Log (MAL) manual*. Birmingham, AL: UAB CI Therapy Research Group.

Summary

POPULATION	Suspected arm/hand impairment
TYPE OF MEASURE	Structured interview questionnaire
WHAT IT ASSESSES	ADL abilities with affected arm
TIME	<20 minutes
COST	Free

Contact

Edward Taub, PhD

University of Alabama—Birmingham

Birmingham, Alabama

Web: www.uab.edu/cas/psychology/psy-fac/33-primary-faculty/63-dr-edward-taub

Examiner's manual: www.uab.edu/citherapy/images/pdf_files/CIT_Training_MAL_manual.pdf

www.uab.edu/citherapy/training-manuals-a-publications

Chapter 77: QuickDASH (Disability of the Arm, Shoulder and Hand) Outcome Measure

Description

The QuickDASH (Disability of the Arm, Shoulder and Hand) is a self-report questionnaire that assesses a person's perceived level of incapacity pertaining to disability of the arm, shoulder, and hand and is based on the 30-item DASH instrument, where each item on the QuickDASH was retained relative to key concepts of upper-limb functioning as well as the selection of the highest ranked items from the original according to their psychometric properties (Kennedy et al., 2013). The assessment explores the ability to perform certain activities as well as symptoms associated with arm, shoulder, and hand impairment and includes such items as (1) opening a tight or new jar; (2) doing heavy household chores (i.e. wash walls, floors); (3) carrying a shopping bag or briefcase; and (4) the presence or absence of tingling (pins and needles) in arm, shoulder, or hand, as well as interference with work or other activities due to injury. Each item of the QuickDASH is rated along a 5-point scale (1 to 5) of various responses (i.e., none to extreme or no difficulty to unable) and like the original assessment has 2 optional modules pertaining to work and sports/performing arts that have 4 items each. The assessment can be completed in less than 5 minutes with higher scores suggestive of greater impairment.

Psychometrics

During development, using data derived from 407 and 200 subjects with various upper extremity limb impairments, test-retest reliabilities were significant at r=0.94, while convergent construct validity ranged from 0.70 to 0.80 for the various domains, and correlation with change ranged from 0.35 to 0.39 (Beaton, Wright, & Katz, 2005). Whalley and Adams (2009) found that when used in an outpatient occupational therapy clinic, QuickDASH showed responsiveness to change as scores were 50.43 (mean) at baseline and 32.13 at discharge. Results of the QuickDASH using a cohort of 255 subjects before and after a physical therapy program determined that the minimum detectable change at the 90% confidence level was determined to be 12.85 points (Franchignoni et al., 2014). A study of 101 persons presenting to physical therapy found test-retest reliability to be r=0.90 with mean scores at baseline of 37.2 and 30.4 at follow up, whereas the correlation coefficients between change in scores with the Numeric Pain Rating Scale and the Global Rating of Change scale were

0.45 and 0.26, respectively (Mintken, Glynn, & Cleland, 2009). A study by Polson, Reid, McNair, and Larmer (2010) of 35 subjects recruited from private physiotherapy practice found mean scores for the QuickDASH at baseline were 37.7, which decreased to 18.5 at discharge or 6 weeks post-baseline, suggesting that the QuickDASH is a responsive questionnaire. A study of persons with Deputryn's syndrome found a statistically significant correlation between the preoperative QuickDASH score and the mean total range of movement at −0.33 (Budd, Larson, Chojnowski, & Shepstone, 2011).

Advantages

There is a good amount of research in support of the QuickDASH for use in clinical practice. The assessment is free to use in certain populations and administration time is less than 5 minutes. Based on the 30-item DASH, it retains only the strongest statistical items. The Institute for Work & Health maintains a website devoted to the QuickDASH measure where information can be found and downloaded. Access to a free online form as well as a score calculation service is also available.

Disadvantages

The QuickDASH is primarily composed of activity items that measure physical disability leaving low impact, non-activity items out. Thus it could be argued that the 11-item short form may not cover all relevant domains associated with arm, shoulder, and hand injury (Gummesson, Ward, & Atroshi, 2006).

Administration

The QuickDASH has clearly outlined instructions as well as scoring interpretations available. During assessment the client is asked to consider and rate each item using various self-perceived rating scales from 1 to 5 relative to issues associated with disability of the arm, shoulder, and hand, with particular regard for function and feeling. An optional sports/performing arts and work section can also be completed. Scoring employs the following algorithm:

$$\frac{[\,(\text{sum of responses}) - 1\,] \times 25}{n}$$

*n=number of response

Permission

The QuickDASH outcome measure is free to use in clinical practice, not-for-profit use, and non-commercial research. Any other use requires permission from the Institute for Work & Health, who holds the copyright to the assessment and can be contacted at the information following. More information can be found in the following journal article:

Gummesson, C., Ward, M., & Atroshi, I. (2006). The shortened Disabilities of the Arm, Shoulder and Hand questionnaire (QuickDASH): Validity and reliability based on responses within the full-length DASH. *BMC Musculoskeletal Disorders, 7*(44), 1-7.

Summary

POPULATION	Suspected shoulder, arm, or hand impairment
TYPE OF MEASURE	Self-report questionnaire
WHAT IT ASSESSES	Self-perceived level of performance
TIME	< 5 minutes
COST	Free

Contact

DASH Outcome Measures

Institute for Work & Health

481 University Avenue, Suite 800

Toronto, Ontario

Canada M5G 2E9

Phone: (416) 927-2027, ext. 2173

Email: dash@iwh.on.ca

Web: http://dash.iwh.on.ca/

CHAPTER 78: WOLF MOTOR FUNCTION TEST (WMFT)

Description

The Wolf Motor Function Test (WMFT), developed by Wolf et al. (1989) and later modified by Taub et al. (1998), is used to assess upper extremity function. The impairment-based test quantifies upper extremity movement and was initially designed to examine the effects of constraint-induced movement therapy for survivors of stroke and traumatic brain injury (TBI); thus the WMFT is particularly sensitive to the level of motor functioning characteristic of those types of conditions (Fritz, Blanton, Uswatte, Taub, & Wolf, 2009). The original form of the test consisted of 21 simple tasks sequenced according to the joint involved (i.e., shoulder to fingers) and level of difficulty (gross to fine motor skill), whereas the current version contains 17 tasks and comprises 3 parts: (1) timing, which is the speed at which the functional task can be completed, (2) functional ability and the movement quality when completing those tasks, and (3) the strength ability to lift against gravity. (Morris, Uswatte, Crago, Cook, & Taub, 2001; Whitall, Savin, Harris-Love, & McCombe Waller, 2006). Example items on the test include the following: (1) forearm to table (side), in which subject attempts to place his or her forearm on the table by abduction at the shoulder; (2) forearm to box (side), where the subject attempts to place his or her forearm on a box by abduction at the shoulder; (3) reach and retrieve (front), where the subject attempts to pull a 1-pound weight across the table by using elbow flexion and a cupped wrist; and (4) lift pencil (front), in which the subject attempts to pick up pencil by using 3-jaw chuck grasp (Taub, Morris, & Crago, 2011). The subject is allowed 2 minutes for each task and is scored along a 6-point ordinal scale from (1) does not attempt to (6) does attempt with movement that appears to be normal. Lower scores are indicative of decreased motor function. The WMFT takes less than 45 minutes to complete.

Psychometrics

Research by Morris et al. (2001) with 24 chronic hemiplegia subjects showed that inter-rater reliability was $r = 0.97$ or greater for performance time and 0.88 or greater for functional ability, whereas test-retest reliability was $r = 0.90$ for performance time and 0.95 for functional ability. Scores were also found to be stable over two test administrations, suggesting that the WMFT is an instrument with good inter-rater reliability, internal consistency, test-retest reliability, and adequate stability (Morris et al., 2001). Another study compared raters of videotape vs direct observation and found that inter-class correlation

coefficients for videotape vs direct observation ranged from 0.96 to 0.99 and test-retest reliability ranged from 0.97 to 0.99, concluding that videotaping was not necessary for accurate scoring. (Whitall et al., 2006). In order to clarify the meaning of scores obtained in both research and clinical settings, researchers attempted to quantify the standard error of measurement (SEM) and minimal detectable change (MDC) from data collected from 96 individuals with subacute stroke where they found that the performance time scores had an SEM of 0.2 seconds and an MDC of 0.7 seconds; however, in individual task timed items MDC ranged from only 1.0 second (turn-key in lock) to 3.4 seconds (Fritz et al., 2009). Overall, they concluded that when assessing the effect of a therapeutic intervention, if an individual experiences an amount of change equal to or greater than the MDC, then with a 95% confidence interval that margin of change is truly larger than measurement error and not a chance occurrence allowing researchers and clinicians to distinguish which results are actual differences vs which results are simply changes resulting from error or chance. (Fritz et al., 2009).

Advantages

A notable amount of literature exists that supports the use of the WMFT in practice and there are established normative scores for most age groups with increased performance times typically seen with increasing age. Also, when comparing upper extremity scores from the WMFT and the Fugl-Meyer Motor Assessment (FMA) researchers found a ceiling effect occurred in the FMA for the less-affected arm as well as low agreement, which was not found in the WMFT suggesting that the WMFT battery is an instrument sensitive to detecting change, even in a supposedly unaffected side (Wolf et al., 2001). Scores of the WMFT also have the ability to show if interventions improve motor performance over time as motor function is a known predictor of motor recovery in individuals after stroke (Wolf et al., 2001).

Disadvantages

The creators of the measure suggest that there is limited usefulness for patients with chronic stroke and TBI who are considered to be very low-functioning in terms of severity of motor deficit or for persons with acute or subacute stroke before spontaneous recovery has completed, as these populations are frequently only able to complete less than half of the items on the WMFT (Taub et al., 2011). Normative data for this crucial population is sparse as well, evidenced by the difficulty in calculating meaningful summary scores when only attempting the WMFT, thus a reduced or graded version of the WMFT was developed for this population. However, evidence pertaining to it is, as of yet, limited (Taub et al., 2011).

Administration

The WMFT includes 15 function-based tasks and 2 strength-based tasks (2 minutes each) that are scored on a 6-point ordinal scale from (1) does not attempt to (6) does attempt with movement that appears to be normal. Lower scores are indicative of lower functioning. The assessment follows a standardized protocol and the manual includes detailed task descriptions, starting positions for subjects and equipment, timing procedures (including criteria for determining completion points), verbal instructions to be read to subjects, and scoring criteria (Morris et al., 2001). Several pieces of equipment are needed and include tables, a chair, box, free-weights, can, pencil, paperclip, checkers, cards, key lock with the key, towel, basket, and a dynamometer.

TABLE 78-1
ACTIVITIES ON THE WOLF MOTOR FUNCTION TEST
• Reach and retrieve
• Lift can
• Lift pencil
• Lift paper clip
• Stack checkers
• Grip strength
• Turn key in lock
• Fold a towel

Adapted from Taub, E., Morris, D., & Crago, J. (2011). *Wolf Motor Function Test (WMFT) manual* (p. 26). Birmingham, AL: UAB CI Therapy Research Group.

Permissions

The WMFT is free to use in clinical practice and a training manual and supporting publications can be found at the University of Alabama—Birmingham Constraint Induced Movement Therapy website that follows. A videotape of the model can also be obtained by contacting Dr. Taub as well as a template for the assessment for an additional fee of $25. To use in research, publication, or practice contact its creators. More information can be found in the following journal article:

Wolf, S., Catlin, P., Ellis, M., Archer, A., Morgan, B., & Piacento, A. (2001). Assessing the Wolf Motor Function Test as an outcome measure for research with patients after stroke. *Stroke, 32*(7), 1635-1639.

Summary

POPULATION	Stroke; TBI
TYPE OF MEASURE	Activity-based rating scale
WHAT IT ASSESSES	Upper extremity motor performance
TIME	<45 minutes
COST	Free

Contact

Edward Taub, PhD

Department of Psychology

University of Alabama—Birmingham

Birmingham, Alabama

Constraint induced movement therapy website/manual: www.uab.edu/citherapy/training-manuals-a-publications

Steven L. Wolf, PhD

Emory University

Center for Rehabilitation Medicine

Atlanta, Georgia

REFERENCES

Ames, E. (2014). Scoring the MHQ. University of Michigan Medical School. Retrieved from http://mhq.lab.medicine.umich.edu/scoring-the-mhq

Atroshi, I., Gummesson, C., Andersson, B., Dahlgren, E., & Johansson, A. (2000). The Disabilities of the Arm, Shoulder and Hand (DASH) outcome questionnaire: Reliability and validity of the Swedish version evaluated in 176 patients. *Acta Orthopaedica Scandinavica, 71*(6), 613-618.

Beaton, D., Katz, J., Fossel, A., Wright, J., Tarasuk V., & Bombardier, C. (2001). Measuring the whole or the parts? Validity, reliability, and responsiveness of the Disabilities of the Arm, Shoulder and Hand outcome measure in different regions of the upper extremity. *Journal of Hand Therapy, 14*(2), 128-146.

Beaton, D., Wright, J., & Katz, K. (2005). Development of the QuickDASH: Comparison of three item-reduction approaches. *Journal of Bone and Joint Surgery, 87*(5), 1038-1046.

Budd, H., Larson, D., Chojnowski, A., & Shepstone, L. (2011). The QuickDASH score: A patient-reported outcome measure for Dupuytren's surgery. *Journal of Hand Therapy, 24*(1), 15-20.

Chae, J., Labatia, I., & Yang, G. (2003). Upper limb motor function in hemiparesis: Concurrent validity of the Arm Motor Ability Test. *American Journal of Physical Medicine and Rehabilitation, 82*(1), 1-8.

Chatterjee, J., & Price, P. (2009). Comparative responsiveness of the Michigan Hand Outcomes Questionnaire and the Carpal Tunnel Questionnaire after carpal tunnel release. *Journal of Hand Surgery, 34A*, 273-280.

Chung, B., & Morris, S. (2014). Reliability and internal validity of the Michigan Hand Questionnaire. Annals of Plastic Surgery, 73(4), 385-389.

Chung, K. Pillsbury, M., Walters, M., & Hayward, R. (1998). Reliability and validity testing of the Michigan Hand Outcomes Questionnaire. *Journal of Hand Surgery-American, 23*(4), 575-587.

Franchignoni, F., Giordano, A., Sartorio, F., Vercelli, S., Pascariello, B., & Ferriero, G. (2010). Suggestions for refinement of the Disabilities of the Arm, Shoulder and Hand Outcome Measure (DASH): A factor analysis and Rasch validation study. *Archives of Physical Medicine and Rehabilitation, 91*(9), 1370-1377.

Franchignoni, F., Vercelli, S., Giordano, A., Sartorio, F., Bravini, E., & Ferriero, G. (2014). Minimal clinically important difference of the Disabilities of the Arm, Shoulder and Hand Outcome Measure (DASH) and its shortened version (QuickDASH). *Journal of Orthopaedic & Sports Physical Therapy, 44*(1), 30-39.

Fritz, S., Blanton, B., Uswatte, G., Taub, E., & Wolf, S. (2009). Minimal detectable change scores for the Wolf Motor Function Test. *Neurorehabilitation and Neural Repair, 23*(7), 662-667.

Gummesson, C., Ward, M., & Atroshi, I. (2006). The shortened Disabilities of the Arm, Shoulder and Hand questionnaire (QuickDASH): Validity and reliability based on responses within the full-length DASH. *BMC Musculoskeletal Disorders, 7*(44), 1-7.

Horng, Y., Lin, M., Feng, C., Huang, C., Wu, H., & Wang J. (2010). Responsiveness of the Michigan Hand Outcomes Questionnaire and the Disabilities of the Arm, Shoulder and Hand Questionnaire in patients with hand injury. *Journal of Hand Surgery, 35,* 430e6.

Impens, A., Chung, K., Maya, M., Buch, H., Schiopu, E., Kotsis, S.,... Seibold, J. (n.d.) Validation of the Michigan Hand Outcomes Questionnaire (MHQ) in systemic sclerosis. University of Michigan, Ann Arbor. Retrieved from www.med.umich.edu/scleroderma/images/MHQValidationAbstract.pdf

Kennedy, C., Beaton, D., Smith, P., Van Eerd, D., Tang, K., Inrig, T.,... Couban, R. (2013). Measurement properties of the QuickDASH (Disabilities of the Arm, Shoulder and Hand) outcome measure and cross cultural adaptations of the QuickDASH: A systematic review. *Quality of Life Research, 22*(9), 2509-2547

Koh, C. L., Hsueh, I. P., Wang, W. C., Sheu, C. F., Yu, T. Y., Wang, C. H., & Hsieh, C. L. (2006). Validation of the Action Research Arm Test using item response theory in patients after stroke. *Journal of Rehabilitation Medicine, 38,* 375-380.

Kopp, B., Kunkel, A., Flor, H., Platz, T., Rose, U., Mauritz, K.,...Taub, E. (1997). The Arm Motor Ability Test: Reliability, validity, and sensitivity to change of an instrument for assessing disabilities in activities of daily living. *Archives of Physical Medicine and Rehabilitation, 78*(6), 615-620.

Lin, K. C., Hsieh, Y. W., & Chang, W. Y. (2010). Responsiveness and validity of three dexterous function measures in stroke rehabilitation. *Journal of Rehabilitation Research & Development, 47*(6), 563–572.

Lyle, R. C. (1981). A performance test for assessment of upper limb function in physical rehabilitation treatment and research. *International Journal of Rehabilitation Research, 4*(4), 483-492.

McCulloch, K., Cook III, E. W., Fleming, W., Novack, T., & Taub, E. (1988). Reliable test of upper extremity ADL function (abstract). *Archives of Physical Medicine and Rehabilitation, 69,* 755. In B. Kopp, A. Kunkel, H. Flor, T. Platz, U. Rose, K. Mauritz, K.,...E. Taub. (1997). The Arm Motor Ability Test: Reliability, validity, and sensitivity to change of an instrument for assessing disabilities in activities of daily living. *Archives of Physical Medicine and Rehabilitation, 78*(6), 615-620.

McDonnell, M. (2008). Action Research Arm Test. *Australian Journal of Physiotherapy, 54,* 220.

Mintken, P., Glynn, P., & Cleland, J. (2009). Psychometric properties of the shortened disabilities of the Arm, Shoulder, and Hand Questionnaire (QuickDASH) and Numeric Pain Rating Scale in patients with shoulder pain. *Journal of Shoulder and Elbow Surgery, 18,* 920-926.

Morris, D., Uswatte, G., Crago, J., Cook III, E., & Taub, E. (2001). The reliability of the Wolf Motor Function Test for assessing upper extremity function after stroke. *Archives of Physical Medicine and Rehabilitation, 82*(6), 750-755.

Nordin, A., Alt-Murphy, M., & Danielsson, A. (2014). Intra-rater and inter-rater reliability at the item level of the Action Research Arm Test for patients with stroke. *Journal of Rehabilitation Medicine, 46*(8), 738-745.

O'Dell, M. W., Kim, G., Rivera, L., Fieo, R., Christos, P., Polistena, C., ...Gorga, D. (2013). A psychometric evaluation of the Arm Motor Ability Test. *Journal of Rehabilitation Medicine, 45*(6), 519-527.

Platz, T., Pinkowski, C., van Wijck, F., Kim, I., di Bella, P., & Johnson, G. (2005). Reliability and validity of arm function assessment with standardized guidelines for the Fugl-Meyer Test, Action Research Arm Test and Box and Block Test: A multicentre study. *Clinical Rehabilitation, 19*(4), 404-411.

Polson, K., Reid, D., McNair, P., & Larmer, P. (2010). Responsiveness, minimal importance difference and minimal detectable change scores of the shortened Disability Arm Shoulder Hand (QuickDASH) questionnaire. *Manual Therapy, 15*(4), 404-407.

Poole, J., Gonzales, I., & Tedesco, T. (2010). Self-reports of hand function in persons with diabetes. *Occupational Therapy in Health Care, 24*(3), 239-248.

Taub, E., McCulloch, K., Uswatte, G., & Morris, D. (2011). *Motor Activity Log (MAL) manual.* Birmingham, AL: UAB CI Therapy Research Group.

Taub, E., Morris, D., & Crago, J. (2011). *Wolf Motor Function Test (WMFT) manual.* Birmingham, AL: UAB CI Therapy Research Group.

Uswatte, G., Taub, E., Morris, D., Light, K., & Thompson, P. (2006). The Motor Activity Log-28: Assessing daily use of the hemiparetic arm after stroke. *Neurology, 67,* 1189–1194.

Uswatte, G., Taub, E., Morris, D., Vignolo, M., & McCulloch, K. (2005). Reliability and validity of the upper-extremity Motor Activity Log-14 for measuring real-world arm use. *Stroke, 36*(11), 2493-2496.

van der Lee, J., Beckerman, H., Knol, D., de Vet, H., & Bouter, L. (2004). Clinimetric properties of the Motor Activity Log for the assessment of arm use in hemiparetic patients. *Stroke, 35*(6), 1410-1414.

van der Lee, J. H., Roorda, L. D., Beckerman, H., Lankhorst, G. J., & Bouter, L. M. (2002). Improving the Action Research Arm Test: A unidimensional hierarchical scale. *Clinical Rehabilitation, 16,* 646-653.

van Kampen, D., Willems, W. J., van Beers, L., Castelein, R. Scholtes, V., & Terwee, C. (2013). Determination and comparison of the smallest detectable change (SDC) and the minimal important change (MIC) of four-shoulder patient-reported outcome measures (PROMs). *Journal of Orthopaedic Surgery and Research, 8*(1), 40-48.

Weinstock-Zlotnick, G., Page, C., Wolff, A., & Ghomwari, H. (2012). Comparing the responsiveness of the Disabilities of the Arm, Shoulder, and Hand Questionnaire (DASH), Michigan Hand Outcomes Questionnaire (MHQ), and Patient Rated Wrist/Hand Evaluation (PRWHE) for hand fractures. *Journal of Hand Therapy, 25*(4), e6.

Whalley, K., & Adams, J. (2009). The longitudinal validity of the quick and full version of the Disability of the Arm, Shoulder and Hand Questionnaire in musculoskeletal hand outpatients. *Hand Therapy, 14*(1), 22-25.

Whitall, J., Savin, S., Harris-Love, M., & McCombe Waller, S. (2006). Psychometric properties of a Modified Wolf Motor Function Test for people with mild and moderate upper-extremity hemiparesis *Archives of Physical Medicine and Rehabilitation, 87*(5), 656-660.

Wolf, S., Catlin, P., Ellis, M., Archer, A., Morgan, B., & Piacentino, A. (2001). Assessing the Wolf Motor Function test as outcome measure for research in subjects after stroke. *Stroke, 32*(7), 1635-1639.

Yozbatiran, N., Der-Yeghiaian, L., & Cramer, S. C. (2008). A standardized approach to performing the Action Research Arm Test. *Neurorehabilitation and Neural Repair, 22*(1), 78-90.

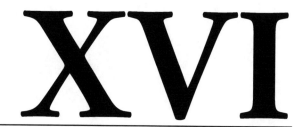

Muscle Tone and Spasticity

CHAPTER 79: MODIFIED ASHWORTH SCALE

Description

The modified Ashworth Scale is designed to measure an individual's muscle tone, which is generally defined as the resistance of muscle as it is being passively lengthened or stretched and occurs as a result of the intrinsic synergies of muscle, tendon, and connective tissue as well as the active contraction of muscle (Blackburn, van Vliet, & Mockett, 2002). As increased resistance to passive stretch (hypertonus) is common in a number of disorders, such as stroke or cerebral palsy, its assessment and management is a major component of many rehabilitation protocols and the modified Ashworth Scale quantifies that resistance (Blackburn et al., 2002). The Ashworth Scale was originally developed by Ashworth in 1964 as a taxonomy to assess the anti-spastic effects of carisoprodol in multiple sclerosis subjects. Through his research he described a 5-point ordinal scale for grading the muscle resistance he encountered when moving a limb through the range of motion during passive stretching of the muscle. Relative to spasticity, the assessment grades the subject's level of muscle tone as follows: (0) normal muscle tone; (1) slight increase in muscle tone, "catch" when limb moved; (2) more marked increase in muscle tone but limb is easily flexed; (3) considerable increase in muscle tone; and (4) limb rigid in flexion or extension. The Ashworth Scale was modified by Bohannon and Smith (1987) by adding the grade of 1+ as well as slightly modifying definitions of muscle tone to render the scale more discrete. The observational assessment takes less than 5 minutes to complete as the person is graded on the ability of his or her limb to move passively through the range of motion.

Psychometrics

Bohannon and Smith (1987) found inter-rater reliability of manual testing of elbow flexor muscle spasticity of 30 patients with intracranial lesions to be r=0.87. Comparing the original and modified assessments using Kappa values, which indicate the measure of agreement corrected for chance (1.0=total agreement between raters, 0=no agreement), Haas, Bergstrom, Jamous, and Bennie (1996) found Kappa values ranged between 0.21 and 0.61 (mean 0.37) with the original scale being slightly more reliable though not statistically significant. A study of 20 patients with chronic spinal cord injury found that intra-rater reliability ranged from fair to almost perfect (0.20 to

1.0) and differed significantly between raters and inter-rater reliability was poor-to-moderate (0.60) for all muscle groups. Inter-session reliability for a single rater was found to be only fair-to-good (0.40 to 0.75) for all muscle groups (Craven & Morris, 2010). While a study by Li, Wu, and Li (2014), using 2 raters, found that kappa values were 0.66 and 0.69 for elbow flexors and 0.48 and 0.48 for plantar flexors in study of 51 subjects with hemiplegic stroke, suggesting that alternative or complimentary measures be considered in conjunction with the modified Ashworth Scale.

Advantages

Both the original and modified versions of the Ashworth Scale are relatively simple and easy assessments to administer and there is a fair amount of research in support of their use in clinical practice. A unique aspect of both versions is that they allow the clinician to isolate the muscle being tested and each muscle test can be completed in only a couple of minutes. Information purveyed from results can also be used to gauge effects of interventions as well as establishing a baseline assessment of an individual's muscle tone.

Disadvantages

Lack of agreement between research studies have been noted, as problems have arisen with the ability to reproduce adequate intra- and inter-rater reliability results (those >0.85) in many studies. Others have noted that the modified Ashworth Scale scoring remains ambiguous and is less reliable than the original version of the assessment and there is some research to suggest that the assessments appear to be more reliable for the upper extremities. (Pandyan et al., 1999). There may be several reasons for this, such as the assessment's construct or that resistance to passive movement is a complex measure that may be influenced by many factors.

Administration

During assessment the subject is placed in the supine position. If testing a muscle that primarily flexes, the joint is placed in a maximally flexed position and moved to a position of maximal extension over a 1 second count of "one thousand one," while keeping in mind to grade the ability of the joint to move through the passive range of motion relative to the patient's muscle tone while considering the inclusion/exclusion criteria of the levels of the scale.

TABLE 79-1

RANK DESCRIPTORS OF THE MODIFIED ASHWORTH SCALE

GRADE	DESCRIPTION
0	No increase in muscle tone.
1	Slight increase in tone; evidenced by a catch or minimum resistance at the end of range of motion when moved through flexion or extension.
1+	Slight increase in tone; evidenced also by a slight catch, followed by minimal resistance throughout the remainder (less than half) of the range of movement.
2	More marked increase in muscle tone through most of the range of movement, but affected part(s) are easily moved.
3	Considerable increase in muscle tone; passive movement difficult.
4	Affected part is rigid in flexion or extension.

Adapted from Bohannon, R., & Smith, M. (1987). Inter-rater reliability of a modified Ashworth Scale of muscle spasticity. *Physical Therapy, 67,* 206-207.

Permissions

The Ashworth scales are free to use in private practice and are wholly contained in several articles as well as other relevant places. Their use in research or publication can be obtained by contacting the creators or where published. More information can be found in the following journal articles:

Ashworth, B. (1964). Preliminary trial of carisoprodol in multiple sclerosis. *Practitioner, 192,* 540-542.

Bohannon, R., & Smith, M. (1987). Inter-rater reliability of a Modified Ashworth Scale of muscle spasticity. *Physical Therapy, 67,* 206-207.

Summary

POPULATION	Muscle tone anomalies; cerebrovascular accident; cerebral palsy; general
TYPE OF MEASURE	Hierarchical rating scale
WHAT IT ASSESSES	Level of muscle tone; spasticity
TIME	<5 minutes
COST	Free

Contact

Richard W. Bohannon, PT, EdD

Department of Kinesiology

University of Connecticut

Storrs, Connecticut

CHAPTER 80: TARDIEU SCALE OF SPASTICITY

Description

The Tardieu Scale of Spasticity is a commonly used measurement of spasticity that explicitly measures the velocity-dependent aspect of the spasticity phenomenon as a limb is moved through the range of motion as opposed to simply measuring resistance to passive movement like the Ashworth Scale and others. The scale was developed by Tardieu, Shentoub, and Delarue (1954). Upon observing the angle of movement at relaxation and upon stretching of the muscle, they suggested that the differences between those two angles could determine the presence of soft tissue changes. The Tardieu Scale was modified by Held et al. (1969) where they improved upon original definitions of speed, positioning of the limb tested, and when the assessment should take place. A further revision took place in 1999 by Boyd et al. that included standardized limb placement as well as limb positioning and speed of movement (Haugh, Pandyan, & Johnson, 2006). Limb speed or velocity are hallmarks of the Tardieu assessment and the data collection procedure involves the use of two speeds of passive movement (one very slow, the other as fast as possible) as well as recording the angle at which a clear catch in the passive movement is felt, thus quality of muscle reaction and angle of muscle reaction are documented (Mehrholz et al., 2005). The assessment across each joint tested takes less than 5 minutes and angles are measured using a goniometer.

Psychometrics

Researchers found exact agreement (i.e., 1.0) between laboratory and Tardieu measurement in identifying the presence or absence of spasticity in the elbow flexors and ankle plantar flexors which contrasted with the Ashworth Scale's 63% agreement. Similar results were found for identifying the presence or absence of contracture with 94% agreement for the Tardieu scale (Patrick & Ada, 2006). A study of 4 experienced therapists using 30 traumatic brain injury (TBI) subjects who were measured across 12 muscle groups found intra-rater reliability of the modified Ashworth Scale to be only moderate to good (0.47 to 0.62), whereas the modified Tardieu Scale was considered moderate to very good, and excluding shoulder external rotation at $r = 0.53$, scores ranged from $r = 0.65$ to 0.87 (Mehrholz et al., 2005). The same study found that overall, inter-rater reliability (i.e., the level of agreement between raters) was considered to be only poor to moderate, ranging from to $r = 0.29$ to 0.53 (Mehrholz et al., 2005). Another study by 2 physiotherapists who performed

Tardieu Scale measurements in elbow flexors of 13 stroke patients found goniometry, test-retest and inter-rater reliability to be 0.86 and 0.66, respectively (Paulis, Horemans, Brouwer, & Stam, 2011). Exploring the two joint angles measured by goniometer, which includes the R1 angle, which is the *angle of catch* after a fast velocity stretch and the R2 angle, defined as the passive joint range of movement following a slow velocity stretch, a study of 91 adult subjects with stroke found intra-rater agreement for elbow flexors for catch R1, R2, and R2-R1 to be $r = 0.99$, 0.98, and 0.99, respectively (Singh, Joshua, Ganeshan, & Suresh, 2011). The same study found that intra-rater agreement for plantar flexors was also good for R1 ($r = 0.99$), R2 (0.99), and R2-R1 (0.91). However, a similar by Li et al. (2014) using the same elbow flexors and plantar flexors found inter-rater and intra-rater agreement to be between $r = 0.58$ to 0.89 for R1 and R2 and between 0.63 to 0.70 for R1-R2 among a sample of 50 subjects post-hemiplegic stroke.

Advantages

There is a fair amount of research in support of its use in clinical practice and it is free to use. The Tardieu Scale is unique in its ability to test the velocity-dependent aspect of spasticity, not simply passive movement through the range of motion like other measures.

Disadvantages

Tardieu Scale administration can be somewhat difficult as exact movements and limb measurements are required using a goniometer. There has also been a lack of stability of the assessment, with several research studies noting low inter-rater reliability scores that may be occurring as a result of an overgeneralization of the scale (i.e., an inability to adequately test all body parts as it would intend). For example, Ben-Shabat, Palit, Fini, Winter, and Holland (2013) found that inter-class correlation coefficients were moderately to highly reliable for the R1 and R2 measurements of affected hamstrings, gastrocnemius, rectus femoris, and soleus with a mean of 0.83, while poor reliability was found for all measurements of the affected adductors (0.48 to 0.59) and quadriceps (0.35 to 0.37). Mehrholz et al. (2005) also found problems with the scoring range of the scale where they noted that with the current 5-point scale a score of 3 or 4 was rarely determined in their study of 30 TBI patients. They argue that a scale of 3 or 4 max might be more appropriate to fit the clinical spectrum of spasticity at proximal and distal joints where the problems were noted.

Administration

The Tardieu scale is always performed at the same time of day and with the subject's body in a constant position for a given limb (Haugh et al., 2005). Upper limb assessment is completed in the sitting position and lower limb assessment in the supine position (Haugh et al., 2005). Other joints, particularly the neck, need remain in a constant position throughout the test and between subtests (Haugh et al., 2005). For each muscle group, reaction to stretch is rated at a specified stretch to velocity where the angle of muscle reaction is also measured at the catch. Different velocity to stretch definitions are used. *V1* is as slow as possible and is used to measure the passive range of motion; *V2* is the speed of the limb segment falling under gravity and is used to rate spasticity; and *V3* is as fast as possible, and is considered faster than the rate of the natural drop of the limb under gravity and is also used to rate spasticity (Haugh et al., 2005). Scoring includes the following as well as goniometry angular measurements:

TABLE 80-1
SCORING GRADES OF THE MODIFIED TARDIEU SCALE
0. No resistance throughout the course of the passive movement.
1. Slight resistance throughout the course of the passive movement with no clear catch at precise angle.
2. Clear catch at precise angle, interrupting the passive movement, followed by release.
3. Fatigable clonus (5 to 10 seconds when maintaining pressure) occurring at precise angle.
4. Indefatigable clonus (4 to 10 seconds when maintaining pressure) occurring at precise angle.
Adapted from Yam, W. K. L., & Leung, M. S. M. (2006). Interrater reliability of modified Ashworth Scale and modified Tardieu Scale in children with spastic cerebral palsy. *Journal of Child Neurology, 21*(12), 1032.

Permissions

The Tardieu Scale is located in the public domain, is free to use in clinical practice, and can be found in its entirety in several journal articles. More information can be found in the following articles:

Tardieu. G., Shentoub, S., & Delarue, R. (1954). A la recherché d'une technique de mesure de la spasticite. *Revue Neurologique, 91*, 143-44.

Haugh, A., Pandyan, A., & Johnson, G. (2006). A systematic review of the Tardieu Scale for the measurement of spasticity. *Disability and Rehabilitation, 28*(15), 899-907.

Summary

POPULATION	Muscle tone anomalies; cerebrovascular accident; cerebral palsy; general
TYPE OF MEASURE	Hierarchical rating scale
WHAT IT ASSESSES	Level of muscle tone; spasticity
TIME	<5 minutes
COST	Free

Contact

Copyright Clearance Center

222 Rosewood Drive

Danvers, MA 01923

Phone: (855) 239-3415

E-mail: info@copyright.com

Web: www.copyright.com

REFERENCES

Ashworth, B. (1964). Preliminary trial of carisoprodal in multiple sclerosis. *Practitioner, 192*, 540-542.

Ben-Shabat, E., Palit, M., Fini, N., Winter, A., & Holland, A. (2011). Intra- and interrater reliability of the modified Tardieu Scale for the assessment of lower limb spasticity in adults with neurologic injuries. *Archives of Physical Medicine and Rehabilitation, 94*, 2494-2501

Blackburn, M., van Vliet, P., & Mockett, S (2002). Reliability of measurements obtained with the Modified Ashworth Scale in the lower extremities of people with stroke. *Physical Therapy, 82*, 25-34.

Bohannon, R., & Smith, M. (1987). Interrater reliability of a Modified Ashworth Scale of muscle spasticity. *Physical Therapy, 67*, 206-207.

Craven, B., & Morris, A. (2010). Modified Ashworth Scale reliability for measurement of lower extremity spasticity among patients with SCI. *Spinal Cord, 48*, 207–213.

Haas, B., Bergstrom, E., Jamous, A., & Bennie, A. (1996). The inter rater reliability of the original and of the Modified Ashworth Scale for the assessment of spasticity in patients with spinal cord injury. *Spinal Cord, 34*, 560-564.

Haugh, A. B., Pandyan, A., & Johnson, G. (2006). A systematic review of the Tardieu Scale for the measurement of spasticity. *Disability and Rehabilitation, 28*(15), 899-907.

Li, F., Wu, Y., & Li, X. (2014). Test-retest reliability and inter-rater reliability of the Modified Tardieu Scale and the Modified Ashworth Scale in hemiplegic patients with stroke. *European Journal of Physical Rehabilitation and Medicine, 50*(1), 9-15.

Mehrholz, J., Wagner, K., Meissner, D., Grundmann, K., Zange, C., Koch, R., & Pohl, M. (2005). Reliability of the Modified Tardieu Scale and the Modified Ashworth Scale in adult patients with severe brain injury: A comparison study. *Clinical Rehabilitation, 19*(7), 751-759.

Pandyan, A., Johnson, G., Price, C., Curless, R., Barnes, M., & Rodgers H. (1999). A review of the properties and limitations of the Ashworth and modified Ashworth Scales as measures of spasticity. *Clinical Rehabilitation, 13*, 373–383.

Patrick, E., & Ada, L. (2006). The Tardieu Scale differentiates contracture from spasticity whereas the Ashworth Scale is confounded by it. *Clinical Rehabilitation, 20*(2), 173-182.

Paulis, W., Horemans, H., Brouwer, B., & Stam, H. (2011). Excellent test–retest and inter-rater reliability for Tardieu Scale measurements with inertial sensors in elbow flexors of stroke patients. *Gait and Posture 33*, 185–189.

Singh, P., Joshua, A. M., Ganeshan, S., & Suresh, S. (2011). Intra-rater reliability of the modified Tardieu Scale to quantify spasticity in elbow flexors and ankle plantar flexors in adult stroke subjects. *Annals of Indian Academy of Neurology, 14*(1), 23–26.

Tardieu. G., Shentoub, S., & Delarue, R. (1954). A la recherché d'une technique de mesure de la spasticite. *Revue Neurologique, 91*, 143-144.

Yam, W. K. L., & Leung, M. S. M. (2006). Interrater reliability of Modified Ashworth Scale and Modified Tardieu Scale in children with spastic cerebral palsy. *Journal of Child Neurology, 21*(12), 1031-1035.

XVII

Occupational Performance

Bortnick, K.
Occupational Therapy Assessments for Older Adults: 100 Instruments for
Measuring Occupational Performance (pp. 237-260).
© 2017 Taylor & Francis Group.

CHAPTER 81: ASSESSMENT OF LIFE HABITS (LIFE-H)

Description

The Assessment of Life Habits (LIFE-H) is a global measure designed to assess the quality of social participation of people with disabilities and its effect on occupational performance and is based on the Disability Creation Process (DCP) model by Fougeyrollas et al. (1989) as well as the Classification of Functioning and Disabilities (ICF) of the World Health Organization (WHO), which argue that as social beings, participation is necessary for health and well-being. Completed as either a self-report or proxy questionnaire, items are grouped into 12 broad categories that include such examinations as nutrition, mobility, and employment (Fougeyrollas & Noreau, 2003). The assessment contains 77 items where each is considered with regard to 3 aspects of performance: (1) the level of accomplishment a person feels he or she has attained scored as no difficulty, with difficulty, accomplished by a proxy, not accomplished, or not applicable; (2) the type of assistance needed for each life habit scored as no assistance, assistive device, adaptation, or human assistance; and (3) the subject's level of satisfaction he or she feels regarding the way each life habit is completed, which is scored as very dissatisfied, dissatisfied, more or less satisfied, satisfied, or very satisfied. Example items include undertaking vocational training (trade school, university, community college); doing major household tasks (spring cleaning, painting, major repairs, etc.); and dressing and undressing the lower half of the body, which includes clothing, accessories and the choice of clothes (Fougeyrollas & Noreau, 2003). LIFE-H generates several scores according to unique algorithms and can be completed in less than 40 minutes.

TABLE 81-1
DOMAINS OF THE ASSESSMENT OF LIFE HABITS MEASURE
1. Nutrition
2. Responsibility
3. Fitness
4. Interpersonal relationships
5. Personal care
6. Community life
7. Communication
8. Education
9. Housing
10. Employment
11. Mobility
12. Recreation

Adapted from Noreau, L., Desrosiers, J., Robichaud, L., Fougeyrollas, P., Rochette, A., & Viscogliosi, C. (2004). Measuring social participation: Reliability of the LIFE-H in older adults with disabilities. *Disability & Rehabilitation, 26*(6), 348

Psychometrics

A study by Noreau, Desrosiers, Robichaud, Fougeyrollas, Rochette, & Viscogliosi (2004) found overall excellent test–retest reliability excluding the employment and education subscales (r = 0.95, range: 0.91 to 0.98), as well as very good inter-rater reliability (r = 0.89, range: 0.80 to 0.93). The same study found that the test–retest intra-class correlation coefficients of the participation total score and its two sub-scores had excellent reliability as well for most life domains (range: 0.79 to 0.93) with the exception of interpersonal relationships, which showed only moderate reliability at 0.60. A structured review by Figueiredo, Korner-Bitensky, Rochette, and Desrosiers (2010) identified 11 cerebrovascular-accident-specific studies where test-retest reliabilities ranged from r = 0.80 to 0.95, whereas the inter-rater reliability range varied between 0.64 and 0.91. Furthermore, the agreement between client and proxy scores was 0.73 to 0.82. Finally, it was determined that correlations between the LIFE-H sub-scores and the Functional Independence Measure were significant at 6 months, ranging from 0.71 to 0.88 and moderate to significant at 2 weeks post-stroke (0.57 to 0.85). Desrosiers et al. (2004) established the validity of the LIFE-H by comparing it with the Craig Handicap Assessment and Reporting Technique (CHART) and the Community Integration Questionnaire (CIQ) among spinal cord and traumatic brain injury populations where results showed that the correlations with the CHART varied from 0.76 (physical independence), 0.36 (occupation), 0.33 (mobility), and 0.14 (social integration), while correlations with the CIQ were more homogeneous (0.43 to 0.83).

Advantages

There is a good amount of research in support of its use in clinical practice. The measure is also available as a short form, 16-item version, or a long form designed for in-depth assessment of specific domains of social participation. LIFE-H is based on the DCP model as well as the ICF by the WHO, which is becoming a more important construct relative to occupational therapy.

Disadvantages

Noreau et al. (2004) found a lack of observed variability of data for the interpersonal relationships domain, which may be a limiting factor relative to the value of the social roles sub-scale. Poulin & Desrosiers (2009) also found the same phenomenon during their study in which most participants scored near the maximum value of the scale (9), suggesting that the domain might not be a good fit or interpersonal relationships may be difficult to quantify.

Administration

The LIFE-H evaluates level of occupational performance (i.e., daily activities and social roles) by considering the degree of difficulty and the type of assistance a person may need to perform activities of daily living and instrumental activities of daily living. Scoring involves adding up the

number of applicable life habits for each domain which are then put through a formula to derive a score along a scale from 0 to 9, where 0 indicates total handicap (i.e., the activity is not accomplished) and 9, which indicates optimal occupational performance (meaning the activity is accomplished) (Desrosiers et al., 2004). The examiner's manual contains detailed instructions for administration, scoring, and referenced norms.

TABLE 81-2
EXAMPLE LEVEL OF ACCOMPLISHMENT SCORING (0 TO 9)
0. Activity not accomplished
1. Accomplished with substitution
2. Accomplished with difficulty, required human assistance, technical aid, or adaptation
3. Accomplished with difficulty, human assistance
4. Accomplished with no difficulty, required human assistance, technical aid, or adaptation
5. Accomplished with no difficulty, required human assistance
6. Accomplished with difficulty, technical aid or adaptation
7. Accomplished with difficulty
8. Accomplished with no difficulty, technical aid, or adaptation
9. Accomplished with no difficulty
Adapted from Desrosiers, J., Noreau, L., Robichaud, L., Fougeyrollas, P., Rochette, A., & Viscogliosi, C. (2004). Validity of the assessment of life habits in older adults. *Journal of Rehabilitation Medicine, 36*(4), 179.

Permissions

The LIFE-H assessment can be purchased from the International Network on the Disability Creation Process (INDCP) website. It comes in several versions and prices vary from $2 to $35. Permission to use in research or for commercial purposes can also be obtained by contacting the INDCP. More information can be found in the following research article:

Desrosiers, J., Noreau, L., Robichaud, L., Fougeyrollas, P., Rochette, A., & Viscogliosi, C. (2004). Validity of the assessment of life habits in older adults. *Journal of Rehabilitation Medicine, 36*(4), 177-182.

Summary

POPULATION	General
TYPE OF MEASURE	Self-report or proxy questionnaire
WHAT IT ASSESSES	Level of social participation
TIME	< 5 minutes
COST	Free

Contact

International Network on the Disability Creation Process

525, boulevard Wilfrid-Hamel Est, Local A-08

Québec, Canada, G1M 2S8

Phone: (418) 529-9141

Web: www.ripph.qc.ca/node/1195

Chapter 82: Canadian Occupational Performance Measure (COPM)

Description

The Canadian Occupational Performance Measure (COPM) is a standardized assessment that is delivered through a semi-structured interview as well as a questionnaire/rating scale designed to assess a client's self-perception of occupational performance and satisfaction with that performance over time. It is based on the Canadian Model of Occupational Performance and is intended to help clients identify, prioritize, and evaluate important issues they encounter in occupational performance (Law et al., 2011). Through discussion, the client first identifies occupational performance issues that he or she would like to work on and then ranks each item (1 to 10) relative to their importance to the individual for the following general categories:

1. Self-care, which includes the following:
   a. Personal care
   b. Functional mobility
   c. Community management
2. Productivity, which is composed of the following:
   a. Paid/unpaid work
   b. Household management
   c. Play/school
3. Leisure, which is further delineated into the following subcategories:
   a. Quiet recreation
   b. Active recreation
   c. Socialization.

The next step of the assessment involves the identification of the 5 most important problems, which are then rated relative to performance and satisfaction and are scored along a scale of 1 to 10 with (1) not being able to do the activity and (10) being able to do the activity extremely well, which is then calculated as a total score (i.e., the sum of each problem area). Along with an overall score, a problem list is generated to focus treatment goals. The COPM can be completed in less than 20 minutes.

Psychometrics

A research study among persons with ankylosing spondylitis (n = 119) listed a total of 1495 occupational performance problems in their COPM interviews and prioritized 569 of them. The most frequent problems cited were associated with

exercise and sports, sleeping, indoor mobility, and socializing (Kjeken et al., 2005). The same study found test-retest reliability, conducted in a number of formats, to be good to excellent with intra-class correlation coefficients for performance and satisfaction at r= 0.92 and 0.93 when rescored by personal interview, r = 0.73 and 0.73 when rescored by telephone interview, and lastly, r = 0.90 and 0.90 when rescored by mail (Kjeken et al., 2005). A study of 138 subjects referred to outpatient occupational therapy departments of an academic medical center found significant differences between the mean COPM assessment and reassessment scores as 78 of the 138 (57%) clients indicated an improvement, 40 clients (29%) indicated no change, and 20 clients (14%) indicated deterioration (Bolt et al., 2011). Another study of 113 with various tendon injuries or Dupuytren's disease found that the correlations between the DASH Outcome assessment and COPM performance and satisfaction subscales were –0.48 and –0.58, whereas correlations with the Michigan Hand Questionnaire-29 were 0.42 and 0.60, respectively (van de Ven-Stevens, Graff, Peters, van der Linde, & Geurts, 2015).

Advantages

There is a significant amount of research in support of its use in clinical practice and it is considered to be a gold standard in the assessment of occupational performance as well as being client centered. The COPM is based on the Canadian Model of Occupational Performance and can deliver unique insights into client-perceived strengths, weaknesses, and goals. No special training or licensing are needed to administer the assessment and the COPM maintains an informative website devoted to the scale.

Disadvantages

The assessment generally takes less than 20 minutes to complete administration; however, time can be longer in certain populations. As the COPM is a loosely designed open-format assessment, its success relies on both input and motivation of the client to perform an honest appraisal of his or her strengths, weaknesses, and goals and to a lesser extent guidance from the clinician.

Administration

During assessment the client is asked to identify and rank problematic issues with everyday activities with regard to three domains of occupational performance outlined on the measure. Step 2 requires the client to further consider those identified areas and select 5 that he or she would like to address or make known to the clinician, which are then rated along a scale of 1 to 10 relative to performance and satisfaction with that performance. Information purveyed from the measure can then be used by the clinician to create treatment goals or to develop interventions. Reassessment using the same methods occurs after intervention where scores are then compared.

Permission

The COPM can be purchased from the Canadian Association of Occupational Therapists e-store and is available in a number of formats including e-delivery. Prices vary from $15 for 100 forms to $500 for 5000 forms. The examiner's manual is $50. Permission to use in research or publication can be obtained by contacting where purchased or the authors of the COPM listed in the Contact section at the end of this chapter. More information can be found in the following journal article:

Law, M., Baptiste, S., Carswell, A., McColl, M., Polatajko, H., Pollock, N., & Opzoomer, A. (1990). The Canadian Occupational Therapy Performance Measure: An outcome measure for occupational therapy. *Canadian Journal of Occupational Therapy, 57*(2), 82-87.

Summary

POPULATION	General
TYPE OF MEASURE	Client-centered rating scale
WHAT IT ASSESSES	Level of occupational performance; satisfaction
TIME	< 20 minutes
COST	≥ $15; varies

Contact

Mary Law, PhD

McMaster University

Faculty of Health Sciences

Hamilton, Ontario, Canada

Web: http://fhs.mcmaster.ca/ceb/faculty_member_law.htm

Canadian Association of Occupational Therapists

CTTC Building 3400-1125

Colonel By Dr

Ottawa, ON K1S 5R1 Canada

Phone: (800) 434-2268

Web: www.thecopm.ca/

Chapter 83: Functional Behavior Profile (FBP)

Description

The Functional Behavior Profile (FBP), developed by Baum, Edwards, and Morrow-Howell (1993), is a standardized assessment used to describe the productive behaviors observed by caregivers of individuals with neurocognitive disorders (NCD) of the Alzheimer's and related types or other disorders, such as stroke, where basic ability to engage in occupational performance is of concern, by recording and examining the recent observations of those individuals (Baum & Edwards, 2000). It is a 27-item questionnaire rating scale that can be completed by the clinician, primary caregiver, or in some instances as a self-report. Theoretically, the FBP explores three concepts: (1) task performance, which is considered the capabilities of the individual for doing and includes taking responsibility for tasks, performing neat and timely work, concentration, and handling tools; (2) social interaction, which is the individual's engagement with others in conversations and social activities; and (3) problem solving, which measures the ability of the person to make decisions and learn new tasks (Baum & Edwards, 2000). The FBP uses a 5-point Likert scale for each item, which is scored from (0) never to (4) always, as well as 1 question pertaining to time (i.e. >25 minutes, 5 to 15 minutes). The maximum score possible is 108 with higher scores being indicative of better performance. The FBP can be completed in less than 15 minutes.

Psychometrics

Early research into the measure found that the following 3 factors were able to explain 70.6% of the variance: (1) task performance, (2) problem solving, and (3) social interaction (Baum et al., 1993). Comparing established research, Burgener, Popovich, and Twigg (2005) found that the FBP subscale Cronbach's alphas scores ranging from 0.94 to 0.96 generally concurred with their results of Cronbach's alpha for the total scale of 0.94, with subscales ranging from 0.83 to 0.85. Also, results were found to be valid through the stages of NCD of the Alzheimer's and related types, supporting the instrument's reliability as the person progresses into the latter stages of disease. Baum and Edwards (2000) examined a stroke population and demonstrated that individuals with scores of 84 or lower were 5 times more likely to need supervision after discharge than those with scores of 85 or higher, and 69% of those patients were considered to be classified correctly into groups based on scores of the FBP alone, highlighting its predictive value. A study by Balli et al. (2014) of 22 subjects with multiple sclerosis (MS) using 2 raters who examined scores of the Italian translation, found that total score inter-rater reliability was $r = 0.73$ with a range of 0.65 to 0.81, while the inter-rater reliability for task performance domain questions was $r = 0.94$, the problem solving domain was 0.87, and the social interaction domain was lowest at 0.77. The same study found excellent overall test-retest reliability at $r = 0.96$ with a range of 0.92 to 0.98. Furthermore, the internal consistency values were also high for the total score ($\alpha = 0.89$) as well as for the 3 domains of task performance, problem solving, and social interaction ($\alpha = 0.90, 0.86,$ and 0.84).

Advantages

No special training or certifications are needed to administer the FBP. It is located in the public domain, thus it is free to use in clinical practice, research, or publication. The assessment can be completed in less than 15 minutes, and because it is relatively quick to administer it may have added value in determining if further investigations are warranted by the clinician. Results of the Italian translation were also in line with established research, suggesting cross-cultural validity.

Disadvantages

There is a limited amount of research in support of its use in varied clinical populations and arguably, when completed by proxy, its answers may rely on subjective observational information from the caregiver or clinician, which may be

TABLE 83-1
DOMAINS OF THE FUNCTIONAL BEHAVIOR PROFILE
• Activities of daily living
• Cognition
• Executive function
• Functional mobility
• Life participation
• Social interactions
• Reasoning/problem solving
• Patient satisfaction
• Social relationship tasks
• Social interactions

Adapted from Balli, E., Giovannelli, T., & Paci, M. (2014). The Italian version of the Functional Behavior Profile: Reliability in a population of persons with multiple sclerosis. *Neurological Sciences, 35*(8), 1294.

different than the client's perceptions of his or her strengths and weaknesses; however, a study by Goverover et al. (2005) found that self-report and proxy scores were closely matched for MS subjects (n = 35) at 88.9 ± 11.3, self and 87.3 ± 13.6, proxy and for healthy controls (n = 39) where scores were 101.3 ± 6.5, self and 102.4 ± 6.7 proxy.

Administration

During assessment, the individual or informant is asked to consider the person's behavior over the past week relative to the 27 items that pertain to basic physical, executive, and social engagement capabilities. The FBP produces 4 separate scores: a total score with a maximum of 108 as well as 3 domain scores where some questions overlap relative to (1) task performance, which includes items 1 to 11; (2) problem solving, which includes items 9, 10, 21 to 27; and (3) social interaction, which includes items 11 to 21. Each domain can be administered separately or the scale can be administered as a whole. Items are scored as either (4) always, 100%; (3) usually, 80%; (2) sometimes, 50%; (1) rarely, 20%; or (0) never, < 10%, where higher score suggest better occupational performance.

TABLE 83-2
EXAMPLE ITEMS OF THE FUNCTIONAL BEHAVIOR PROFILE
• Can use tools or instruments in performing tasks (kitchen, hobby, razor)
• Can manipulate small items (hand work, buttoning, makeup)
• Activities are appropriate to the time of day (sleeps at night, alert during the day)
• Can respond to a one-step command
• Shows enjoyment in activities
• Participates in activities
• Performs activities without frustration
• Can identify familiar persons
• Initiates conversation with family
• Socializes when others initiate the interactions
• Expresses him- or herself appropriate to the situation
• Is able to make a decision when presented with choices
• Can learn a simple activity without difficulty
Adapted from Baum, C., Edwards, D. F., & Morrow-Howell, N. (1993). Identification and measurement of productive behaviours in senile dementia of the Alzheimer type. *The Gerontologist, 33*(3), 403-408

Permissions

The FBP is located in the public domain and is free to use in clinical practice as well as in research or publication. More information can be obtained by contacting its author or where it was published at the information that follows. The FBP is wholly contained in the following journal article as well as other places such as the web:

Baum, M., Edwards, D. F., & Morrow-Howell, N. (1993). Identification measures and measurement of productive behaviors in senile dementia of the Alzheimer's type. *The Gerontologist, 33*(3), 403-408.

Summary

POPULATION	Neurocognitive disorders; cerebrovascular accident; general
TYPE OF MEASURE	Proxy questionnaire; self-report
WHAT IT ASSESSES	Basic occupational performance
TIME	< 15 minutes
COST	Free

Contact

Carolyn Baum, PhD, OTR, FAOTA

Washington University—St. Louis

St. Louis, Missouri

Web: www.ot.wustl.edu/about/our-people/faculty/carolyn-m-baum-254

CHAPTER 84: IN-HOME OCCUPATIONAL PERFORMANCE EVALUATION (I-HOPE)

Description

The In-Home Occupational Performance Evaluation (I-HOPE) is an assessment developed to target activities performed in the home that are essential for aging in place whereby a multistep procedure establishes current activity patterns, identifies activities that are difficult but important to the older adult, and identifies the environmental barriers that influence specific activities (Stark, Somerville, & Morris, 2010). It does this by inventorying current and desired activity patterns using photographic images as visual cues that the client views as activity cards. Content for the cards are considered activities that occur naturally in the home and during assessment they serve as a visual cue to recall current and previous participation in those activities and include such items as carrying items, getting in or out of bed, opening jars, talking on the phone, reading/writing, washing and drying clothes, getting dressed, opening or closing doors, getting in or out of the car, preparing a meal, and ironing clothes. During assessment the activity cards are viewed and sorted by the client into four categories of occupational performance: (1) I do not do and don't want to do; (2) I do now with no problem; (3) I do now with difficulty; and (4) I do not do but would like to do (Stark et al., 2010). The result is that activities that are important, difficult, or impossible to perform within the client's current context are able to be identified and prioritized. The unique scoring system is also able to determine the magnitude of the environment's influence on those performance activities deemed important. The I-HOPE includes 44 stimulus cards and can be completed in less than 30 minutes. A revised version by Keglovits, Somerville, and Stark (2015) combines 8 new activities as well as the removal of several activities to create a final card sort deck of 43 activities. The revised version uses a similar but more complex scoring system in which data produces the same four sub-scores relative to activity participation, performance, satisfaction, and severity of environmental barriers.

Psychometrics

Early research into the original I-HOPE items by Stark et al. (2010) found internal consistencies for the various subscales to be r=0.85 for participation, 0.78 for satisfaction, 0.77 for performance, and 0.77 for severity of environmental barriers. That research also established good reliability as intra-class correlation coefficients (ICCs) of the I-HOPE subscales were 0.99 for participation, 0.94 for performance, 1.0 for satisfaction, and 0.99 for environmental barriers.

The measure was also found to correlate positively with the Functional Independence Measure scale—daily activities subscale at r=0.53 and with the satisfaction with performance of daily activities subscale at r=0.43. Also, the two were negatively correlated relative to the environmental barrier severity subscale at r=−0.46. ICCs of the I-HOPE subscales also showed good reliability for activity participation at 0.99, whereas performance was 0.94, satisfaction 1.0, and environmental barriers at 0.99. That study also found that a comparison of pre- and post-test scores showed significant change (5.70 to 7.38) suggesting good discriminant ability of the measure. A study by Keglovits et al. (2015) found that all subscales of the revised I-HOPE demonstrated good internal consistency with a range of α=0.82 to 0.90 and like the original ICCs were also high with a range of 0.94 to 1.0 demonstrating good reliability.

Advantages

Both I-HOPE versions are relatively easy to administer, require no special training, and are unique in that they use a photographic picture interface with the client allowing him or her to decide on his or her ability to engage in home-bound occupations as well as which of those occupations are deemed important. Information purveyed also addresses the person–environment fit when performing daily activities in the home (Keglovits et al., 2015).

Disadvantages

There is a limited amount of peer-reviewed research pertaining to the I-HOPE in support of its use in clinical practice. Another potential limitation is the fact that the client must be evaluated in his or her current living environment which is in contrast to a number of other assessments (Stark et al., 2010).

Administration

During assessment of the revised I-HOPE the client first views stimulus activity cards (>40) and is then asked to sort the cards into 1 of 5 performance categories, such as those that he or she would like to do but are problematic. Next, an activity participation score is produced, which is the proportion of difficult activities divided by the total number of activities. This is followed by a sorting activity where the stimulus cards are ranked from most to least important. Then, using the 10 most problematic activities, the subject provides ratings relative to performance, satisfaction, and self-efficacy along variable 5-point Likert scales (1 to 5), where higher scores suggest better ability. In the final step, the clinician observes and rates client performance relative to the identified problem areas as well as those environmental barriers that make performance difficult or unsafe (Keglovits et al.,2015).

Permissions

Use of the assessment in practice as well as research or publication can be obtained by contacting the creators at the information that follows. More information can be found in the following journal articles:

Stark, S. L., Somerville, E. K., & Morris, J. C. (2010). In-Home Occupational Performance Evaluation (I-HOPE). *American Journal of Occupational Therapy, 64*(4), 580-589.

Keglovits. M., Somerville, E., & Stark, S. (2015). In-Home Occupational Performance Evaluation for Providing Assistance (I-HOPE Assist): An assessment for informal caregivers. *American Journal of Occupational Therapy, 69*, 1-10.

Summary

POPULATION	General; community dwelling
TYPE OF MEASURE	Stimulus-based hierarchy rating of activities in the home
WHAT IT ASSESSES	Desired occupations; supports and barriers; environment
TIME	< 30 minutes
COST	n/a

Contact

Susan L. Stark, PhD, OTR/L

Washington University School of Medicine

St. Louis, Missouri

Web: www.ot.wustl.edu/about/ourpeople/faculty/susy-stark-271

Chapter 85: Independent Living Scales (ILS)

Description

The Independent Living Scale (ILS) is an observational task analysis tool in which data about the client is collected over a 7-day period by examining 3 domains of occupational performance: (1) activities of daily living (ADLs), (2) behavior and, (3) initiation. The ILS is composed of 5 scales: (1) memory-orientation, which examines orientation, recall, and recognition; (2) managing money; (3) managing home and transportation; (4) health and safety; and (5) social adjustment, which explores one's interpersonal relationships (Revheim & Medalia, 2004). The assessment is composed of 68 items that are graded relative to subject performance along a 3-point scale from 0 to 2 (Fish, 2011). Results of the ILS yield 5 subscale scores and a total score (0 to 100) as well as 2 additional subscales whose scores are derived from those of the 68 items: a performance-information factor subscale, which reflects the skills needed for task performance, such as using a telephone book or making change, and a problem-solving factor subscale, which comprises 33 items that evaluate abstract reasoning and judgment required for daily living and explores such questions as, "What would you do if your lights and television went out simultaneously?" (Revheim & Medalia, 2004). ILS scoring uses a factor system where each item is uniquely weighted relative to its importance. For example, dressing has a value of 5 points out of the 61 subscale points where it resides, whereas leisure only has a value of 2 points (Revheim & Medalia, 2004). The assessment can be completed in less than 45 minutes.

Psychometrics

A study by Ashley, Persel, and Clark (2001) of 5290 traumatic brain injury (TBI) subjects admitted to a post-acute rehabilitation facility over a 15-year period demonstrated a test-retest reliability of $r = 0.72$. While citing prior work with the ILS of 77 subjects, they found total inter-rater reliability to be good at $r = 0.85$, whereas inter-rater reliability was 0.7 for the behavior sub-scale, and 0.93 for the ADL subscale. Good convergent validity was also noted as well between 0.82 to 0.87 as significant correlations were found with the Vineland Adaptive Behaviour Scale (0.82), and with the American Association for Mental Deficiency Adaptive Behavior Scales (0.87). Finally, statistical fit using a four-factor model, they determined that for the self-care model the fit was 0.50, directed aggression was 0.79, environmental care was 0.80, and for protective task avoidance it was 0.65, suggesting that these four factors are consistent with clinical observations of skill necessary for independent living (Ashley et al., 2001). Among 40 clients of mixed diagnoses (TBI, cerebrovascular accident, multiple sclerosis) in an acute neurological rehabilitation hospital, the ILS had a modest correlation with Functional Independence Measure (FIM) discharge scores at 0.39 (Gillen & Gernert-Dott, 2000). The same study found that correlations between individual subtests of the ILS with FIM discharge scores varied from 0.47 for the management of home and transportation scale, 0.44 for health and safety scale, to minimal ($r = 0.80$, $p = 0.673$) for the memory/orientation scale (Gillen & Gernert-Dott, 2000). Assessing the validity of the ILS among persons with schizophrenia ($n = 162$), Revheim and Medalia (2004) determined that scores on the ILS problem solving subscale differed significantly across 3 levels of care for persons requiring maximum, moderate, and minimal supervision when compared with scores on the Global Assessment of Functioning measure, which was only able to discriminate between 2 levels of care.

Table 85-1			
Problem Solving Factor Subscale by Living Status, Among Subjects With Schizophrenia* and Established Norms			
VARIABLE	**MAXIMUM SUPERVISION (N = 87)**	**MODERATE SUPERVISION (N = 54)**	**MINIMUM SUPERVISION (N = 21)**
ILS-PB scores*	29 (SD: 10.6)	38.4 (11.5)	48.9 (6.2)
Norms	20 to 39	40 to 49	50 to 63
$n = 162$; ages 18 to 52 years old			
Adapted from Revheim, N., & Medalia, A. (2004). The Independent Living Scales as a measure of functional outcome for schizophrenia. *Psychiatric Services, 55*(9), 1053.			

Advantages

The ILS allows for a valid comparison of individual scores over time, as well as highlighting areas of occupational competence and those requiring assistance (Persel, 2012). Its results can also purvey information required for independent living as well as guidelines for the appropriate supervision requirements of individuals to remain independent.

Originally developed for adults with neurocognitive disorders (NCD) of the Alzheimer's and related types, it has also been validated across a number of patient populations including those with a diagnosis of a psychiatric illness (Baird, 2006). Finally, there is a fair amount of research in support of its use in clinical practice and it can be purchased from Pearson Inc., who owns the copyright.

Disadvantages

The ILS can be rather complicated and time consuming to administer and it may require the analysis of many tasks over a 7-day period. There is also some research to suggest that person traits relative to disablement, such as physical or sensory disabilities, should be considered during testing as many potential respondents may be penalized because of the way items are administered and scored (Cohen, 2001).

Administration

The examiner's manual, when purchased, provides detailed instructions as well normative data for the different scales including cutoff scores to establish criterion validity with adults 65 years old and older who are living independently, semi-independently, or dependently. Sample data is also provided for those with psychiatric diagnosis, NCD of the Alzheimer's and related types, and TBI. Several items are needed such as a telephone, telephone book, money, envelope, scratch paper, pen, pencil, and stopwatch. Domain items are weighted as follows: (1) ADLs—17 items (61 points); (2) behavior—11 items (30 points); and (3) initiation—16 items (9 points) (Persel, 2012).

Permissions

The ILS can be purchased from Pearson for a cost of $360. Use of the battery in research or publication can be obtained by contacting Pearson or its author at the information following. More information can be found in the following journal article:

Ashley, M., Persel, C., & Clark, M. (2001). Validation of an independent living scale for post-acute rehabilitation applications. *Brain Injury, 15*(5), 435-442.

Summary

POPULATION	General
TYPE OF MEASURE	Activity-based rating scale
WHAT IT ASSESSES	Occupational performance; independent living skills
TIME	<45 minutes; across therapy days
COST	$360

Contact

Pearson Inc.

Attn: Inbound Sales and Customer Support

P.O. Box 599700

San Antonio, TX 78259

Phone: (800) 627-7271

Email: clinicalcustomersupport@pearson.com

Web: www.pearsonclinical.com/therapy/ products/100000181/independent-living-scales-ils. html

CHAPTER 86: KITCHEN TASK ASSESSMENT (KTA)

Description

Developed by Baum and Edwards (1993), the Kitchen Task Assessment (KTA) is an activity-based observational tool designed to measure executive, organizational, planning, and judgment skills of impaired adults. Originally validated within the neurocognitive disorder (NCD) population, it has shown to be valid across a number of settings where its results purvey information regarding the level of assistance a subject may need to perform everyday activities as well as his or her occupational performance, and in particular, as it relates to those that are kitchen based. All activities are performed in the kitchen, thus the measure requires access to a kitchen counter, stove, refrigerator, and sink. During assessment the client performs two activities: (1) a pre-test washing hands activity along with (2) making a cooked pudding. If the person is unable to wash his or her hands with or without assistance, then no further testing is needed. If the subject is able to wash his or her hands independently he or she is then instructed to begin the cooked pudding task where the person is scored relative to his or her ability to adequately perform the following 6 cognitive components necessary for task completion: (1) initiation, (2) organization, (3) performance of all steps, (4) sequencing, (5) judgment, and (6) safety and completion (Josman & Birnboim, 2001). Scores are based on observations of the clinician and can range from (0) independent to (3) totally incapable for each of the 6 cognitive components. Total KTA scores range from 0 to 18. A modified scoring system is also available that rates items from 0 to 5 with a total range of 0 to 25. For both, higher scores are associated with more assistance. The KTA can be completed in 15 minutes.

Psychometrics

Initial research by its creators of 106 subjects with NCD Alzheimer's established excellent internal consistency at $\alpha = 0.96$, whereas inter-rater reliability of the KTA total score was $r = 0.85$, ranging from 0.62 for the safety component to perfect agreement (1.0) for initiation (Baum & Edwards, 1993). High correlation coefficients were also achieved (0.72 to 0.84), suggesting that all of the domains measured contributed to the cognitive dimension of task performance (Baum & Edwards, 1993). A study of 126 healthy controls and persons with NCD using a canonical analysis methodology, which is a type of statistical measure of correlations between variables, determined that 4 factors existed; however, the loading on the first factor relative to each of the 6 cognitive components were able to explain 67% to 81% of the total variance with the exception of initiation at 0.55, suggesting good uni-dimensionality of the measure (Baum, Edwards, Yonan, & Storandt, 1996).

Advantages

The KTA is unique in that it evaluates the cognitive processes that affect task performance as well as recording the level of cognitive support necessary for successful task completion (Josman & Birnboim, 2001). No training or certifications are needed and the assessment can be completed in 15 minutes. A children's version of the KTA is also available, which may have some value in certain older populations, and can be readily downloaded from the Washington University—St. Louis occupational therapy website.

Disadvantages

There is a limited amount of research pertaining to the assessment and it requires the use of a kitchen, which may not be available in many therapy departments. Some have also suggested that gender bias could enter into the equation with regard to a kitchen activity.

Administration

During assessment, the examiner is instructed to cue only after determining that the client cannot perform without help (i.e., after 5 seconds), unless safety is an issue (Josman &Birnboim, 2001). Total scores range from 0 to 18, where a mean score of 4.65 indicates that verbal cueing is necessary to support performance, while a score of 9.18 to 13.88 indicates the need for physical assistance (Josman & Birnboim, 2001).

Permissions

The KTA is free to use in clinical practice. To use in research or publication contact its authors at the information that follows or where it has been published. The KTA is wholly contained in the following journal article:

Baum, C., & Edwards, D. (1993). Cognitive performance in senile dementia of the Alzheimer's type: The Kitchen Task Assessment. *American Journal of Occupational Therapy,* (47), 431-436.

Summary

POPULATION	General
TYPE OF MEASURE	Activity-based rating scale
WHAT IT ASSESSES	Cognitive skills necessary for occupational performance; kitchen-based activity
TIME	20 minutes
COST	Free

Contact

Carolyn Baum PhD, OTR, FAOTA

Washington University—St. Louis

St. Louis, Missouri

Web: www.ot.wustl.edu/about/ourpeople/faculty/carolyn-m-baum-254

CHAPTER 87: KOHLMAN EVALUATION OF LIVING SKILLS (KELS)—FOURTH EDITION

Description

The Kohlman Evaluation of Living Skills (KELS), 4th Edition, developed by Kohlman-Thompson (1992), is an evaluation tool used to determine an individual's ability to function with basic life skills and combines both a structured interview and the performance of various tasks to determine those life skills (Kohlman-Thompson, 1992). The assessment comprises five domains: (1) self-care, (2) safety and health, (3) money management, (4) transportation and telephone, and (5) work and leisure, and has 17 tasks/items (Kohlman-Thompson, 1992). KELS uses two scoring categories: (0) independent or (1) assistance/unable to complete task successfully, with the exception of work and leisure where half points are also possible. Each item on the scale has its own inclusion/exclusion criteria for correct scoring. For example, the item relating to knowledge of emergency numbers would be administered through a standardized interview outlined in the manual in which the subject would be scored as independent if he or she is able give local emergency numbers or the operator's number and would be scored as needs assistance if he or she is unable to give those numbers, or if they look in the phone book and do not find the number(s) without assistance (Kohlman-Thompson, 1992). Total scores are summarized with higher scores being more problematic. A short qualitative summary, prepared by the clinician, may also be included with results. KELS can be completed in less than 45 minutes.

TABLE 87-1	
DOMAIN AND TASK ITEMS OF THE KOHLMAN EVALUATION OF LIVING SKILLS	
DOMAIN	**TASK ITEMS**
Self-care	Appearance
	Frequency of self-care activities
Safety and health	Awareness of dangerous household situations
	Identification of appropriate action for sickness and accidents
	Knowledge of emergency numbers
	Knowledge and location of medical/dental facilities
Money management	Use of money in purchasing items
	Obtain and maintain source of income
	Budgeting of money for food
	Budgeting monthly income
	Use of banking forms
	Paying bills
Transportation and telephone	Mobility within community
	Basic knowledge of transit system
	Use of phone book and telephone
Work and leisure	Plans for future employment
	Leisure activity involvement

Adapted from Kohlman-Thompson, L. (1992). *The Kohlman Evaluation of Living Skills* (3rd ed., pp. 14-38). Bethesda, MD: AOTA Press.

Psychometrics

Inter-rater reliability of the previous edition, as outlined in the manual, has values ranging from $r = 0.74$ to 0.94 (Kohlman-Thompson, 1992). A study of 92 community-dwelling older adults established the concurrent validity of the KELS 3rd edition with the Global Assessment Scale and the Bay Area Functional Performance Evaluation where significant correlations were found at 0.78 to 0.89 and -0.84, respectively (Zimnavoda, Weinblatt, & Katz, 2002). A predictive validity study of 20 post-discharge patients (40 to 60 days) determined that results of the KELS 3rd edition were able to accurately predict (1.0) which geriatric patients would be successful in community placements (Kohlman-Thompson, 1992). A cross-sectional study by Burnett, Dyer, and Naik (2009) of 200 community-dwelling older adults found strong correlations between the KELS 3rd edition and the Executive Cognitive Test at $r = 0.71$, and the Executive Clock Drawing Test 1 at $r = 0.63$, suggesting that KELS may provide an indication of potential limitations in the ability to plan, sequence, execute, and/or monitor behaviors necessary for safe and independent living.

Advantages

KELS is an established assessment that has shown continued relevance to the profession of occupational therapy. The test addresses a range of essential aspects of daily living skills and no special training is needed outside of the testing manual. The 4th edition (Kohlman-Thompson & Robnett, 2016), which was developed from a normative sample of 200 subjects, includes several updates that incorporate the use of technology such as the use of cell phones, and electronic banking, as well as the removal of obsolete items. An accompanying flash drive includes electronic banking items and forms for administration.

Disadvantages

The amount of supporting research for the latest edition is limited and standardized reproduction of testing procedures is required along with the use of outside materials. The manual recommends that testing may not be appropriate for individuals who have been hospitalized for over 30 days as their perceived abilities may have changed. KELS is also based on the urban North American culture thus when used in rural settings some items may not be applicable.

Administration

KELS involves the use of a structured interview along with the performance of specific tasks to help the clinician grade the daily living skills thought necessary for independent living as well as to develop interventions to allow clients to function as independently as possible. The assessment has three possible scoring categories: 0 if the person is determined to be independent, and 0.5 or 1 if he or she needs assistance to complete the task, which varies depending on the domain. Items not applicable receive a score of 0. A total score of 5.5 or less suggests that the client is able to live independently, whereas a score of 6 or more indicates the person is considered to need assistance to live in the community (Kohlman-Thompson, 1992). Materials needed include but are not limited to a telephone, bar of soap, pencil, deck of cards, and $2 and change. A further example of the test is basic knowledge of the transit system where the clinician examines a person's skills, through interview, to successfully choose and take a bus to a place he or she has not been before. The client would be scored independent if he or she is able to (1) give or check the number of a bus route near where they live, (2) ask the bus driver for route number, (3) reads route from bus stop signs, (4) call transit information to get route information, or (5) gets route information from bus schedule (Kohlman-Thompson, 1992). Assistance would be needed if he or she did not know how to or could not find out what bus to ride or gives answers that would not enable him or her to take the correct bus.

Permissions

The KELS assessment is published by the American Occupational Therapy Association (AOTA) Press where the test book and instructions can be purchased at a cost of $99 to $149. Permission to use the scale for other purposes can be obtained by contacting the author or the AOTA Press. More information can be found in the following:

Kohlman-Thompson, L. (1992). *The Kohlman Evaluation of Living Skills (KELS)*. Rockville, MD: American Occupational Therapy Association.

Summary

POPULATION	General
TYPE OF MEASURE	Interview/activity-based rating scale
WHAT IT ASSESSES	Occupational performance skills necessary for independent living; activities of daily living/instrumental activities of daily living
TIME	<45 minutes
COST	$99 to $149

Contact

Regula H. Robnett, PhD, OTR/L

University of New England

Biddeford, Maine

Web: www.une.edu/people/regula-h-robnett

KELS 4th edition manual: https://myaota.aota.org/shop_aota/prodview.aspx?TYPE=D&PID=277716288&SKU=900374

Chapter 88: Measure of the Quality of the Environment (MQE)

Description

The Measure of the Quality of the Environment (MQE) is a standardized measure based on the Disability Creation Process model and is designed to evaluate the influence that environmental factors have on occupational performance by exploring such issues as the quality of a person's participation and his or her functional capabilities (Fougeyrollas, Tremblay, Noreau, St-Onge, & Dumont, 2006). Administered as a self-report questionnaire, the person is asked to estimate the impact the environment exerts upon his or her daily life through an examination of his or her successes and failures relative to their occupational performance within those environments (Fougeyrollas, Noreau, St-Michel, & Boschen, 2008). The MQE comprises six domains: (1) social support and attitudes, (2) income, labor, and income security, (3) government and public services, (4) equal opportunities and political orientations, (5) physical environment and accessibility, and (6) technology. The MQE has 109 questions, 40 of which address the physical environment in which the subject is presently operating and 69 that address his or her social environment (Fougeyrollas et al., 2008). An example vignette of the MQE includes a list of situational factors intended to explore the influence of such things as winter climatic conditions (snow, ice, cold); public transportation services in the community (schedule, stops, frequency, route); work hours and social networks (support from others); income (availability, financial programs, services); and physical accessibility (Fougeyrollas et al., 2008). Each item is rated along a 7-point Likert scale ranging from -3 major obstacle to +3 major facilitator where unique criteria relative to obstacles and facilitators are used for each item. The MQE can be completed in less than 30 minutes with higher scores associated with better occupational performance within client context. A short 26-item version is also available that uses the same scoring system and can be completed in less than 10 minutes.

Psychometrics

Test-retest reliability results of a study done with young adults with cerebral palsy (n = 28) showed that 85% of the items obtained an agreement above 60%, whereas a test-retest reliability study done by its creators showed moderate to high kappa's for 57% of the items (Fougeyrollas et al., 2008). A convenience sample of persons aged 40 to 97 years (n = 51) 6 months post-discharge from an intensive functional rehabilitation unit found the association between the total MQE barrier scores and the Assessment of Life Habits scores to be significant at 0.42, although, results showed that the MQE category support and attitudes was not statistically significant and was considered an outlier in the study (Rochette, Desrosiers, & Noreau, 2001). A study of persons over 65 years of age (mean age: 80.7 years) who had been registered for home-based rehabilitation (n = 91) found that the top facilitators chosen on the MQE were support from members of the family, 76 (83.5%); television media services, 76 (83.5%); health services, 70 (76.9%); and rehabilitation services, 66 (72.5%), whereas the top barriers to occupational performance were family situation, 16 (17.6%); rehabilitation services, 15 (16.5%); the availability of businesses, 12 (13.2%); and the attitudes of the service providers, 11 (12.1%) (Vik, Nygard, & Lilja, 2007).

Advantages

The MQE is based on the conceptual model of the Disability Creation Process and both a short and long versions are available (26 and 109 items). It has also been translated into several languages, which suggests cross-cultural relevance. There is an interactive website (in French that can be translated) dedicated to the MQE that is maintained by the International Network on the Disability Creation Process (INDCP).

Disadvantages

There is a limited amount of direct peer-reviewed research available regarding the assessment. Also, there is a lack of established norms as well, and because its results only yield an item score the clinician must interpret domain and total scores according to clinical judgment.

Administration

During assessment the client is asked to consider situational vignettes and then decide if the item facilitates or hinders occupational performance. An example item asks the person to consider his or her abilities and personal limits and to indicate to what extent the following influences affect his or her daily life: the attitudes of family, friends, and colleagues (Fougeyrollas et al., 2008).

TABLE 88-1
SCORING CONTINUUM OF THE MEASURE OF THE QUALITY OF THE ENVIRONMENT

-3	Major obstacle; completely prevents accomplishment of the activity
-2	Medium obstacle; largely hinders accomplishment of the life activity
-1	Minor obstacle; mildly hinders accomplishment of a life activity or slightly increases its level of difficulty
0	No influence
1	Minor facilitator; compensates a little for the impairments or disabilities and allows partial accomplishment of the life activity or slightly decreases its difficulty
2	Medium facilitator; partially compensates for the impairments or disabilities and allows partial accomplishment of the life activity or accomplishment with difficulty
3	Major facilitator; fully compensates for the impairments or disabilities and allows full accomplishment of the life activity without constraint nor difficulty

Adapted from Fougeyrollas, P., Noreau, L., St-Michel, G., & Boschen, K. (2008). *Measure of the Quality of the Environment—version 2.0* (pp. 4-7). Quebec, Canada: RIPPH/INDCP.

Permissions

The MQE assessments can be purchased from the INDCP website where prices range from $16 to $24. Permission to use in research or for commercial purposes can also be obtained by contacting the INDCP. More information can be found in the following research article:

Fougeyrollas, P., Noreau, L., St-Michel, G., & Boschen, K. (2008). *Measure of the Quality of the Environment—Short Version.* Quebec, Canada: RIPPH/INDCP

Summary

POPULATION	General
TYPE OF MEASURE	Self-report questionnaire
WHAT IT ASSESSES	Contextual factors that support or hinder occupational performance
TIME	< 30 minutes
COST	$16 to $24

Contact

International Network on the Disability Creation Process

525, boulevard Wilfrid-Hamel Est, Local A-08

Québec, Canada G1M 2S8

Phone: (418) 529-9141, poste 6202

Web site for the MQE—long form: www.ripph.qc.ca/37-assessment-tool-long-form-mqe

MQE—short form: www.ripph.qc.ca/38-assessment-tool-short-form-mqe

Chapter 89: Model of Human Occupation Screening Tool 2.0 (MOHOST)

Description

The Model of Human Occupation Screening Tool (MOHOST) is based on the Model of Human Occupation (MOHO) by Kielhofner, (1980), and was developed to assess the primary concepts of that theory, which argue that occupational participation is influenced by several factors such as (1) volition, which is considered a client's motivation to engage in occupation; (2) habituation, or the way in which a client patterns activities and engages in daily habits and routines; (3) performance capacity, which is thought to be a client's available motor, process, and communication skills; and (4) environment, which refers to what extent a client's physical and social environments support or inhibit occupational functioning and engagement (Kielhofner et al., 2010). The assessment is composed of six domains: (1) volition, (2) habituation, (3) communication and interaction skills, (4) process skills, (5) motor skills, and (6) the environment. Each domain supports 4 questions for a total of 24 items where information is gathered through observation, interview, and assessment of performance and includes such rated observations as the client's expectations of success, non-verbal skills, posture and mobility, and physical resources. MOHOST items are scored along a 4-point letter rated scale to guide the selection of appropriate choices as follows: (F) facilitates occupational participation, (A) allows occupational participation, (I) inhibits occupational participation, and (R) restricts occupational participation. Scoring uses an algorithm to convert letter scores to numbers where final domain and total scores are then able to generate a profile of a person's strengths and weaknesses, which may include such items as his or her motivation and patterns of occupation and how they affect participation (Forsyth et al., 2011). Administration times vary but the MOHOST could be completed in as little as 20 minutes if the clinician is familiar with the client.

Psychometrics

When comparing admission and discharge sores for an inpatient rehabilitation unit (n = 54), average MOHOST discharge scores were significantly greater (1.10, SD = 1.35) than measures at admission (0.79, SD = 1.98), indicating an ability of the measure to track client progress over time with motor skills and environment subscales showing the largest increases (Kramer, Kielhofner, Lee, Ashpole, & Castle, 2009). A study of 1039 adult psychiatric service users determined the MOHOST to have moderate correlations with the Volitional Questionnaire motivation for occupation subscale at r = 0.58, while significant correlations were found with the Assessment of Communication and Interaction Skills communication and interaction subscale at r = 0.82 (Kielhofner et al., 2010). A statistical analysis by Forsyth et al. (2011) by 9 occupational therapists of scores of 163 clients with both physical and mental health disabilities indicated a misfit of 2 items: physical space and physical resources and concluded that overall, most items worked well to define a single construct of occupational participation with roles, responsibility, occupational demands, and appraisal of abilities representing the highest levels of occupational participation.

Advantages

Scoring for the MOHOST is unique in that it yields client strengths and weaknesses as opposed to a numeric value. A random survey of 1000 occupational therapists (259 replies) found that more than 80% indicated that they have used MOHO theory in their practices, which suggests that the MOHOST tool is relevant to current occupational therapy practice (Lee, Taylor, Kielhofner, & Fisher, 2008).

Disadvantages

One limitation of MOHOST involves the gathering of client data, which is not standardized, as it is done through clinical observation, assessment, watching the subject engage in activities, as well as discussions with client, caregivers, and staff, and as such, it influences both the inter-rater and intra-rater reliability of the assessment, which can affect other areas of its statistical properties as well.

Administration

During assessment, information is elicited with regard to the 24 occupational participation specific items through a variety of ways (including standardized and non-standardized) where each is then scored relative to the acronym FAIR. The choice of each letter is considered with regard to the extent to which personal or environmental factors support or detract from an individual's participation in occupations where (F) facilitates occupation and (R) restricts. It is also suggested that the clinician should use MOHO theory to further interpret the meaning of the ratings and to individualize goals and intervention plans accordingly (Kramer et al., 2009).

Permissions

The MOHOST standardized assessment can be purchased through the MOHOST Clearinghouse at the address that follows for $40. Permission to use in research or commercial purposes can be obtained by contacting the MOHOST Clearinghouse as well. More information can be found in the following research article:

Kielhofner, G., Fan, C., Morley, M., Garnham, M., Heasman, D., Forsyth, K.,...Taylor, R. (2010). A psychometric study of the Model of Human Occupation Screening Tool (MOHOST). *Hong Kong Journal of Occupational Therapy, 20*(2), 63-70.

Summary

POPULATION	General
TYPE OF MEASURE	Rating scale
WHAT IT ASSESSES	Factors that support or hinder occupational performance and participation
TIME	≥20 minutes
COST	$40

Contact

Model of Human Occupation Clearinghouse

Attn: MOHO Clearinghouse

Fax: (312) 413-0256

Web: www.cade.uic.edu/moho/productDetails.
aspx?aid=4

REFERENCES

Ashley, M., Persel, C., & Clark, M. (2001). Validation of an independent living scale for post-acute rehabilitation applications. *Brain Injury, 15*(5), 435-442.

Baird, A. (2006). Fine tuning recommendations for older adults with memory complaints: Using the Independent Living Scales with the Dementia rating scale. *Clinical Neuropsychologist, 20*(4), 649-661.

Balli, E., Giovannelli, T., & Paci, M. (2014). The Italian version of the Functional Behavior Profile: Reliability in a population of persons with multiple sclerosis. *Neurological Sciences, 35*(8), 1293-1298.

Baum, C., & Edwards, D. (1993). Cognitive performance in senile dementia of the Alzheimer's type: The Kitchen Task Assessment. *American Journal of Occupational Therapy, (47)*, 431-436.

Baum, M., & Edwards, D. (2000). Documenting productive behaviors. Using the Functional Behavior Profile to plan discharge following stroke. *Journal of Gerontological Nursing, 26*(8), 54.

Baum, M., Edwards, D., & Morrow-Howell, N. (1993). Identification measures and measurement of productive behaviors in senile dementia of the Alzheimer's type. *Gerontologist, 33*(3), 403-408.

Baum, C., Edwards, D., Yonan, C., & Storandt, M. (1996). The relation of neuropsychological test performance to performance of functional tasks in dementia of the Alzheimer type. *Archives of Clinical Neuropsychology, 11*(1), 69-75

Bolt, E., Dekker, J., Eyssen, I., Maasdam, A., Oud, T., & Steultjens, M. (2011). Responsiveness of the Canadian Occupational Performance Measure. *Journal of Rehabilitation Research and Development, 48*(5), 517-528.

Burgener, S., Popovich, A., & Twigg, P. (2005). Measuring psychological well-being in cognitively impaired persons. *Dementia, 4*(4), 463-485.

Burnett, J., Dyer, C., & Naik, A. (2009). Convergent validation of the Kohlman Evaluation of Living Skills (KELS) as a screening tool of older adults' capacity to live safely and independently in the community. *Archives of Physical Medicine and Rehabilitation, 90*(11), 1948-1952.

Cohen, L. (2001). Review of the Independent Living Scales. In R. A. Spies & B. S. Plake (Eds.). *The Fourteenth Mental Measurements Yearbook*. Lincoln, NE: Buros Institute of Mental Measurements.

Desrosiers, J., Noreau, L., Robichaud, L., Fougeyrollas, P., Rochette, A., & Viscogliosi, C. (2004). Validity of the assessment of life habits in older adults. *Journal of Rehabilitation Medicine, 36*(4), 177-182.

Figueiredo, S., Korner-Bitensky, N., Rochette, A., & Desrosiers, J. (2010). Use of the LIFE-H in stroke rehabilitation: A structured review of its psychometric properties. *Disability & Rehabilitation, 32*(9), 705-712.

Fish, J. (2011). Independent Living Scales. In J. Kreutzer, J. DeLuca, & B. Caplan. (eds). *Encyclopedia of Clinical Neuropsychology* (p. 1305). New York, New York: Springer Verlage.

Fougeyrollas, P., & Noreau, L. (2003). *Assessment of Life Habits (LIFE-H 3.1) General Short Form*. Quebec, Canada: INDCP.

Fougeyrollas, P., Noreau, L. St-Michel, G., & Boschen, K. (2008). *Measure of the Quality of the Environment—version 2.0*. Quebec, Canada: RIPPH/INDCP.

Fougeyrollas, P., Tremblay, J., Noreau, L., St-Onge, M., & Dumont, S. (2006). Subjective measurement of participation and environmental barriers and facilitators in population surveys: Use of standardized tools with a sub-sample of the Quebec Activity Limitations Survey (QALS). Living in our Environment. 12th annual North American Collaborating Conference on ICF; June 5-7, 2006. Vancouver, British Columbia, Canada.

Forsyth, K., Parkinson, S., Kielhofner, G., Kramer, J., Mann, L., & Duncan, E. E. (2011). The measurement properties of the Model of Human Occupation Screening Tool and implications for practice. *New Zealand Journal of Occupational Therapy, 58*(2), 5-13.

Gillen, R., & Gernert-Dott, P. (2000). Relationship of independent living scales to a functional outcome measure and neuropsychological tests. *Abstracts/Archives of Clinical Neuropsychology, 15*, 663.

Goverover, Y., Kalmar, J., Gaudino-Goering, E., Shawaryn, M., Moore, N.,...DeLuca, J. (2005). The relation between subjective and objective measures of everyday life activities in persons with multiple sclerosis. *Archives of Physical Medicine and Rehabilitation, 86*(12), 2303-2308.

Josman, N., & Birnboim, S. (2001). Measuring kitchen performance: What assessment should we choose? *Scandinavian Journal of Occupational Therapy, 1*(8), 193-202.

Keglovits, M., Somerville, E., & Stark, S. (2015). In-Home Occupational Performance Evaluation for Providing Assistance (I-HOPE Assist): An assessment for informal caregivers. *American Journal of Occupational Therapy, 69*(5), 1-10.

Kjeken, I., Dagfinrud, H., Uhlig, T., Mowinckel, P., Kvien, T. K., & Finset, A. (2005). Reliability of the Canadian Occupational Performance Measure in patients with ankylosing spondylitis. *The Journal of Rheumatology, 32*(8), 1503–1509.

Kielhofner, G., Fan, C., Morley, M., Garnham, M., Heasman, D., Forsyth, K.,...Taylor, R. (2010). A psychometric study of the Model of Human Occupation Screening Tool (MOHOST). *Hong Kong Journal of Occupational Therapy, 20*(2), 63-70.

Kohlman-Thompson, L. (1992). *The Kohlman Evaluation of Living Skills* (3rd ed.). Bethesda, MD: AOTA Press.

Kohlman-Thompson, L., & Robnett, R. (2016). *Kohlman Evaluation of Living Skills* (4th Ed.). Bethesda, MD: AOTA Press.

Kramer, J., Kielhofner, G., Lee, S., Ashpole, E., & Castle, L. (2009). Utility of the Model of Human Occupation Screening Tool for detecting client change. *Occupational Therapy in Mental Health, 25*(2), 181-191.

Law, M., Baptiste, S., Carswell, A., McColl, M, Polatajko, H., & Pollock N. (2011). *Canadian Occupational Performance Measure* (4th ed.). Toronto, Canada: Canadian Association of Occupational Therapists. In I. Eyssen, M. Steultjens, T. Oud, E. Bolt, A. Maasdam, & J. Dekker. (2011). Responsiveness of the Canadian Occupational Performance Measure. *Journal of Rehabilitation Research and Development, 48*(5), 517-528

Lee, S., Taylor, R., Kielhofner, G., & Fisher, G. (2008). Theory use in practice: A national survey of therapists who use the Model of Human Occupation. *American Journal of Occupational Therapy, 62*(1), 106-117.

Noreau, L., Desrosiers, J., Robichaud, L., Fougeyrollas, P., Rochette, A., & Viscogliosi, C. (2004). Measuring social participation: Reliability of the LIFE-H in older adults with disabilities. *Disability & Rehabilitation, 26*(6), 346-352.

Persel, C. (2012). *The Independent Living Scale*. The Center for Outcome Measurement in Brain Injury. Retrieved from www.tbims.org/combi/ils

Poulin, V., & Desrosiers, J. (2009). Reliability of the LIFE-H satisfaction scale and relationship between participation and satisfaction of older adults with disabilities. *Disability & Rehabilitation, 31*(16), 1311-1317

Revheim, N., & Medalia, A. (2004). The Independent Living Scales as a measure of functional outcome for schizophrenia. *Psychiatric Services, 55*(9), 1052-1054.

Rochette, A., Desrosiers, J., & Noreau, L. (2001). Association between personal and environmental factors and the occurrence of handicap situations following a stroke. *Disability and Rehabilitation, 23*(13), 559- 569.

Stark, S., Somerville, E., & Morris, J. (2010). In-Home Occupational Performance Evaluation (I-HOPE). *American Journal of Occupational Therapy, 64*(4), 580-589.

van de Ven-Stevens, L., Graff, M., Peters, M., van der Linde, H., & Geurts, A. (2015). Construct validity of the Canadian Occupational Performance Measure in participants with tendon injury and Dupuytren disease. *Physical Therapy, 95*(5), 750-757.

Vik, K., Nygard, L., & Lilja, M. (2007). Perceived environmental influence on participation among older adults after home-based rehabilitation. *Physical and Occupational Therapy in Geriatrics, 25*(4), 1-20.

Zimnavoda, T., Weinblatt, N., & Katz, N. (2002). Validity of the Kohlman Evaluation of Living Skills (KELS) with Israeli elderly individuals living in the community. *Occupational Therapy International, 9*(4), 312-325.

XVIII

Pain Assessment

90. McGill Pain Questionnaire (MPQ)

91. Mini Suffering State Exam (MSSE)

92. Pain Assessment Checklist for Seniors With Limited Ability to Communicate (PACSLAC)

Bortnick, K.
Occupational Therapy Assessments for Older Adults: 100 Instruments for Measuring Occupational Performance (pp. 261-269).
© 2017 Taylor & Francis Group.

CHAPTER 90: McGILL PAIN QUESTIONNAIRE (MPQ)

Description

The McGill Pain Questionnaire (MPQ), developed by Melzack (1987), is a self-report rating scale intended to quantify the severity of pain a person may be experiencing. The main instrument is composed of 20 subcategories in which the subject is asked to describe his or her pain by choosing, from a list of several, single-word verbal pain descriptors (1 to 5) for each subcategory. The descriptors (76) encompass 4 major domains: (1) sensory, (2) affective, (3) evaluative, and (4) miscellaneous (Melzack, 2005). The descriptors in each subcategory are of a hierarchical design such that they are ranked in value relative to their position in the word set. For example, the person may choose either (1) jumping, (2) flashing, or (3) shooting to describe spatial pain. A subsequent section of the measure includes an exploration of items that may exacerbate pain (20 choices) such as heat, cold, damp, or stimulants (coffee), as well as a 6-item section similar to the first to further describe the client's pain. The total score is termed the Pain Rating Index (PRI) and ranges from 0 to 78, with higher scores associated with more pain. Scoring also provides for a unique Present Pain Index (PPI), which measures overall pain intensity drawn from six indicators (Strand, Ljunggren, Bogen, Ask, & Johnsen, 2008). A short form (MPQ-SF) derived from the original is also available, which consists of only 15 descriptors of pain, 11 from the sensory and 4 from the affective categories (Strand et al., 2008). The MPQ can be completed in less than 30 minutes with higher scores suggestive of more pain.

Psychometrics

Examination of internal consistency of the original MPQ by Melzack (1975) reported significant correlations (≥ 0.89) with the PRI, the number of words chosen, and the PPI; however, only fair to moderate test-retest reliability (0.70) was determined. Using the short form in an osteoarthritis cohort, one study found high intra-class correlation coefficients (ICCs) of reliability for the total, sensory, affective, and average pain scores at $r = 0.96$, 0.95, 0.88, and 0.89, respectively, whereas the current pain component demonstrated only a moderate ICC of $r = 0.75$ (Grafton, Foster, & Wright, 2005). Using the MPQ-SF, Strand et al. (2008) established that test–retest reliability values for the total and sensory scores of patients with musculoskeletal pain were $r = > 0.74$, however, it was poor for the affective score (0.63). In patients with inflammatory rheumatic pain the ICC values for the total score ($r = 0.93$) and sensory score (0.95) were excellent as well as acceptable for the

affective scores at (0.79). The same study explored MPQ-SF responsiveness to clinically important change as defined by a score of 63 on the Patients Global Impression of Change was 92% in rheumatic patients and 52% in patients with musculoskeletal pain. Comparing the MPQ-SF and the Visual Analog Scale (VAS), scores were found responsive to change, showing mostly large (>0.80) SRM values in patients who reported to have improved. An SRM, or *statistical region merging*, is an algorithm that evaluates the grouping of values based on merging of criteria.

Advantages

Both MPQ versions are client-centered, clinician-directed outcome measures that are easy to administer. They assess a number of pain indicators and do not require any specialized training. The MPQ can also provide the clinician with valuable information about an individual's perception, reaction, and cognition of his or her pain state, which are important factors to consider when choosing treatment modalities and interventions (Strand et al., 2008).

Disadvantages

The MPQ's role as a self-administered assessment may be limited in certain populations due to the complicated adjectives used by some descriptors. The long-version MPQ can take up to 30 minutes to complete.

Administration

The MPQ is self-administered tool in which the client circles the most appropriate pain descriptor for each of the categories addressed where the pain descriptors are organized in a hierarchical fashion. For example, the evaluative item choices would be as follows: (1) annoying, (2) troublesome, (3) miserable, (4) intense, and (5) unbearable. There is also a 6-item section in which a person attempts to identify how strong his or her pain is. An example would be, "Which word describes your pain right now? (1) Mild, (2) discomforting, (3) distressing, (4) horrible, or (5) excruciating." There is also a section relating to items that may exacerbate pain (20 choices) such as loud noises, going to work, or fatigue. Similarly, the MPQ-SF is composed of only 15 pain descriptors that are rated as either (0) none, (1) mild, (2) moderate, or (3) severe; however, the short form derives 3 pain scores from the sum of the intensity rank values of the words chosen for sensory, affective, and total descriptors and the PPI index of the standard MPQ as well as a VAS rating (Melzack, 1987). Higher scores for both assessments are associated with more pain.

Permissions

The MPQ and the MPQ-SF can be accessed through the MAPI Research Trust: Education Information Dissemination website and can be used in clinical practice if requested first. There are user agreements and royalty fees if the scale is to be used for commercial or research purposes and distribution fees may be requested according to study design and context of use of the questionnaire. The following reference publications will give further insight into this assessment:

Melzack, R. (1975). The McGill Pain Questionnaire: Major properties and scoring methods. *Pain*, (3), 277 99.

Melzack. R. (1987). The short-form McGill Pain Questionnaire. *Pain, 30*, 191-197.

Summary

POPULATION	General
TYPE OF MEASURE	Hierarchical rating scale
WHAT IT ASSESSES	Pain levels
TIME	< 30 minutes
COST	Free for private practice

Contact

MAPI Research Trust

27, rue de la Villette

69003 Lyon, France

Phone: +33 (0) 472-13-65-75

Email: contact@mapi-trust.org

Website: www.mapi-trust.org

Ronald Melzack, PhD,

Department of Psychology

McGill University

Montreal, Ontario, Canada

CHAPTER 91: MINI SUFFERING STATE EXAM (MSSE)

Description

The Mini Suffering State Exam (MSSE) is a relatively quick observational measure developed to assess pain for people with limited ability to communicate as well as the level of suffering a person may be in, which are associated with many late or end stage disease processes. The MSSE is composed of 10 items relating to the person's characteristics, as well as the perception of his or her condition as interpreted by the clinician or caregiver. Each item is scored as either 0 (no) or 1 (yes) with totals ranging from 0 to 10. The MSSE can be completed in less than 10 minutes with higher scores reflecting higher degrees of suffering.

TABLE 91-1
ITEMS ON THE MINI SUFFERING STATE EXAM
• Not calm
• Screams
• Pain
• Presence of decubitus ulcers
• Malnutrition
• Eating disorders
• Invasive actions
• Unstable medical condition
• Suffering according to medical opinion
• Suffering according to family opinion
Adapted from Aminoff, Z (2007). Mini-Suffering State Examination scale: Possible key criterion for 6-month survival and mortality of critically ill dementia patients. *American Journal of Hospice and Palliative Care, 24*(6), 472.

Psychometrics

Research by its creators of 103 consecutive bedridden clients found inter-rater reliability to be r = 0.74 and 0.72 using 2 physician raters (Aminoff, Purits, Noy, & Adunsky, 2004). High agreement was also determined for 7 items of the assessment with a range of 0.88 to 0.97 and substantial agreement for the remaining 3 at 0.62 to 0.68, suggesting good concurrent validity (Aminoff et al., 2004). A significant negative correlation was found between the MSSE and the Comfort Assessment in Dying with Dementia at r = −0.80 (Aminoff et al., 2004). When determining when a person should enter hospice and mortality rates, research found that after 6 months of follow up, mortality rates of patients with low, intermediate, and high MSSE scores were 24.3% (9/37), 67.5% (27/40), and 84.6% (22/26), respectively, making the MSSE a useful predictor of mortality in end-stage dementia clients and when a person should enter hospice as well (Aminoff, 2007).

Advantages

The MSSE is a simple and quick assessment to administer, less than 10 minutes, and is particularly useful for people with limited verbal skills. It does not require any specialized training and can be a good initial screen to decide if further testing is warranted. The MSSE scale has also shown to be a reliable and valid clinical tool for evaluating the severity of the patient's condition and his or her level of suffering when severity of symptoms otherwise makes it difficult to quantify. It may also have some usefulness in determining when a person should enter hospice.

Disadvantages

The amount of peer-reviewed research pertaining to the scale is limited and there may be limited discriminatory value between types of suffering because it only comprises 10 items.

Administration

The MSSE is an observational check list in which the clinician or caregiver observes the client and notes the presence or absence of the 10 items on the measure, which can be based on professional opinion or according to caregiver or family opinion. The test uses a straightforward dichotomous scoring system of 0 (no) or 1 (yes) with a range of 0 to 10 with higher scores suggestive of more suffering.

Permissions

The MSSE is located in the public domain and is free to use in both clinical practice and research. It requires no special permissions and is discussed further in the following journal articles:

Aminoff, Z. (2007). Mini-Suffering State Examination scale: Possible key criterion for 6-month survival and mortality of critically ill dementia patients. *American Journal of Hospice and Palliative Care, 24*(6), 470-474.

Aminoff, B., Purits, E., Noy, S., & Adunsky A. (2004). Measuring the suffering of end-stage dementia: Reliability and validity of the Mini-Suffering State Examination. *Archives of Gerontology and Geriatrics, 38*(2), 123-130

Summary

POPULATION	General; persons with limited verbal skills
TYPE OF MEASURE	Rating scale
WHAT IT ASSESSES	Pain levels
TIME	≥10 minutes
COST	Free

Contact

Bechor Zvi Aminoff, MD, PhD

Chaim Sheba Medical Center

Ramat Gan, Israel

Chapter 92: Pain Assessment Checklist for Seniors With Limited Ability to Communicate (PACSLAC)

Description

The Pain Assessment Checklist for Seniors with Limited Ability to Communicate (PACSLAC) is an observational assessment designed to quantify the level of pain a person may be in and is particularly useful for individuals with a limited ability to communicate. The measure consists of 60 items covering various domains pertaining to (1) facial expressions, (2) activity/body, (3) social/personality, and (4) mood, as well as several other non-verbal indicators that also quantify pain levels. During assessment the clinician or caregiver completes the PACSLAC by observing the individual and noting whether any of the 60 items are present or observed by way of a checklist. Examples of behaviors included in the PACSLAC are grimacing, fidgeting, agitation, and shaking/trembling. Each item is scored as 1 point and the presence of higher scores is indicative of more pain descriptors and more severe pain. The assessment can be completed in less than 10 minutes and yields only a total standardized score; however, subscale scores are available for individual interpretation by the clinician.

Psychometrics

By comparing results from persons who experienced painful incidents Zwakhalen, Hamers, Abu-Saad, and Berger (2006) established high levels of internal consistency for total scores at $\alpha = 0.82$ to 0.92, although Cronbach's alpha values for the subscales were lower at 0.55 to 0.73. Also, the correlations calculated between Global Intensity Ratings and PACSLAC scores were moderate at $r = 0.39$ to 0.54. A study of 50 subjects with neurocognitive disorders of the dementia type who had a mean Mini Mental State Exam score of 7.5 showed that total PACSLAC scores ranged from 1 to 22 with a mean of 5.7 (SD = 4.0). Results also showed that the correlation coefficient was significant at 0.83 for scores rated by the researcher and those rated by caregivers (Cheung & Choi, 2008). A study of 40 raters who completed the PACSLAC relative to 2 situations during which a patient under their care experienced a clearly identifiable painful event (i.e., a fall or a painful medical procedure) found that results showed substantial correlations between those painful events at $r = 0.39$ for event 1 and $r = 0.54$ for pain event 2 (Fuchs-Lacelle & Hadjistavropoulos, 2004). The average total PACSLAC score for pain event 1 was 20.3 (SD = 7.5), and for pain event 2 it was 17.9 (SD = 8.3) (Fuchs-Lacelle & Hadjistavropoulos, 2004).

Advantages

The PACSLAC is easy to administer and is excellent for people with limited or no verbal skills making it particularly relevant for certain patient populations. It also does not require specialized training and can be completed in less than 10 minutes.

Disadvantages

There is a limited amount of supporting research pertaining to the PACSLAC. One reason for this might be the fact that it is a relatively newer assessment.

Administration

During assessment the clinician observes the subject and denotes the presence of any pain indicators as outlined on the assessment. In the form of a checklist, developers recommend that only the total score be interpreted, because reliability has been established for the whole assessment and not for the subscale scores (Hadjistavropoulos, Fitzgerald, & Marchildon, 2010).

Table 92-1		
Example Activity/Body Movement Domain Items		
Fidgeting	Pulling away	Flinching
Restless	Pacing	Wandering
Trying to leave	Refusing to move	Thrashing
Adapted from Fuchs-Lacelle, S., & Hadjistavropoulos, T. (2004). Development and preliminary validation of the Pain Assessment Checklist for Seniors with Limited Ability to Communicate (PACSLAC). *Pain Management Nursing, 5*(1), 48.		

Permissions

To use the PACSLAC in clinical practice, research, or for commercial purposes contact the copyright holders at the email that follows. The PACSLAC is generally free for private practice as well as some other entities, but it may not be reproduced without permission. The assessment and supporting information can also be viewed at the website following. More information can be found in the following journal article:

Fuchs-Lacelle, S., & Hadjistavropoulos, T. (2004). Development and preliminary validation of the Pain Assessment Checklist for Seniors with Limited Ability to Communicate (PACSLAC). *Pain Management Nursing*, 5(1), 37-49.

Summary

POPULATION	General; persons with limited verbal skills
TYPE OF MEASURE	Rating scale
WHAT IT ASSESSES	Pain levels
TIME	≥ 10 minutes
COST	Free for private practice

Contact

Thomas Hadjistavropoulos, ABPP, FCAHS

Research Chair in Aging and Health

Professor

University of Regina

Regina, Saskatchewan, Canada

Web: www.geriatricpain.org/Content/Assessment/ Impaired/Pages/PACSLAC.aspx

REFERENCES

Aminoff, Z. (2007). Mini-Suffering State Examination scale: Possible key criterion for 6-month survival and mortality of critically ill dementia patients. *American Journal of Hospice and Palliative Care, 24*(6), 470-474.

Aminoff, Z., Purits, E., Noy, S., & Adunsky A. (2004). Measuring the suffering of end-stage dementia: Reliability and validity of the Mini-Suffering State Examination. *Archives of Gerontology and Geriatrics, 38*(2), 123-130.

Cheung, G., & Choi, P. (2008). The use of the Pain Assessment Checklist for Seniors with Limited Ability to Communicate (PACSLAC) by caregivers in dementia care. *New Zealand Medical Journal, 121*(1286), 21-29.

Fuchs-Lacelle, S., & Hadjistavropoulos, T. (2004). Development and preliminary validation of the Pain Assessment Checklist for Seniors with Limited Ability to Communicate (PACSLAC). *Pain Management Nursing, 5*(1), 37-49.

Grafton, K., Foster, N., & Wright, C. (2005). Test-retest reliability of the short-form McGill Pain Questionnaire: Assessment of intraclass correlation coefficients and limits of agreement in patients with osteoarthritis. *Clinical Journal of Pain, 21*(1), 73-82.

Hadjistavropoulos, T., Fitzgerald, T., & Marchildon, G. (2010). Practice guidelines for assessing pain in older persons with dementia residing in long-term care facilities. *Physiotherapy Canada, 62*(2), 104-113.

Melzack, R. (1975). The McGill Pain Questionnaire: Major properties and scoring methods. *Pain, 1*, 277–299.

Melzack, R. (1987). The Short-Form McGill Pain Questionnaire. *Pain, 30*, 191-197.

Melzack, R. (2005). The McGill Pain Questionnaire from description to measurement. *Anesthesiology, 103*, 199–202.

Strand, L., Ljunggren, A., Bogen, B., Ask, T., & Johnsen, B. (2008). The Short-Form McGill Pain Questionnaire as an outcome measure: Test–retest reliability and responsiveness to change. *European Journal of Pain, 12*, 917–925.

Zwakhalen, S., Hamers, J., Abu-Saad, H., & Berger, M. (2006). Pain in elderly people with severe dementia: A systematic review of behavioural pain assessment tools. *BMC Geriatrics, 6*(3). doi: 10.1186/1471-2318-6-3

XIX

Quality of Life (QoL)

Bortnick, K.
Occupational Therapy Assessments for Older Adults: 100 Instruments for Measuring Occupational Performance (pp. 271-282).
© 2017 Taylor & Francis Group.

Chapter 93: DEMQOL and DEMQOL-Proxy

Description

The DEMQOL is a standardized questionnaire designed to quantify the quality of life (QoL) of individuals with mild to moderate neurocognitive disorders (NCD) of the Alzheimer's and related types through the measurement of behavioral and psychological symptoms known to effect well-being and explores such symptomology as agitation, depression, anxiety, disinhibition, and irritability (Banerjee et al., 2006). The DEMQOL can be administered either as a self-report or interview as well as through information gathered from an informant (Rowen et al., 2012). The self-report/interview and informant-based instruments differ slightly and contain 28 and 31 items, respectively, that are designed to address three main concerns: (1) an individual's thoughts toward his or her feelings; (2) thoughts toward memories; and (3) everyday life. During administration the respondent is asked to consider his or her feeling over the previous week. An example question of the DEMQOL is, "How worried have you been about not having enough company?" The assessment uses 2 4-point ordinal scales (1 to 4) with example possible scoring choices being (1) a lot to (4) not at all. The self-report/interview format total scores range from 28 to 112 and the proxy version scores have a range of 31 to 124. The measure can be completed in less than 10 minutes with higher scores indicating better QoL.

Psychometrics

A factor analysis of the 28-item self-report version displayed a 4-factor model composed of daily activities, memory, negative emotion, and positive emotion that accounted for 49.9% of the variance, whereas analysis of the DEMQOL-Proxy yielded only a 2-factor model of functioning and emotion, which accounted for 35.2% of the variance (Smith et al., 2007). The same study found that the self-report DEMQOL had an internal consistency of $\alpha = 0.87$ and test–retest reliability was of $r = 0.76$ (Smith et al., 2007). Furthermore, it was determined that the discriminant validity between the DEMQOL and Quality of Life in Alzheimer's disease (QOLAD) assessment was 0.39 and convergent validity was 0.54 (Smith et al., 2007). A literature review of six instruments, which included the QOLAD, DEMQOL, Quality of Life in Late-Stage Dementia, Dementia Quality of Life instrument, Cornell Brown Scale for Quality of Life in Dementia, and the Alzheimer Disease-Related Quality of Life, concluded that the DEMQOL and QOLAD were the most suitable for use across a range of disease stages and have the advantage of having both

patient and proxy versions available (King, Zapart, Sansoni, & Marosszeky, 2008).

Advantages

The DEMQOL assessments are both relatively quick and simple measures that require no special training or permissions. There is also a good amount of research in support of their use for both clinical and research applications. The DEMQOL is unique in that it is specifically designed for those with NCD of the Alzheimer's and related types and may be particularly useful for those with mild to moderate impairment. The self-report and caregiver versions can be used separately or in conjunction with each other, allowing the clinician to gain further insights into client QoL.

Disadvantages

Quantifying QoL can be vague and ill-defined for individuals with NCD, as accurate assessment of one's own QoL is predicated on intact cognitive processes and the ability to retrieve and integrate information into a wider context as well as an awareness of one's life circumstances (Gertz & Berwig, 2008). Assessment by proxy can be challenging as well because the assessment of another may be influenced by subjective characteristics, such as personality, nature of the relationship, the amount of time spent together, and level of impairment. A study by Barroso-Sousa et al. (2013) found that statistically significant differences existed between self-reported ratings and caregivers' ratings of subjects' QoL, as caregivers often rated the person's QoL lower than the patient did. Results of a study by Gomez-Gallego, Gomez-Garcia, and Ato-Lozano (2015) generally concurred. They found that QoL evaluations of an informant group seemed to be influenced by their own emotional state and the inner experience, often about the effects of the disease process and overall, suggested that caregiver ratings might be more useful for monitoring the efficacy of treatment when burden is low.

Administration

The DEMQOL, when used as either caregiver proxy or self-report, has specific instructions to follow for accurate administration, thus ensuring standardization. The DEMQOL-Proxy version contains 31 questions as well as 1 practice question that address memory, feelings, and everyday life, where each item is scored as either (1) a lot, (2) quite a bit, (3) a little, and (4) not at all. One final item on each test is scored as either (1) very good, (2) good, (3) fair, or (4) poor. Similar to the caregiver version, the self-report has the same responses but only 28 overall questions. Some items need to be reversed when scoring where total scores range from 31 to 124 (proxy version) and 28 to 112 (self-report/interview version), with higher scores for both indicating better QoL.

TABLE 93-1
EXAMPLE ITEMS OF THE DEMQOL
FEELINGS
In the last week, have you felt…
• Worried or anxious?
• That you are enjoying life?
MEMORY
In the last week, how worried have you been about…
• Forgetting who people are?
• Forgetting what day it is?
EVERYDAY LIFE
How worried have you been about…
• Getting help when you need it?
• Getting to the toilet in time?
• Not having company?
• People not listening to you?
• Getting the affection you want?
Adapted from Mulhern, B., Rowen, D., Brazier, J., Smith, S., Romeo, R., Tait, R.,…Banerjee, S. (2013). Development of DEMQOL-U and DEMQOL-PROXY-U: Generation of preference-based indices from DEMQOL and DEMQOL-PROXY for use in economic evaluation. *Health Technology Assessment, 17*(5), 26-27.

Permissions

The DEMQOL assessments and the manual can be downloaded from the Dementia Collaborative Research Centres website, as well as the Brighton and Sussex Medical school website at the information that follows and are free to use in clinical practice. To use in research or publication contact its creators at the information that follows. More information can be found in the following research article:

Smith, S., Lamping, D., Banerjee, S., Harwood, R., Foley, B., Smith, P.,…Knapp, M. (2007). Development of a new measure of health-related quality of life for people with dementia: DEMQOL. *Psychological Medicine, 37*(5), 737-46.

Summary

POPULATION	NCD Alzheimer's and related type; cognitive impairment
TYPE OF MEASURE	Self-report/interview; proxy questionnaire
WHAT IT ASSESSES	QoL
TIME	≥10 minutes
COST	Free

Contact

Sube Banerjee, MD, FRCPsych

Director of Centre for Dementia Studies

Brighton and Sussex Medical School

Brighton, United Kingdom

Web: www.bsms.ac.uk/about/contact-us/staff/ professor-sube-banerjee.aspx

Website for copies of the assessment: www.bsms.ac.uk/ research/cds/research/demqol.aspx

CHAPTER 94: EQ-5D AND EQ-VAS

Description

The EQ-5D and EQ-VAS are both utility-based questionnaires and visual analog scales (VAS) of health-related quality of life (HRQoL), which, according to Patrick and Erickson (1993), is the particular value assigned to the duration of survival as modified by impairments, functional states, perceptions, and social opportunities influenced by disease, injury and treatment. Developed by the EuroQol Group, the EQ-5D is a 5-item, 3-choice response assessment of an individual's HRQoL and is based according to a person's subjective view of the following attributes: mobility, self-care, usual activities, pain, anxiety, and depression (Davis, Liu-Ambrose, Richardson, & Bryan, 2013). Although, it seems to be a relatively simple 5-item assessment, the EQ-5D employs a distinctive scoring algorithm that has the ability to describe 243 unique health states, which, in turn, yields a single summary score between –1 and +1 that defines a person's health state. The summary scores can then be used to facilitate comparisons across different health conditions and patient population norms, with higher scores indicative of a better quality of life (QoL). A 5-response assessment, as opposed to the to 3-response system discussed previously, is also available in the EQ-5D-5L, which is designed to have better discriminative capacity and sensitivity to change than the EQ-5D, as well as smaller ceiling effects (Davis et al., 2013). Like the original, respondents record their level of problems experienced in the same 5 questions of health; however, they choose between 5 levels of health outcomes: (1) no problem, (2) slight problem, (3) moderate problem, (4) severe problem, or (5) extreme problem. Based on the new combination of responses, respondents can be classified into one of 3125 unique health-state profiles (Fogarty et al., 2013). The accompanying EQ-VAS of both outcome measures is a simple VAS where a client is asked to gauge his or her current health state between *best* and *worst* imaginable, which can then be used by the practitioner as a subjective quantitative measure of well-being. Example items of the 3-response test are as follows:

- Mobility
  - (1) I have no problems in walking about
  - (2) I have some problems in walking about
  - (3) I am confined to bed
- Pain/discomfort
  - (1) I have no pain or discomfort
  - (2) I have moderate pain or discomfort
  - (3) I have extreme pain or discomfort.

The EQ-5D battery can be completed in less than 5 minutes.

Psychometrics

Results from a multinational study of healthy individuals found that test–retest agreement from an Italian sample was r = 0.83 with a range of 0.70 to 0.94 for each dimension. The highest score was for looking after oneself and the lowest was for pain or discomfort. Results from a Spanish study were similar with test-retest agreement of r = 0.94 and a range of 0.86 (pain or discomfort) to 0.99 (looking after oneself). A study of subjects with a major neurocognitive disorder found that item intra-class correlation coefficients of the test were r = 0.72, with an internal consistency Cronbach's alpha of α = 0.64, while item/total correlation ranged from 0.33 to 0.53 (Diaz-Redondo, Rodriguez-Blazquez, Ayala, Martinez-Martin, & Forjaz, 2014). A study by Fogarty et al. (2013) of multiple sclerosis patients, found that the EQ-5D-5L (5-response assessment) displayed good discriminatory capacity with performance differing between the various domains of health; however, evidence of a ceiling effect was noted for self-care and anxiety/depression. A stepwise regression model by Hurst, Kind, Ruta, Hunter, and Stubbings (1997) showed that EQ-5D utility values and VAS were explained best as a function of pain, disability, disease activity, and mood while other variables (side-effects, years of education) were needed to explain the VAS.

Advantages

The EQ-5D and associated scales are simple and easy to administer and can be completed in less than 5 minutes. There is also a large amount of research in support of their use in clinical practice. Both the EQ-5D and EQ-5D-5L (3- and 5-response assessments) and EQ-VAS have shown to be culturally relevant measures with published norms available for many countries. The EQ-5D and EQ-5D-5L employ unique scoring systems that are able to deliver 243 and 3125 different possible health states according to a designed algorithm. The EQ assessments can also be used across various patient populations as well as research settings. Finally, the EuroQol Group has an excellent interactive website devoted to these and other standardized assessments they have created.

Disadvantages

The EQ-5D batteries contain only 5 health-related questions and although they use unique scoring systems they may be considered by some to be only quick screens to determine if a more thorough investigation is warranted. Fees are required to use either EQ-5D versions in private practice depending on the size of the entity where it is to be used as well as the mode(s) of administration (i.e., paper covering telephone scripts, PDA, tablet or Web-based).

Administration

During testing, the respondent is asked to indicate his or her present health state by placing a mark in the box against the most appropriate statement in each of the 5 dimensions, which results in a number expressing the level selected for that dimension (Rabin, de Charro, & Szende, 2004). The EQ-VAS records the respondent's self-rated health on a vertical, 20-cm VAS where the endpoints are labelled *best imaginable health state* and *worst imaginable health state*, allowing an individual to quantify his or her health along a continuum that can then be used as a quantitative measure by the clinician (Rabin et al., 2004). The EQ-5D scores are converted to a single summary index by applying a formula that attaches weights to each of the levels in each dimension based on the valuation of health states from general population samples (EuroQol, 2015). The 5 dimension scores can then be combined to produce a large number of possible health states. A utility index, ranging from –1 to +1, is then calculated and assigned to each health state through an algorithm (Diaz-Redondo et al., 2014).

Permissions

In order to use the EQ-5D and EQ-VAS assessments in practice, research or publication the developers ask that you first register your study, trial, or project by completing a registration form located on the EuroQol website at the information following. Once registered, the EuroQol group will then contact you concerning the type of use and scope of your project. Licensing fees apply and can range from €600 for a small clinical practice to €2800 for a hospital or other unit (with more than 10,000 annual patients). More information can be found in the following publication:

Szende, A., & Williams, A. (2004). *Measuring self-reported population health: An international perspective based on EQ-5D*. Rotterdam, Netherlands: EuroQol Group.

Summary

POPULATION	General
TYPE OF MEASURE	Self-report questionnaire
WHAT IT ASSESSES	HRQoL
TIME	< 5 minutes
COST	Varies

Contact

EuroQol Executive Office

Marten Meesweg 107

3068 AV Rotterdam

The Netherlands

Phone: 31 884400190

Web: www.euroqol.org/eq-5d-products/how-to-obtain-eq-5d.html

Chapter 95: Stroke Specific Quality of Life Scale (SS-QOL)

Description

The Stroke Specific Quality of Life Scale (SS-QOL) is an instrument designed to measure the quality of life (QoL) of stroke populations and is intended to identify common areas that affect health-related QoL (HRQoL). The assessment is composed of 49 items within 12 domains that include such items as energy, family roles, mobility, and self-care. The scale is administered either as a self-report or by proxy where during assessment the person answers questions relating to each of the 12 domains. For example, a question relating to energy would be, "Do you feel tired all of the time?" while an item relating to family roles would be, "I felt I was a burden to my family." Each of the 49 items are then ranked along 1 of 3 possible 5-point Likert scales The first relates to the amount of help needed ranked as either (1) total help, (2) a lot of help, (3) some help, (4) a little help, or (5) no help at all. Another scale relates to one's ability to engage in the activity. Lastly is a response giving the level of agreement with a particular statement. The SS-QOL has a score range of 49 to 245 with higher scores indicating a better HRQoL (Teixeira-Salmela, Neto, Magalhaes, Lima, & Faria, 2009) A shorter 8-domain version is also available and is considered a combination of 4 original domains: mobility, upper-extremity function, self-care, and work/productivity as well as 4 new domains slightly different than the original (energy, language, mood, and social roles) (Hsueh, Jeng, Lee, Sheu, & Hsieh, 2011). A 12-item version exists as well that takes one question from each of the original assessment's 12 domains. The original SS-QoL can be completed in 10 minutes.

TABLE 95-1	
THE 12 DOMAINS OF THE STROKE SPECIFIC QUALITY OF LIFE SCALE	
1. Energy	7. Self-care
2. Family roles	8. Social roles
3. Language	9. Thinking
4. Mobility	10. Upper extremity functioning
5. Mood	11. Vision
6. Personality	12. Work and productivity
Adapted from Williams, L., Weinberger, M., Harris, L., Clark, D., & Biller, J. (1999). Development of a stroke-specific quality of life scale. *Stroke, 30*(7), 1364.	

Psychometrics

Original research of the SS-QOL of 34 ischemic stroke survivors demonstrated good uni-dimensional construct, as each of 12 domains had excellent internal consistency where Cronbach's alpha values for each domain were $\alpha = \geq 0.73$ (range: 0.73 to 0.89). It was also shown to correlate with the Short-Form 36 Health Survey at 0.65 (Williams, Weinberger, Harris, Clark, & Biller, 1999). The same study found that the SS-QOL domains that were most frequently identified as most affected were hand/arm function (56%), family roles (56%), language (56%), mobility (31%), work/productivity (28%), cognitive (19%), mood (19%), and energy (13%) (Williams et al., 1999). A study of 33 stroke survivors with chronic hemiparesis recruited from an outpatient physical therapy clinic by Silva, Ishida Correa, De Morais Faria, and Ferrari Correa (2015) estimated the internal consistency SS-QOL to be quite high at $\alpha = 0.91$, indicating good stability with regard to item calibration; however, their Rasch analysis detected the following three items with erratic behavior:

1. Item 14: Did you need help to use the toilet?

2. Item 15: I did my hobbies and recreation for shorter periods of time than I would like.

3. Item 17: I had less sex than I would like to.

Another study of 56 subjects with chronic hemiparesis compared the construct of the SS-QOL with the International Classification of Functioning, Disability, and Health (ICF) and identified 54 concepts embedded within the SS-QOL, and of those 51 were linked to ICF categories: 22 (41%) relating to body functions; 26 (48%) activities and participation; and 3 (5.5%) comprised of environmental factors (Teixeira-Salmela et al., 2009).

Advantages

The SS-QOL is a relatively quick and easy scale to administer and there is also a good amount of literature in support of its use in clinical practice. The SS-QOL is located in the public domain, thus it is free to use in research and publication. Also, no special training or certifications are needed.

Disadvantages

Although, the SS-QOL has been validated in several stroke patient populations, a study by Boosman, Passier, Visser-Meily, Rinkel, and Post (2010) of subjects with intracerebral hemorrhage demonstrated the presence of both ceiling and floor effects with substantial ceiling effects for 10 of the 12 domains, most notably for the domains of self-care and vision, on which more than half of all respondents chose the highest possible score. This suggests that the SS-QOL may have limited use for this population or may lack sensitivity for higher functioning individuals.

Administration

During assessment, the subject is asked to consider several questions or statements relative to his or her personal experience and then rate his or her answer using one of the three possible scoring scales. Subscales for each of the domains can be examined as well as the total score by the clinician to gain insight into client QoL.

TABLE 95-2
EXAMPLE ITEMS OF THE STROKE SPECIFIC QUALITY OF LIFE SCALE
MOOD
• I was discouraged about my future.
• I wasn't interested in other people or activities.
• I slept more than I would like.
PERSONALITY
• I was irritable.
• I was impatient with others.
• My personality has changed.
UPPER EXTREMITY FUNCTION
• Did you have trouble putting on socks?
• Did you have trouble buttoning buttons?
• Did you have trouble dialing a telephone number?
Adapted from Williams, L., Weinberger, M., Harris, L., Clark, D., & Biller, J. (1999). Development of a stroke-specific quality of life scale. *Stroke, 30*(7), 1368.

Permissions

The SS-QOL is located in the public domain and is free to use in clinical practice as well as research or publication. It is wholly contained in the following journal article and is also available from various websites. The authors ask that the citation that follows be used when referenced.

Williams, L. S., Weinberger, M., Harris, L. E., Clark, D. O., & Biller, J. (1999). Development of a stroke-specific quality of life scale. *Stroke, 30*(7), 1362-1369.

Summary

POPULATION	CVA
TYPE OF MEASURE	Self-report questionnaire
WHAT IT ASSESSES	HRQoL
TIME	< 10 minutes
COST	Free

Contact

Linda S. Williams, MD

Indiana University

Center for Health Services and Outcomes Research

VA HSR&D Center of Innovation

Roudebush VA Medical Center

Indianapolis, Indiana

Chapter 96: World Health Organization Quality of Life—Abbreviated Version (WHOQOL-BREF)

Description

The World Health Organization Quality of Life Abbreviated Version (WHOQOL-BREF) is a quality of life (QoL) assessment whose creation was sponsored by the World Health Organization (WHO) in order to develop an instrument that would be applicable across many patient populations and more importantly, many cultures. The initiative arose in part because measures of health status that have been developed in western countries have been constrained by cultural expectations and developer bias, thus the goal was to create as broad an assessment as possible concerning QoL (Garcia-Rea & LePage, 2010; Harper, 1996). The WHOQOL–BREF, which has been translated into 50 languages, contains 26 items that encompass 4 domains: physical (7 items), psychological (6 items), social relationships (3 items), and environmental (8 items). There are also 2 global questions that address overall QoL and health satisfaction (Kalfoss, Low, &Molzahn, 2008). Derived from data compiled from the original 100-item assessment, 1 highly relevant item from each of its 24 dimensions were included in the creation of the new short version as well as 2 new items (Mas-Expósito, Amador-Campos, Gómez-Benito, & Lalucat-Jo, 2011). Administered as either a self-report or interview, each question is scored along a 5-point Likert scale with respect to the person's QoL over the last 2 weeks. Scoring uses a weighted framework with higher scores indicating better QoL. The WHOQOL-BREF can be completed in less than 10 minutes.

TABLE 96-1
EXAMPLE DOMAIN ITEMS OF THE WORLD HEALTH ORGANIZATION QUALITY OF LIFE ABBREVIATED VERSION
PHYSICAL
• Pain and discomfort
• Sleep and rest
• Energy and fatigue
PSYCHOLOGICAL
• Positive feelings
• Body image and appearance
• Negative feelings
SOCIAL RELATIONSHIPS
• Personal relationships
• Social support
• Sexual activity
ENVIRONMENT
• Freedom, physical safety, and security
• Financial resources
• Opportunities for acquiring new information and skills
Adapted from Harper, A., & Power, M. (1998). Development of the World Health Organization WHOQOL-BREF Quality of Life Assessment. *Psychological Medicine, 28*(3), 552.

Psychometrics

Twenty-four data centers representing 23 countries with 11,830 respondents established the psychometric properties of the WHOQOL-BREF where factor analysis of the 4 domains found that internal consistency was highest for the 7-item physical domain at α = 0.82, followed by the psychological domain at 0.81, the environment domain at 0.80, and lowest for the social domain at 0.68 (Skevington, Lotfy, & O'Connell, 2004). The same cohort determined that the mean scores of the 4 domains were physical at 16.2, psychological at 15.0, environment at 13.5, and social at 14.3 (Skevington et al., 2004). Another study involving data sets of 300 people determined that domain scores produced by the WHOQOL-BREF correlated highly with the original WHOQOL-100 with a range of 0.89 to 0.95 (Harper & Power, 1998). A study among patients with schizophrenia showed excellent internal consistency of α = 0.88 at baseline and 0.89 at 1-year follow-up (Mas-Expósito et al., 2011). Internal consistencies and test–retest coefficients, in a homeless substance-dependent veteran population were above 0.70 for all domains (Garcia-Rea & LePage, 2010). Divergent validity of WHOQOL–BREF showed that domain scores were negatively correlated with the Global Deterioration Scale with coefficients ranging from –0.47 to –0.76 for a Canadian sample of 192 older adults, and –0.46 to –0.59 for a Norwegian sample of 469 older adults. The same study found correlations with the Short Form 12 (an instrument that measures health and functioning status) were also statistically significant with

a range from r = 0.24 to 0.78 for the Canadian sample and r = 0.21 to 0.76 for the Norwegian (Kalfoss et al., 2008).

Advantages

The WHOQOL-BREF is a relatively simple assessment that has a large amount of research in support of its use in clinical practice. It has been shown to support a world model of QoL that is defined by one's perceptions of *position in life* in the context of the culture and value systems in which the person lives, in relation to his or her goals, expectations, standards, and concerns (Mas-Expósito et al., 2011). The WHO maintains an excellent interactive website devoted to the WHOQOL assessments where it and other information can be downloaded.

Disadvantages

The weighted scoring system may be complicated and a study of healthy older adults from Canada and Norway found that ceiling effects were present among items in the physical and environmental domains (Kalfoss et al., 2008).

Administration

The WHOQOL-BREF can be completed as either a self-report or interview in which each item is scored along a 5-point Likert scale (1 to 5). Scores are computed using an algebraic formula to produce both a domain score and total score. Three items of the WHQOL-BREF must be reversed before scoring as well.

TABLE 96-2
DISCRIMINANT VALIDITY OF T-TEST DOMAIN SCORES FOR ILLNESS VS WELL SAMPLES

DOMAIN	PHYSICAL	PSYCHOLOGICAL	SOCIAL	ENVIRONMENT
Mean, sick	13.1	13.7	14.0	13.8
Mean, well	15.4	14.8	14.8	14.1

Adapted from Skevington, S., Lotfy, M., & & O'Connell, K. (2004). The World Health Organization's WHOQOL-BREF quality of life assessment: Psychometric properties and results of the international field trial: A Report from the WHOQOL Group. *Quality of Life Research, 13,* 299–310,

TABLE 96-3

EXAMPLE ITEMS ON THE WORLD HEALTH ORGANIZATION QUALITY OF LIFE ABBREVIATED VERSION

- Do you have enough energy for everyday life?
- Are you able to accept your bodily appearance?
- Do you have enough money to meet your needs?
- How available to you is the information that you need in your day-to-day life?
- To what extent do you have the opportunity for leisure activities?
- How satisfied are you with your sleep?

Adapted from The World Health Organization. (2004). *The World Health Organization Quality of Life (WHOQOL)-BREF* (pp. 3-4). Geneva, Switzerland.

Permissions

The WHOQOL-BREF is free to use in clinical practice but must be requested first at the WHO website. Use in research, publication, or for commercial purposes can also be obtained by contacting the WHO or its affiliates at the information following, as well as the original publications which contain the assessment. More information can be found in the following journal article:

Harper, A., & Power, M. (1998). Development of the World Health Organization WHOQOL-BREF Quality of Life Assessment. *Psychological Medicine, 28*(3), 551-558.

Summary

POPULATION	General
TYPE OF MEASURE	Self-report questionnaire
WHAT IT ASSESSES	QoL
TIME	< 10 minutes
COST	Free

Contact

United States World Health Organization Quality of Life Center

Attn: Instrument Distribution Coordinator

University of Washington Department of Health Services

Box 359455

Seattle, Washington, USA 98195-9455

Phone: (800) 291-2193

Email: seaqol@u.washington.edu

Web: http://depts.washington.edu/seaqol/WHOQOL

World Health Organization

Email: WHOQOL@who.int

Web: www.who.int/substance_abuse/research_tools/whoqolbref/en/

REFERENCES

Banerjee, S., Smith, S. C., Lamping, D. L., Harwood, R. H., Foley, B., Smith, P.,...Knapp, M. (2006). Quality of life in dementia: More than just cognition. An analysis of associations with quality of life in dementia. *Journal of Neurology, Neurosurgery and Psychiatry, 77*(2), 146-148.

Barroso-Sousa, M., Luiza-Santos, R., Arcoverde, C., Simões, P., Belfort, T., Adler, I.,...Nascimento-Dourado, M. (2013). Quality of life in dementia: The role of non-cognitive factors in the ratings of people with dementia and family caregivers. *International Psychogeriatrics, 25*(7), 1097–1105.

Boosman, H., Passier, P., Visser-Meily, J., Rinkel, G., & Post, M. (2010). Validation of the Stroke Specific Quality of Life scale in patients with aneurysmal subarachnoid haemorrhage. *Journal of Neurology Neurosurgery and Psychiatry, 81*, 485-489.

Davis, J., Liu-Ambrose, T., Richardson, C., & Bryan, S. (2013). A comparison of the ICECAP-O with EQ-5D in a falls prevention clinical setting: Are they complements or substitutes? *Quality of Life Research, 22*(5), 969-977.

Diaz-Redondo, A., Rodriguez-Blazquez, C., Ayala, A., Martínez-Martín, P., & Forjaz, M. J. (2014). EQ-5D rated by proxy in institutionalized older adults with dementia: Psychometric pros and cons. *Geriatrics and Gerontology International, 14*(2), 346-353.

EuroQol. (2015). Valuation of EQ-5D. Retrieved from www.euroqol.org/about-eq-5d/valuation-of-eq-5d.html

Fogarty, E., Walsh, C., Adams, R., McGuigan, C., Barry, M., & Tubridy, N. (2013). Relating health-related Quality of Life to disability progression in multiple sclerosis, using the 5-level EQ-5D. *Multiple Sclerosis Journal, 19*(9), 1190-1196.

Garcia-Rea, E., & LePage, J. (2010). Reliability and validity of the World Health Organization Quality of Life: Brief Version (WHOQOL-BREF) in a homeless substance dependent veteran population. *Social Indicators Research, 99*(2), 333-340.

Gertz, H., & Berwig, M. (2008). Critical observations on measuring quality of life of persons suffering from dementia. *Nervenarzt, 79*, 1023–1035. In M. Berwig, H. Leicht, K. Hartwig, & H. J. Gertz. (2011). Self-rated quality of life in mild cognitive impairment and Alzheimer's disease: The problem of affective distortion. *GeroPsych: The Journal of Gerontopsychology and Geriatric Psychiatry, 24*(1), 45-51.

Gomez-Gallego, M., Gomez-Garcia, J., & Ato-Lozano E. (2015). Addressing the bias problem in the assessment of the quality of life of patients with dementia: Determinants of the accuracy and precision of the proxy ratings. *Journal of Nutrition, Health and Aging, 19*(3), 365-372.

Harper, A. (1996). *WHOQOL-BREF: Introduction, administration, scoring and generic version of the assessment*. Geneva, Switzerland: World Health Organization.

Harper, A., & Power, M. (1998). Development of the World Health Organization WHOQOL-BREF Quality of Life Assessment. *Psychological Medicine, 28*(3), 551-558.

Hsueh, I. P., Jeng, J. S., Lee, Y., Sheu, C. F., & Hsieh, C. L. (2011). Construct validity of the Stroke-Specific Quality of Life Questionnaire in ischemic stroke patients. *Clinical Rehabilitation, 21*, 620–627.

Hurst, N., Kind, P., Ruta, D., Hunter, M., & Stubbings, A. (1997). Measuring health-related quality of life in rheumatoid arthritis: Validity, responsiveness and reliability of EuroQol (EQ-5D). *Rheumatology, 36*(5), 551-559.

Kalfoss, M., Low, G., & Molzahn, A. (2008). The suitability of the WHOQOL–BREF for Canadian and Norwegian older adults. *European Journal on Ageing, 5*, 77–89.

King, M., Zapart, S., Sansoni, J., & Marosszeky, N. (2008). Measuring health related quality of life in persons with dementia, facilitating knowledge exchange and transfer for a dynamic future. Thirteenth Annual National Health Outcomes Conference, April 29-May 1, 2008. Canberra, Australia.

Mas-Expósito, L., Amador-Campos, J., Gómez-Benito, J., & Lalucat-Jo, L. (2011). The World Health Organization Quality of Life Scale Brief Version: A validation study in patients with schizophrenia. *Quality of Life Research, 20*(7), 1079-1089.

Mulhern, B., Rowen, D., Brazier, J., Smith, S., Romeo, R Tait, R.,...Banerjee, S. (2013). Development of DEMQOL-U and DEMQOL-PROXY-U: Generation of preference-based indices from DEMQOL and DEMQOL-PROXY for use in economic evaluation. *Health Technology Assessment, 17*(5), 1-160.

Patrick, D. L., & Erickson, P. (1993). Concepts of health related quality of life. In D. L. Patrick & P. Erickson. *Health Status and Health Policy* (p. 419). Oxford, United Kingdom: Oxford University Press.

Rabin, R., de Charro, F., & Szende, A. (2004). Introduction. In A. Szende & A. Williams. (2004). *Measuring Self-reported population health: An international perspective based on EQ-5D*. Rotterdam, Netherlands: EuroQol Group.

Rowen, D., Mulhern, B., Banerjee, S., van Hout, B., Young, T., Knapp, M.,...Brazier, D. (2012). Estimating preference-based single index measures for dementia using DEMQOL and DEMQOL-Proxy. *Value in Health, 15*(2), 346–356.

Silva, S., Ishida Correa, F., De Morais Faria, C., & Ferrari Correa, J. (2015). Psychometric properties of the Stroke Specific Quality of Life scale for the assessment of participation in stroke survivors using the Rasch model: A preliminary study. *Journal of Physical Therapy Science, 27*(2), 389-392.

Skevington, S., Lotfy, M., & O'Connell, K. (2004). The World Health Organization's WHOQOL-BREF quality of life assessment: Psychometric properties and results of the international field trial: A Report from the WHOQOL Group. *Quality of Life Research, 13*, 299–310,

Smith, S. C., Lamping, D. L., Banerjee, S., Harwood, R. H., Foley, B., Smith, P.,...Knapp, M. (2007). Development of a new measure of health-related quality of life for people with dementia: DEMQOL. *Psychological Medicine, 37*(5), 737-746.

Teixeira-Salmela, L., Neto, M., Magalhães, L., Lima, R., & Faria, C. (2009). Content comparisons of stroke-specific quality of life based upon the international classification of functioning, disability, and health. *Quality of Life Research, 18*(6), 765-773.

Williams, L., Weinberger, M., Harris, L., Clark, D., & Biller, J. (1999). Development of a stroke-specific quality of life scale. *Stroke, 30*(7), 1362-1369.

World Health Organization. (2004). *The World Health Organization Quality of Life (WHOQOL)-BREF*. Geneva, Switzerland

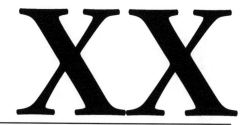

Vision and Visual Perceptual Measures

Bortnick, K.
Occupational Therapy Assessments for Older Adults: 100 Instruments for Measuring Occupational Performance (pp. 283-303).
© 2017 Taylor & Francis Group.

CHAPTER 97: BEERY-BUKTENICA DEVELOPMENTAL TEST OF VISUAL MOTOR INTEGRATION—SIXTH EDITION (BEERY VMI-6)

Description

The Beery-Buktenica Developmental Test of Visual Motor Integration—Sixth Edition (Beery VMI-6) is a standardized assessment used to identify those individuals having difficulty with visual-motor integration as well as to measure the extent of integration of visual and motor abilities (McCrimmon, Altomare, Matchullis, & Jitlina, 2012). Designed for use across the lifespan, ages 2 to 100 years old, the most recent edition has principally represented a normative update from the fifth edition (Beery & Beery, 2010). Published by Pearson Inc., the Beery VMI-6 consists of one core task, Visual-Motor Integration (VMI), and two supplemental tasks, Visual Perception (VP) and Motor Coordination (MC). The VMI section evaluates an individual's integration of visual perception and motor skills whereby the person is asked to copy a series of geometric forms using pencil and paper in which items are arranged in developmental sequence, from less to more complex; whereas the VP task evaluates an individual's visual abilities without the use of any motor skills where the person is presented with various similar visual figures, of which one is the correct target stimuli (McCrimmon et al., 2012). The MC task is used to evaluate fine motor skills and often can be scored based on prior observations by the clinician during the previous subtest assessments, which includes such observations as whether or not the individual was able to hold a pencil correctly (McCrimmon et al., 2012). The VMI has both a short (21-item) and full (30-item) version where both take less than 15 minutes to complete. The administration time for the supplemental VP and MC tasks is approximately 5 minutes each. Higher scores and number of items passed indicate better performance.

TABLE 97-1
EXAMPLE VISUAL MOTOR INTEGRATION MAIN SCALE HIERARCHY OF ITEMS
• Open square and circle
• Three-line cross
• Directional arrows
• Two-dimensional rings
• Six-circle triangle
• Circle and tilted square
• Vertical diamond
• Tilted triangles
• Eight-dot circle
• Wertheimer's hexagons
• Horizontal diamond
• Three-dimensional rings
• Necker cube
• Tapered box
• Three-dimensional star

Adapted from Brown, T., Unsworth, C., & Lyons, C. (2009). An evaluation of the construct validity of the Developmental Test of Visual-Motor Integration using the Rasch Measurement Mode. *Australian Occupational Therapy Journal, 56*(6), 394.

Psychometrics

The Beery VMI, has remained relatively stable over time and its content validity is evidenced by the fact that the original 72 geometric items have now been reduced to 30 forms arranged in a developmental sequence (McCrimmon et al., 2012). The examiner's manual reports internal consistency for the VMI adult sample to be good to excellent with a coefficient alpha value of $\alpha = 0.89$ (range 0.83 to 0.91); however, Brown, Chinner, and Stagnitti (2010) found only moderate internal consistency at $\alpha = 0.66$ in a study of 61 healthy adults. The same study found only fair test-retest reliability as well at $r = 0.61$, while inter-rater reliability was good at 0.79 and intra-rater reliability excellent at 0.95, suggesting that overall, the VMI exhibited moderate to high levels of reliability. A subsequent study by, Brown, Chinner, and Stagnitti (2011) established the convergent validity of the VMI-5 with the Range Test of Visual Motor Integration assessment at $r = 0.70$ where the mean VMI-5 score for the adult population (n=61) was 26.64 (2.37).

TABLE 97-2			
MEAN SCORES AND CORRELATIONS WITH THE ADULT SAMPLE** INDICATING THE MEASUREMENT OF SIMILAR CONSTRUCTS ACROSS THE LIFESPAN			
AGE	**N**	**MEAN SCORE (SD)**	**CORRELATION**
≥ 18 years old	61	26.64 (2.37)	**
11 to 17 years old	19	24.90 (2.33)	0.77
5 to 10 years old	73	20.56 (3.54)	0.70
mean age = 32 years ± 11			
Adapted from Brown, T., Chinner, A., & Stagnitti, K. (2011). Convergent validity of two visual motor integration tests. *British Journal of Occupational Therapy, 74*(6), 295, 299.			

Advantages

There is a significant amount of research in support of the VMI for use in clinical practice and, since its development in the early 60s, it has gone through numerous refinements. The VMI also has well-established norms which are based on a standardized national sample of 1021 adults ages 19 to 100 years old (Beery, Buktenica, & Beery, 2015). The main test has both short and full versions along with the supplemental tests that are relatively quick to administer. Finally, the VMI is maintained by Pearson Inc. and could be considered much less expensive than some other visual perceptual measures at $145.

Disadvantages

Results of a study of children ages 5 to 12 years old, which may have some implications for older adult populations, found that although the VMI displayed uni-dimensionality there may be some redundancy relative to items 4/5/11, items 18/22/24, as well as items 26/27/29, which can present scoring implications as the VMI test is terminated when 3 consecutive items are not passed (Brown et al., 2009). The same study also found that item 9 (copied circle) may exhibit differential bias based on gender (Brown et al., 2009)

Administration

As the VMI employs drawing of shapes, various measurements and degrees of angles may need to be applied to determine a score, suggesting careful analysis by the examiner; however, the manual includes detailed instructions and suggests that if in doubt the item should be scored as passed (McCrimmon et al., 2012). For the VP supplemental section, one point is awarded for each correct item based on first response, not those given after teaching or correcting, and for the MC supplemental, one point is awarded for each item where there are pencil marks between all dots and within the borders (McCrimmon et al., 2012). Specific additional rules are also outlined in the manual, which provides scoring guidelines and examples for all three tasks as well as standard scores, percentiles, and age equivalents (McCrimmon et al., 2012).

Permissions

The Beery VMI-6 is a standardized assessment kit that can be purchased from Pearson as well as other therapy supply stores. The kit contains the examiner's manual, 10 short-form tests, 10 long-form tests, 10 supplementary visual tests, and 10 supplementary motor tests for roughly $145. A separate manual can also be purchased for $70. Permission to use in research or publication can be obtained by contacting the copyright holders or its creators at the information that follows. More information can be found in the following publication:

Beery, K. E., & Beery, N. A. (2010). *Administration, scoring, and teaching manual for the Beery-VMI.* (6th ed.). San Antonio, TX: Pearson.

Summary

POPULATION	General; ages 2 to 99 years
TYPE OF MEASURE	Activity based
WHAT IT ASSESSES	Visual motor integration/skills
TIME	15 to 30 minutes
COST	$145

Contact

Natasha Beery, MA

Director of BSEP and Community Relations

Berkley, California

Web: www.berkeleyschools.net/departments/bsep/

Pearson Clinical

Inbound Sales and Customer Support

P.O. Box 599700

San Antonio, TX 78259

Phone: (800) 627-7271

Email: clinicalcustomersupport@pearson.com

Web: www.pearsonclinical.com/therapy/ products/100000663/the-beery-buktenica- developmental-test-of-visual-motor-integration- 6th-edition-beery-vmi.html

Chapter 98: Developmental Test of Visual Perception—Adolescent and Adult (DTVP-A)

Description

The Developmental Test of Visual Perception—Adolescent and Adult (DTVP-A), by Reynolds, Pearson, and Voress (2002), is a standardized battery designed to measure the visual-perceptual and visual-motor abilities of persons aged 11 to 75 years and has shown to be especially useful in the evaluation of traumatic brain injury and stroke patients where right-hemisphere function is of primary concern. The assessment consists of 6 different but interrelated subscales: (1) copying, (2) figure-ground, (3) visual motor search, (4) visual closure, (5) form constancy, and (6) visual motor speed. Three subscales of the DTVP-A are considered motor-free (figure-ground, visual closure, and form constancy), while three involve the use of visual motor skills to complete task items (copying, visual–motor search, and visual motor speed) (Brown, Mapleston, Nairn, & Molloy, 2013). An example item of the assessment is visual motor speed, in which the subject is first shown four different geometric designs, two of which have special marks, where he or she must then find them on a page filled completely with the four similar designs that have no marks (DTVP-A, 2012). Scoring employs unique algorithms for all subscales to produce several scores including a general visual-perceptual index, a motor-reduced visual perception index, and a visual-motor integration index. The DTVP-A can be completed in less than 30 minutes.

Psychometrics

The examiner's manual reports test-retest reliability coefficients involving 3 subjects for the 3 motor-free subscales to be r = 0.71 for figure ground, 0.71 for visual closure, and 0.74 for form constancy; whereas the composite scale was found to have a test-retest reliability coefficient of r = 0.81, while inter-rater reliability coefficients for the same sample were r = 0.98 for figure-ground, 0.99 for visual closure, and 0.99 for form constancy with the coefficient for the composite scale excellent at 0.99 (Reynolds et al., 2002). The manual report of internal consistency of the 3 motor-free subscales were figure ground (α = 0.77), visual closure (0.81), and form constancy (0.89), while the composite score for the visual perceptual scale was 0.92 (Reynolds et al., 2002). A study by Brown, Elliott, et al. (2011) showed that subjects with neurological impairment scored 16.0 points lower (maximum 49) on the DTVP-A than persons without impairment with statistically significant mean differences for the 3 subscales of figure-ground (with impairment 10.86 and 6.91 without), visual closure (with impairment 15.47 and 11.73 without), and form constancy (with impairment 18.24 and 11.73 without), suggesting good discriminant validity. A study of 229 individuals 49 with neurological impairment and 172 without, found that DTVP-A (non-motor) total scores were significantly correlated with the Motor Visual Perception Test (MVPT-3) total scores at r = 0.73, whereas the DTVP-A subscales of figure-ground, visual closure and form constancy correlated with MVPT-3 total scores at r = 0.59, 0.68, and 0.65, respectively (Bourne et al., 2012). The DTVP-A total score was also significantly correlated with subscales 1 to 7 of the Test of Visual-Perceptual Skills with coefficients ranging from r = 0.48 to 0.68. The figure-ground subscale ranged from 0.36 to 0.56, visual closure ranged from 0.43 to 0.64, and form constancy range from 0.51 to 0.64 (Bourne et al., 2012). The study discussed earlier by Reynolds et al. (2002) also established correlations with the Draw a Person Test, and the Comprehensive Trail Making Test at 0.39 and 0.40, respectively.

Advantages

The DTVP-A has been in use since the mid-1960s and there is a good amount of research in support of the current version in clinical practice. The DTVP-A also has the ability to document if intervention is necessary as well as the effectiveness of those interventions relative to visual-perceptual or visual-motor difficulties The normative sample in the manual consists of 1664 adolescents and adults residing in 19 states in the United States with scores normed through age 75 years old.

Disadvantages

A factor analysis by Brown (2011) found that although the majority of the 49 items of the 3 motor reduced scales exhibited moderate uni-dimensionality, when all 3 motor-reduced subscales were analyzed as one Total Motor-Reduced Visual Perception Composite Scale (TMRVPCS), several items exhibited Rasch model misfit, as well as gender bias at 14.3% and 8.2% according to the TMRVPCS model, respectively.

Administration

During assessment the subject is asked to attempt tasks of varying degrees of difficulty with instructions clearly outlined in the examiner's manual. The motor-enhanced subscales of the DTVP-A require the respondent to use his or her motor skills to complete test items, whereas the motor-reduced items require participants to analyze 49 black-and-white designs and respond appropriately, using a multiple choice format (Brown, 2011). Scores are obtained by adding the standard scores of the subtests creating a composite score, which is then converted to an indexed norm that can then be compared with standardized norms in the manual in a variety of ways (Brown, 2011).

TABLE 98-1
EXAMPLE SUBSCALES OF THE DEVELOPMENTAL TEST OF VISUAL PERCEPTION—ADOLESCENT AND ADULT

Copying	Subjects are asked to draw a figure the same as the one shown.
Figure-ground	Subjects are asked to find as many stimuli in a complex background the same as the one presented.
Visual-motor search	Subjects must connect random numerical circles in sequence.
Visual closure	Subjects must find a stimulus from a series that has been incompletely drawn.
Form constancy	Subjects must find the stimulus figure out of a series that has a different size, position, or color or is hidden in the background.

Adapted from Pro-Ed Inc. (2012). DTVP-A: Developmental Test of Visual Perception–Adolescent and Adult. Austin, TX. Retrieved from www.proedinc.com/customer/productView.aspx?ID=900

Permissions

The DTVP-A is a test kit that, when purchased, includes an examiner's manual, picture book, 25 profile/examiner record forms, and 25 response booklets in a storage box and is available from numerous therapy supply companies. For example, at Pro-Ed the cost for the assessment battery is $239. Permission to use in research or publication can be obtained by contacting where purchased or its creators. More information can be found in the following publication:

Reynolds, C., Pearson, N., & Voress, J. (2002). *Developmental Test of Visual Perception: Adolescent and Adult*. Austin, TX: Pro-Ed.

Summary

POPULATION	General; ages 11 to 75 years
TYPE OF MEASURE	Activity based; motor and non-motor components
WHAT IT ASSESSES	Visual-perceptual and visual-motor abilities
TIME	< 30 minutes
COST	$239

Contact

Judith K. Voress, EdD
Hammill Institute on Disabilities
Austin, Texas
Email: info@hammill-institute.org

Cecil Reynolds, PhD
Professor Emeritus
Educational Psychology
Texas A & M University
College Station, Texas

CHAPTER 99: MOTOR-FREE VISUAL PERCEPTION TEST— THIRD AND FOURTH EDITIONS (MVPT-3 AND 4)

Description

The Motor-Free Visual Perception Test—Third and Fourth Editions (MVPT-3 and MVPT-4) are standardized assessments designed to measure overall visual perceptual ability by employing a multiple-choice format of simple black-and-white drawings as stimulus items and answer choices. As its name suggests it does not place any demands upon a person's motor-skills (Brown & Elliot, 2011). Both versions assess 5 theoretical visual perceptual constructs: (1) spatial relationships, (2) visual discrimination, (3) figure-ground (4) visual closure, and (5) visual memory. The MVPT-4 represents a reorganization of 45 items from the MVPT-3 (65 items) including new norms for ages 4 through 80 years old or older in which data was collected from 2012 to 2014 on a national, stratified sample of more than 2700 individuals. (Canivez, 2005; Colarusso & Hammill, 2003, Colarusso & Hammill, 2013). The MVPT batteries takes less than 30 minutes to administer and 10 minutes to score and yield single-item and total-scale scores, which can then be converted to a standard score, percentile rank, and age equivalent scores using the norms tables provided in their respective test manuals (Colarusso & Hammill, 2003). When purchased, each manual provides complete instructions and scoring tables that are divided into 5-year intervals for ages 20 to 49 years old and 2-year intervals for ages 50 to 93 years old, and as hypothesized, MVPT scores continue to improve up until a certain age (39 years old for the MVPT-3), after which they then began to decline at a slow but steady, rate (Brown & Elliot, 2011; Canivez, 2005). An example of the assessment includes the subject being shown a drawing and then asked to choose the matching drawing from a set of four.

Psychometrics

Test-retest reliability of the MVPT-3 using a 34-day retest interval of 75 subjects 11 to 84 years old or older was r=0.92, suggesting that the test is relatively stable over time. Internal consistency computed for each age group, ranged from α=0.69 to 0.90, which included those aged 4 to 11 years (Colarusso & Hammill, 2003). Results of a study of 49 subjects with a diagnosed neurological impairment and 172 without showed a statistically significant lower score for those with impairment than those without at 59.91 and 43.96, respectively, suggesting that the MVPT-3 was able to discriminate between the two groups (Brown, Elliott, et al., 2011). Another study using the same group cohort found that MVPT-3 total scores significantly correlated with the Test of Visual Perceptual Skills-3 non-motor total score at r=0.79 and the Developmental Test of Visual Perception-Adolescent and Adult at r=0.73, suggesting that although these tests assess visual perception markedly different they are measuring the same phenomenon (Brown et al., 2012).

Advantages

Originally developed by Colarusso and Hammill in 1972, the MVPT battery has undergone numerous revisions and refinement, thus the present scale has a large amount of evidence in support of its use in clinical practice. The assessments can be purchased from a number of therapy supply stores and when purchased includes detailed instructions for administration and scoring.

Disadvantages

The revised MVPT-4, which was published in 2015, has little direct research in support of its use outside of that done by its creators. Also, work by Brown and Elliott (2011) found that the MVPT-3 total scale was observed to exhibit multidimensionality with scale items loaded on 11 viable factors. In other words, rather than measuring a single construct (i.e., overall visual perceptual abilities), the MVPT-3 total scale actually appeared to measure 11 different constructs or dimensions, which accounted for 58.15% of the test's total variance.

Administration

During assessment the subject is shown a stimulus drawing where her or she must pick the most correct or matching drawing from four scoring choices. The manuals for both the MVPT-3 and MVPT-4 contain detailed instructions and norm tables to be used for converting raw scores to standard scores, percentile ranks, and age equivalents. For example, the MVPT-3 standard scores range from 55 to 145, with a distribution mean of 100 and a standard deviation of 15.

Permissions

The MVPT batteries can be purchased from Academic Therapy Publications, the copyright holder, at a cost of $160 for the complete MVPT-4 kit, $45 for the manual, $75 for only test plates, and $40 for record forms. Questions regarding the use of either test in research or publication should be directed toward the copyright holders or their creators at the information following. More information can be found in the following journal article:

Brown, T., & Elliott, S. (2011). Factor structure of the Motor-Free Visual Perception Test—3rd edition (MVPT-3). *Canadian Journal of Occupational Therapy, 78*(1), 26-36.

Summary

POPULATION	General; ages 4 to 80 years
TYPE OF MEASURE	Non-motor; multiple choice and matching
WHAT IT ASSESSES	Visual-perceptual abilities
TIME	< 30 minutes
COST	$160

Contact

Donald D. Hammill, PhD

Hammill Institute on Disabilities

Austin, Texas

Email: info@hammill-institute.org

Academic Therapy Publications

20 Leveroni Court

Novato, CA 94949-5746

Phone: (800) 422-7249

Email: customerservice@academictherapy.com

Web: www.academictherapy.com/

CHAPTER 100: NATIONAL EYE INSTITUTE 25-ITEM VISUAL FUNCTION QUESTIONNAIRE (VFQ-25)

Description

The 25-Item National Eye Institute Visual Functioning Questionnaire (VFQ-25) is designed to measure vision-related functioning and the influence of vision-related problems across a number of conditions associated with poor vision. Based on the original 51-item assessment, it can be administered in either interview or self-report format where its results can be used to identify problems with vision-related function, the influence of visual disability on emotional well-being and social functioning, and a person's ability to engage in activities of daily living (ADLs) (Mangione, 2000). The VFQ-25 represents 11 vision-related constructs and contains up to 39 items, plus an additional single-item general health rating question, which has been shown to be a robust predictor of future health and mortality in population-based studies (Mangione, 2000). An example question on the assessment is, "How much of the time do you worry about your eyesight?" which is then scored as either (1) none of the time, (2) a little of the time, (3) some of the time, (4) most of the time, or (5) all of the time. Scoring involves raw scores being converted to a 100-point scale with higher scores associated with worse performance. Subscale scores can also be generated. The assessment can be completed in less than 15 minutes.

TABLE 100-1
SUBSCALES OF THE 25-ITEM VISUAL FUNCTION QUESTIONNAIRE
• Global vision rating
• Difficulty with near vision activities
• Difficulty with distance vision activities
• Limitations in social functioning due to vision
• Role limitations due to vision
• Dependency on others due to vision
• Mental health symptoms due to vision
• Driving difficulties
• Limitations with peripheral vision
• Limitations with color vision
• Ocular pain

Adapted from Mangione, C. (2000). *The National Eye Institute 25-Item Visual Function Questionnaire (VFQ-25). NEI VFQ-25 Scoring Algorithm—Version 2000.* (p. 3). Bethesda, MD: The National Eye Institute.

Psychometrics

Mangione (2000) found that each VFQ-25 subscale was able to predict 92% of the variance in the corresponding 51-item original subscale score. Further research involving 246 subjects found that internal consistency estimates of the 11 constructs were between α=0.66 and 0.94 with lows for expectations at 0.66 and ocular pain at 0.73, and highs for near activities at 0.94 and distance activities at 0.92. Test-retest reliability of the subscales ranged from r=0.68 for ocular pain and expectations to r=0.91 for near activities and distance activities. The same study was able to identify 2623 problems with vision-related functioning. Those mentioned most frequently were reading problems, driving problems, problems with seeing clearly, and mental health complaints caused by vision (Mangione, Berry, et al., 1998). Furthermore, the mean number of problems/person ranged from 13.5 for those with diabetic retinopathy to 7.9 for persons with glaucoma, and the 3 most common descriptors associated with each problem were difficulty or ease of performance (13%), psychological distress associated with performance of the activity (11%), and complete inability to participate in a visual activity (11%) (Mangione, Berry, et al., 1998). A study by Klein, Moss, Klein, Gutierrez, and Mangione (2001) established the discriminant validity of the assessment by comparing individuals with 20/10 visual acuity who had a composite score of 96.1 with those with 20/800 vision who only scored 62.8. A similar study of participants diagnosed with low vision at tertiary public eye clinics found that subjects achieved overall scores ranging from 11.49 to 62.50 with a mean of 42.14, also suggesting good discriminant ability of the measure (Marella et al., 2010).

Advantages

The VFQ-25 is a relatively quick and easy to administer assessment, and there is a good amount of research in support of its use in clinical practice as well as in research. It has also shown to be relevant in a number of settings as well as across a number of conditions that effect the eye. One of its core constructs is the measurement of ADL ability, making it particularly useful for occupational therapy populations. The assessment is free to use in practice, research, or publication with prior consent. The National Eye Institute maintains a website devoted to the measure.

Disadvantages

Research by Marcella et al. (2010) found that the VFQ-25 had only satisfactory psychometric properties and, according to their Rasch analysis, the assessment could be improved be removing 3 items: general health, pain around the eyes, and driving, as they did not fit into the overall scale for most populations. In their study, the item of pain around the eyes displayed high skewedness and deviation from the expected model and more than 80% of the subjects did not drive, which resulted in high levels of missing data.

Administration

The VFQ-25 is delivered as a self-report or interview format with scoring being a process where original numeric values are re-coded following particular scoring rules creating an overall composite score from 0 to 100, which is the average of all subscale scores. Each item of the subscales can also be averaged to create a subscale score. The manual includes detailed instructions for administration and scoring as well as an appendix of additional items from the 51-item version that the clinician can use to expand the scale up to 39 items in order to gain further insight into client performance (Mangione, 2000). An example question on the VFQ-25 is, "How much pain or discomfort have you had in and around your eyes (for example, burning, itching, or aching)?" which is scored as either (0) none, (1) mild, (2) moderate, (3) severe, or (4) very severe.

Permissions

The VFQ-25 assessment was developed by the National Eye Institute and the Rand Corporation and is free to use in clinical practice, research, or publication if requested. It can also be downloaded from the National Eye Institute website where it and other useful material is available. More information can be found in the following publication:

Mangione, C. (2000). The National Eye Institute 25-Item Visual Function Questionnaire (VFQ-25). NEI VFQ-25 *Scoring Algorithm Version 2000*, 1-15.

Summary

POPULATION	General
TYPE OF MEASURE	Self-report or interview questionnaire
WHAT IT ASSESSES	Vision-related problems
TIME	< 15 minutes
COST	Free

Contact

National Eye Institute

Information Office

31 Center Drive MSC 2510

Bethesda, MD 20892-2510

Phone: (301) 496-5248

Email: 2020@nei.nih.gov

Web: https://catalog.nei.nih.gov/p-300-visual-
function-questionnaire-25.aspx

CHAPTER 101: OCCUPATIONAL THERAPY ADULT PERCEPTUAL SCREENING TEST (OT-APST)

Description

The Occupational Therapy Adult Perceptual Screening Test (OT-APST), developed by Cooke (1992) and further revised in 2001, was created to quantify visual perceptual acuity which is considered the dynamic process of receiving and perceiving the environment through the senses. The measure has proved to be valid in a number of patient populations because disorders of visual perception can occur as a result of acquired brain injury, stroke, or disease often resulting in difficulties organizing, processing, and interpreting information perceived and acting appropriately on that information (Cooke, McKenna, & Fleming, 2005). The OT-APST is an amalgamation of several previously published tests in an inclusive battery format that measures functional skill level in areas commonly impacted by visual perceptual impairment and has 25 items across 7 domains. An example item of the assessment is *shape constancy*, where the subject must identify 4 common shapes in a mixed array of 10 shapes of varying sizes, positioned at differing angles (Cooke, McKenna, & Flemming, 2005). The design of the OT-APST requires test completion using only simple cueing and all of the test items are administered and scored according to standardized format. Achieving a score inside of normal limits is considered to be within two standard deviations of the norm, thus the OT-APST is not intended to gauge the upper limits of functioning (Cooke, McKenna, & Flemming, 2005). The OT-APST can be completed in less than 30 minutes, where only the subtest scores are used to interpret results. However, the authors suggest that the battery be completed in its entirety to maintain a reliable and valid interpretation of its results (Cooke, McKenna, & Flemming, 2005).

TABLE 101-1	
DOMAINS OF THE OCCUPATIONAL THERAPY ADULT PERCEPTUAL SCREENING TEST	
DOMAIN	**DESCRIPTION**
Agnosia	Inability to recognize and classify objects shapes, people, words, and colors
Visuospatial relations	Ability to relate oneself to the position, direction, or movement of objects, or direction of points in space, including unilateral neglect
Body schema	Body awareness
Visuoconstructional skills	Ability to organize a number of parts into a whole, including two three-dimensional building and assembly tasks
Apraxia	Inability to perform learned and skilled purposeful movements in the absence of loss of motor power, sensation, coordination, or language comprehension problems
Acalculia	Difficulty calculating arithmetic problems as a result of confusion in understanding the relative position of numbers and the meaning of mathematical symbols
Functional skills	Reading, writing, ability to complete simple mathematical calculations, tell the time, and use a stapler

Adapted from Cooke, D., McKenna, K., & Fleming, J. (2005). Development of a standardized occupational therapy screening tool for visual perception in adults. *Scandinavian Journal of Occupational Therapy, 12,* 66.

Psychometrics

Inter-rater reliability established in a study of 15 subjects following stroke found that singular results for each of the 25 items ranged from r=0.66 to 1.0, while intra-rater reliabilities for the same 25 items were r=0.64 to 1.0 (Cooke, McKenna, Flemming, & Darnell, 2005). The same study found test-retest reliabilities to have a range of r=0.76 to 0.95 (Cooke, McKenna, Flemming, & Darnell, 2005). A validity study post-stroke compared the OT-APST and the Loewenstein Occupational Therapy Cognitive Assessment (LOTCA) and its geriatric version (LOTCA-G) and found significant correlations between 5 of the related subscales for either the LOTCA at 0.36 to 0.70 or the LOTCA-G at 0.33 to 0.80 (Cooke, McKenna, Fleming, & Darnell, 2006). Furthermore, the study found that correlations between the Functional Independence Measure motor scores and cognitive scores and OT-APST scores ranged from 0.29 to 0.40 and 0.36 to 0.50, respectively (Cooke et al., 2006). A study involving 16 occupational therapy students, 15 practicing therapists, and 50 subjects post-cerebrovascular accident determined that results from the clock drawing activity on the OT-APST, which screens for unilateral neglect and impairments in constructional skills, demonstrated good reliability with intra-class correlation coefficients of r=0.83 and 0.84 between student and therapist interpretations as well as a kappa statistic of reliability at 0.58 and 0.59, suggesting that persons with minimal training can score the subtest and that it is a valid tool that may be used in place of other clock drawing assessments such as those found on the Mini Mental State Exam, The Montreal Cognitive Assessment, or the Mini Cog assessment (Eggins, Gustafsson, & Cooke, 2010)

Advantages

The OT-APST is an occupational therapy specific assessment that has a fair amount of research in support of its use in clinical practice. Delivered in a standardized format, it has normative scoring data and detailed instructions whose results can provide the clinician with a valid assessment of a person's perceptual impairment.

Disadvantages

An investigative study on the use of the OT-APST as a screening tool of visual perception among people with neurocognitive disorders (NCD) of the Alzheimer's and related types found that subjects performed significantly worse than the normative sample on all subscales and only recorded moderate correlations between performance and NCD severity suggesting that results should be interpreted cautiously in populations outside of validated populations such as stroke (Bialy, McKenna, & Cooke, 2007)

Administration

The test kit includes a manual, assessment book, reading card, assessment forms, stopwatch, blocks, stapler, puzzle pieces, detailed instructions, and score interpretations according to age-stratified normative data from 356 adults aged 16 to 97 years. A screening is completed prior to administration to determine if the further testing is warranted. A further example of the measure is a directions and position in space question that involves items being evaluated by requiring the person to move colored blocks to different positions in relation to each other, or to describe the color or point to the block that is furthest away from as well as nearest to or on the tabletop (Cooke, McKenna, Flemming, & Darnell, 2005). Scoring uses various numerical scales/descriptors for each task. For example, a drawing activity might be scored as (0) for gross distortion to (4) no distortion with no elements missing.

Permissions

The OT-APST is a testing battery that can be purchased for roughly $650. Inquiries to use in research or publication or feedback on the use of the OT-APST can be directed toward Deirdre Cooke at the information that follows. More information can be found in the following journal article:

Cooke, D., McKenna, K., & Fleming, J. (2005). Development of a standardized occupational therapy screening tool for visual perception in adults. *Scandinavian Journal of Occupational Therapy, 12*, 59-71.

Contact

Deirdre M. Cooke, PhD

Rehabilitation Coordinator

Occupational Therapist

Mater Private Hospital

Web: www.functionforlife.com.au

Summary

POPULATION	General; ages 16 to 97 years
TYPE OF MEASURE	Activity-based rating scale of performance
WHAT IT ASSESSES	Visual perception and praxis
TIME	<30 minutes
COST	$650

Chapter 102: Ontario Society of Occupational Therapists Perceptual Evaluation (OSOT)

Description

The Ontario Society of Occupational Therapists Perceptual Evaluation (OSOT) (1972) is a standardized assessment developed to test the perceptual capabilities of impaired individuals and its results can provide a measure of an individual's perceptual dysfunction in areas related to basic living skills, determine his or her degree of impairment, monitor change, and measure the effects of treatment and/or spontaneous recovery (Boys, Fisher, & Holzberg, 1991; Toglia & Kirk, 2000). The OSOT consists of 18 tasks organized into 6 functional areas that measure (1) scanning neglect, (2) apraxia, (3) body awareness, (4) visual agnosia, (5) spatial relations, (6) and stereognosis. Each subtest is in the form of behavioral performance tasks that test an individual's motor skills, eye-hand coordination, and visual recognition (Boys, Fisher, Holzberg, & Reid, 1988). The test involves several activities such as recognizing an object using only touch (stereognosis), scanning items for elimination (visual scanning), solving a puzzle of a human figure (body awareness), and stacking blocks (spatial relations). The assessment uses variable 5-point interval scoring systems (0 to 4) that are unique for each item. For example, the ability to manipulate wire grommet devices would be scored as (4) 30 seconds or less to complete 3 tasks, (3) 31 to 60 seconds, (2) 61 to 90 seconds, or (1) unable to complete in less than 91 seconds. The OSOT can be completed in less than 30 minutes with lower scores suggesting more severe impairment.

Psychometrics

When Desrosiers, Mercier, and Rochette (1999) translated the OSOT into French, using a sample of 32 subjects post-traumatic brain injury (TBI), they found overall test-retest reliability to be $r = 0.93$ and intra-rater reliability to be $r = 0.98$. A study of 76 subjects who were either residents of long-term care facilities or older adults living in the community referred to for occupational therapy assessment found inter-rater reliability to be $r = 0.84$ while perceptual status, as measured by the OSOT was highly correlated with the Physical Self-Maintenance Scale at 0.44, the Instrumental Activities of Daily Living (IADL) scale at 0.44, and the Mini-Mental Status Examination (MMSE) at 0.43 (Boyd & Dawson, 2000). Further results found that mean scores for the experimental group were 60.80 (range: 32 to 71) and for controls they were 69.37 (range: 101 to 112), suggesting an ability to detect impairment (Boyd & Dawson, 2000). Early research into the OSOT using a sample of 46 subjects determined inter-rater reliability to be $r = 0.93$ using 2 raters with item total correlations ranging from 0.63 to 0.85 with the exceptions of parts recognition at 0.23, ideomotor at 0.24, ideational apraxia at 0.29, right stereognosis at 0.33, and laterality at 0.46 (Boys et al., 1988). The same study found that mean total scores for the experimental group were 88.1 whereas control group scores were 108.38, also suggesting that the test is able to detect impairment. Additionally, at a score of 110 the sensitivity of the instrument was 100% and specificity was 40% (Boys et al., 1988). At a cutoff score of 100, the sensitivity was 63.7% and the specificity was 100% indicating that a score of 100 optimizes specificity, whereas 110 may optimize its sensitivity (Boys et al., 1988).

Advantages

The OSOT perceptual battery has been able to demonstrate high inter- and intra-rater reliabilities in light of the fact that there are 18 varying items. It has also shown to correlate well with other measures such as the IADL scale and the MMSE, which is the gold standard of cognitive testing. It is also an occupational therapy specific outcome measure.

Disadvantages

There is a limited amount of research in support of its use in clinical practice and that which is available is dated. Also, population studies have so far been limited to only TBI patients. The assessment can be time consuming requiring both an amount of time to set up and administer. Alas, it is costly at $\geq \$900$.

Administration

The OSOT is a standardized assessment that when purchased includes a detailed manual for its administration and scoring. The OSOT consists of 18 activities and uses several 5-point-interval scoring systems (0 to 4) unique for each item. A total score of 91 to 100 suggests mild impairment, 81 to 90 suggests moderate impairment, and a score of 80 or below indicates severe impairment.

Permissions

The OSOT Perceptual Evaluation Kit can be purchased from Nelson Education or other therapy equipment suppliers for $925. Permission to use in research and publication can be obtained by contacting the copyright holders of the measure or where purchased. More information can be found in the following journal article:

Boys, M., Fisher, P., Holzberg, C., & Reid, D. W. (1988). The OSOT Perceptual Evaluation: A research perspective. *American Journal of Occupational Therapy, 42*(2), 92-98.

Summary

POPULATION	Validated in TBI
TYPE OF MEASURE	Activity-based rating scale of performance
WHAT IT ASSESSES	Perceptual dysfunction in daily skills
TIME	< 30 minutes
COST	$925

Contact

Nelson Education

1120 Birchmount Road

Toronto, ON, Canada M1K 5G4

Phone: (800) 914-7776 ext. 2222

Email: Nelson.Clinical@nelson.com

Web: www.nelson.com/assessment/

The Ontario Society of Occupational Therapists

55 Eglinton Ave. E, Suite 210

Toronto, ON, Canada M4P 1G8

Phone: (877) 676-6768

Email: osot@osot.on.ca

Web: www.osot.on.ca/imis15/

Chapter 103: Rivermead Perceptual Assessment Battery (RPAB)

Description

The Rivermead Perceptual Assessment Battery (RPAB) by Whiting et al. (1985), was developed for use by occupational therapists to evaluate a person's ability to engage in visual perceptual tasks following a stroke or head injury (Donnelly, 2002). The RPAB can be used to establish an occupational profile or to measure treatment effect and is composed of 16 subtests across 8 domains, which include (1) form constancy, (2) object copying, (3) spatial awareness, (4) sequencing, (5) cube copying, (6) figure ground, (7) body image, and (8) inattention (Donnelly, 2002). Example test items range from simple color recognition to complex three-dimensional (3D) copying (Friedman & Leong, 1992). The RPAB has both standardized administration and scoring procedures as well as normative data available for adults aged 16 to 97 years. When administered, a failure on 3 or more subtests is suggestive of a visual perceptual deficit (Donnelly, 2002). The RPAB can be completed in less than 60 minutes.

TABLE 103-1
SUBTESTS OF THE RIVERMEAD PERCEPTUAL BATTERY

• Picture matching	• Missing article
• Right/left copying shapes	• Figure-ground discrimination
• Object matching	• Animal halves
• Cube copying	• Sequencing-pictures
• Size recognition	• Right/left copying words
• 3D copying	• Body-image self-identification
• Series	• Body image
• Cancellation	• Color matching

Adapted from Rivermead Perceptual Assessment Battery. (2015). GL Assessment. Retrieved from www.gl-assessment.co.uk/products/rivermead-perceptual-assessment-battery

Psychometrics

A study by Matthey, Donnelly, and Hextell (1993) discussing norms as outlined in the manual, found that although the inter-rater reliability of the 16 subtests was excellent at r = 0.93 with a range of 0.72 to 1.0, the sample used to derive that statistic was only 60 subjects. Similarly, test-retest reliability was moderate at r = 0.73 with a range of 0.27 to 0.83 and was based on a sample of 19 subjects. Early research involving 6 traumatic brain injury subjects and 3 occupational therapist raters found that item inter-rater reliability ranged from r = 0.46 to 1.0 with the lowest ratings for size recognition and animal halves (both at 0.46), self-identification/demonstration (0.56), series (0.57),and picture matching at (0.58) (Bhavnani, Cockburn, Whiting, & Lincoln, 1983). The correlation between 3 functional tasks (upper limb dressing, making a sandwich/packing a lunch box, and setting the table) and the number of subtests passed on the RPAB was calculated in a study of 35 subjects post-cerebrovascular accident where results demonstrated a considerable relationship between a person's performance on the RPAB and his or her performance on the 3 chosen functional tasks at 0.76 for upper limb dressing, 0.44 for making a sandwich/packing a lunch box, and 0.70 for setting the table, suggesting that the RPAB was able to identify the presence of a perceptual deficits during functional tasks (Donnelly, Hextell, & Matthey, 1998). Another study of 80 post-stroke subjects, involving 2 approaches to treatment, found that RPAB total scores were able to show improvement over time for both groups where the transfer of training group improved between initial and final assessments on all except 5 subtests (picture matching, series, animal halves, missing article, and 3D copying); whereas the functional group showed an improvement between initial and final assessments on all except 7 subtests (color matching, size recognition, animal halves, missing article, sequencing pictures, 3D copying, and self-identification) (Edmans & Webster, 2000). A study by Jesshope, Clark, and Smith (1991) compared RPAB scores and activity of daily living (ADL) performance using the Australian ADL Index upon admission to and discharge from rehabilitation and found that patients identified by the RPAB as having perceptual deficits performed more poorly at both admission and discharge than patients without deficits did. However, scores on individual RPAB categories and cognate ADLs were not consistently related, suggesting that there was some disagreement between RPAB scores and expert opinion.

Advantages

Several studies have noted that many of the 16 subtests have demonstrated excellent psychometric properties. The RPAB is also an assessment battery that is available for purchase from a number of therapy supply companies.

Disadvantages

There is a limited amount of current research in support of its use in clinical practice. Also, Friedman and Leong (1992) argued that although the RPAB is a sensitive instrument of perceptual impairment it has two disadvantages: (1) it is time-consuming, often requiring 60 minutes for elderly or stroke patients to complete and (2) the test can be tiring, thus the test cannot be completed within one session for many subjects. Lincoln and Edmans (1989) identified the same problems and found that the test often must be divided into two shorter periods to avoid the effects of fatigue and lack of concentration and arguably, in a busy clinical setting this may not be practical. Matthey et al. (1993) also noted that assessments need to have high stability over time if a clinician is going to be able to estimate the significance of change in score on retesting. Thus the moderate test-retest reliability coefficient of the RPAB (0.73) requires a greater change in score before a clinician can conclude that such change is due to a therapeutic interventions or rather the normal fluctuation inherent in the test. Early research by Lincoln and Clarke (1987) indicated that age and gender were significantly correlated with performance on two subtests: right/left copy and cube copying. Finally, developed in the United Kingdom, the battery is expensive at > $1500 dollars and can be difficult to find in the United States.

Administration

During assessment the subject is asked to perform several activities and is scored according to his or her ability to complete item tasks that are designed to determine the presence or absence of a perceptual deficit. A failure on 3 or more subtests is suggestive of a visual perceptual deficit, whereas a failure of 1 subtest is considered 2 standard deviations away from the mean for the subject's intelligence level (Matthey et al., 1993). The examiner's manual has clearly outlined instructions as well as scoring interpretations.

Permission

The RPAB is a standardized assessment that can be purchased from several therapy supply companies. The cost of the assessment can range from $1500 to $2000. Permission to use in research or publication can be obtained by contacting where purchased or its creators at the information that follows. More information can be found in the following journal articles:

Matthey, S., Donnelly, S. M., & Hextell, D. L. (1993). The clinical usefulness of the Rivermead Perceptual Assessment Battery: Statistical considerations. *British Journal of Occupational Therapy, 56*(10), 365-370.

Whiting, S., Lincoln, N. B. Bhavnani, G., & Cockburn, J. (1986). Rivermead Perceptual Assessment Battery. *Occupational Therapy in Health Care, 3*(3-4):209-10.

Summary

POPULATION	General; ages 16 to 97 years
TYPE OF MEASURE	Activity-based rating scale of performance
WHAT IT ASSESSES	Visual perceptual deficit
TIME	≥60 minutes
COST	$1500 to $2000

Contact

Nadina Lincoln, PhD

University of Nottingham

Nottingham, United Kingdom

Web: www.nottingham.ac.uk/medicine/people/nadina.lincoln

The GL Education Group

Freepost London 16517

Swindon, SN2 8BR

Email: info@gl-assessment.co.uk

Web: www.gl-assessment.co.uk/products/rivermead-perceptual-assessment-battery

REFERENCES

Beery, K. E., & Beery, N. A. (2010). *Administration, scoring, and teaching manual for the Beery-VMI* (6th ed.). San Antonio, TX: Pearson.

Beery, K., Buktenica, N., & Beery, N. (2015). *Beery-Buktenica Developmental Test of Visual-Motor Integration* (6th ed.). San Antonio, TX: Pearson Clinical. Retrieved from: www.pearson clinical.com

Bhavnani, G., Cockburn, J., Whiting, S., & Lincoln, N. (1983). The reliability of the Rivermead Perceptual Assessment and implications for some commonly used assessments of perception. *British Journal of Occupational Therapy, 46*(1), 17-19.

Bialy, A., McKenna, K., & Cooke, D. (2007). Performance of people with dementia on the Occupational Therapy Adult Perceptual Screening Test (OT-APST). *Physical and Occupational Therapy in Geriatrics, 26*(2), 1-21.

Bourne, R., Brown, T., Elliot, S., Glass, S., Lalor, A., Morgan, D.,... Wigg, S. (2012). The convergent validity of the Developmental Test of Visual Perception—Adolescent and Adult, Motor-Free Visual Perception Test—Third Edition and Test of Visual Perceptual Skills Non-Motor—Third Edition when used with adults. *British Journal of Occupational Therapy, 75*(3), 134-143.

Boyd, A., & Dawson, D. (2000). The relationship between perceptual impairment and self-care status in a sample of elderly persons. *Physical and Occupational Therapy in Geriatrics, 17*(4), 1-16.

Boys, M., Fisher, P. & Holzberg, C. (1991). *OSOT Perceptual Evaluation kit.* Toronto, Canada: Nelson A. Thomson Co.

Boys, M., Fisher, P., Holzberg, C., & Reid, D. (1988). The OSOT Perceptual Evaluation: A research perspective. *American Journal of Occupational Therapy, 42*(2), 92-98.

Brown, T. (2011). Construct validity of the three motor-reduced subscales of the Developmental Test of Visual Perception—Adolescent and Adult (DTVP-A): A Rasch analysis model evaluation. *British Journal of Occupational Therapy, 74*(2), 66-77.

Brown, T., Chinner, A., & Stagnitti, K. (2010). The reliability of two visual motor integration tests used with healthy adults. *Occupational Therapy in Health Care, 24*(4), 308-319.

Brown, T., Chinner, A., & Stagnitti, K. (2011). Convergent validity of two visual motor integration tests. *British Journal of Occupational Therapy, 74*(6), 295-303.

Brown, T., & Elliott, S. (2011). Factor structure of the Motor-Free Visual Perception Test—3rd edition (MVPT-3). *Canadian Journal of Occupational Therapy, 78*(1), 26-36.

Brown, T., Elliott, S., Bourne, R., Sutton, E., Wigg, S., Morgan, D.,...Lalor, A. (2011). The discriminative validity of three visual perception tests. *New Zealand Journal of Occupational Therapy, 58*(2), 14-22.

Brown, T., Elliot, S., Bourne, R., Sutton, E., Wigg, S., Morgan, D.,... Lalor, A. (2012). The convergent validity of the Developmental Test of Visual Perception—Adolescent and Adult, Motor-Free Visual Perception Test—Third Edition and Test of Visual Perceptual Skills (Non-Motor)—Third Edition when used with adults. *British Journal of Occupational Therapy, 75*(3), 134-143.

Brown, T., Mapleston, J., Nairn, A., & Molloy, A. (2013). Relationship of cognitive and perceptual abilities to functional independence in adults who have had a stroke. *Occupational Therapy International, 20*(1), 11-22.

Brown, T., Unsworth, C., & Lyons, C. (2009). An evaluation of the construct validity of the Developmental Test of Visual-Motor Integration using the Rasch measurement model. *Australian Occupational Therapy Journal, 56*(6), 393-402.

Canivez, G. L. (2005). Review of the Motor-Free Visual Perception Test–Third Edition. In R. A. Spies and B. S. Plake (Eds.). *The Sixteenth Mental Measurements Yearbook* (pp. 635-638). Lincoln, NE: Buros Institute of Mental Measurements

Colarusso, R., & Hammill, D. (2003). *Motor-Free Visual Perception Test—Third edition.* Novato, CA: Academic Therapy Publications

Colarusso, R., & Hammill, D (2013). *Motor-Free Visual Perception Test-4 (MVPT-4).* Novato, CA: Academic Therapy Publications. Retrieved from www.academictherapy.com/

Cooke, D., McKenna, K., & Fleming, J. (2005). Development of a standardized occupational therapy screening tool for visual perception in adults. *Scandinavian Journal of Occupational Therapy, 12,* 59-71.

Cooke, D., McKenna, K., Fleming, J., & Darnell, R. (2005). The reliability of the Occupational Therapy Adult Perceptual Screening Test (OT-APST). *British Journal of Occupational Therapy, 68*(11), 509-517.

Cooke, D., McKenna, K., Fleming, J., & Darnell, R. (2006). Criterion validity of the Occupational Therapy Adult Perceptual Screening Test (OT-APST). *Scandinavian Journal of Occupational Therapy. 13*(1), 38-48.

Desrosiers, J., Mercier, L., & Rochette, A. (1999). Test-retest and interrater reliability of the French version of the Ontario Society of Occupational Therapy (OSOT) Perceptual Evaluation. *Canadian Journal of Occupational Therapy, 66*(3), 134-39.

Donnelly, S. (2002). The Rivermead Perceptual Assessment Battery: Can it predict functional performance? *Australian Occupational Therapy Journal, 49*(2), 71-81

Donnelly, S. M., Hextell, D., & Matthey, S. (1998). The Rivermead Perceptual Assessment Battery: Its relationship to selected functional activities. *British Journal of Occupational Therapy, 61*(1), 27-32.

Edmans, J., & Webster, J. (2000). A comparison of two approaches in the treatment of perceptual problems after stroke. *Clinical Rehabilitation, 14,* 230-243.

Eggins, W., Gustafsson, L., & Cooke, D. (2010). Interrater reliability of the clock drawing task in the Occupational Therapy Adult Perceptual Screening Test. *British Journal of Occupational Therapy, 73*(2), 77-83.

Friedman, P., & Leong, L. (1992). The Rivermead Perceptual Assessment Battery in acute stroke. *British Journal of Occupational Therapy, 55*(6), 233-237.

Jesshope, H., Clark, S., & Smith, D. (1991). The Rivermead Perceptual Assessment Battery: Its application to stroke patients and relationship with function. *Clinical Rehabilitation, 5*(2), 115-122.

Klein, R., Moss, S., Klein, B., Gutierrez, P., & Mangione C. (2001). The NEI-VFQ-25 in people with long-term type 1 diabetes mellitus: The Wisconsin epidemiologic study of diabetic retinopathy. *Archives of Ophthalmology, 119*(5), 733-740.

Lincoln, N., & Clarke, D. (1987). The performance of normal elderly people on the Rivermead Perceptual Assessment Battery. *The British Journal of Occupational Therapy, 50*(5), 156-157.

Lincoln, N., & Edmans J. (1989). A shortened version of the Rivermead Perceptual Assessment Battery? *Clinical Rehabilitation, 3,* 199-204.

Mangione, C. (2000). The National Eye Institute 25-Item Visual Function Questionnaire (VFQ-25). *NEI VFQ-25 Scoring Algorithm—Version 2000,* 1-15.

Mangione, C., Berry, S., Spritzer, K., Janz. N., Klein, R., Owsley, C., & Lee, P. (1998). Identifying the content area for the 51-Item National Eye Institute Visual Function Questionnaire: Results from focus groups with visually impaired persons. *Archives of Ophthalmology, 116*(2), 227-233.

Mangione, C., Lee, P., Pitts, J., Gutierrez, P., Berry, S., & Hays, R. (1998). Psychometric properties of the National Eye Institute Visual Function Questionnaire. *Archives of Ophthalmology, 116,* 1496-1504.

Marella, M., Pesudovs, K., Keeffe, J., O'Connor, P., Rees, G., & Lamoureux, E. (2010). The psychometric validity of the NEI VFQ-25 for use in a low-vision population. *Clinical and Epidemiologic Research, 51*(6), 2878-2884.

Matthey, S., Donnelly, S., & Hextell, D. (1993). The clinical usefulness of the Rivermead Perceptual Assessment Battery: Statistical considerations. *British Journal of Occupational Therapy, 56*(10), 365-370.

McCrimmon, A., Altomare, A., Matchullis, R., & Jitlina, K. (2012). Test review. *Journal of Psychoeducational Assessment, 30*(6), 588–592.

Pro-ED Inc. (2012). *DTVP-A: Developmental Test of Visual Perception–Adolescent and adult.* Austin, TX. Retrieved from www.proedinc.com/customer/productView.aspx?ID=900

Reynolds, C., Pearson, N., & Voress, J. (2002). *Developmental Test of Visual Perception: Adolescent and adult.* Austin, TX: Pro-Ed. In T. Brown. (2011). Construct validity of the three motor-reduced subscales of the Developmental Test of Visual Perception—Adolescent and Adult (DTVP-A): A Rasch analysis model evaluation. *British Journal of Occupational Therapy, 74*(2), 66-77.

Rivermead Perceptual Assessment Battery (2015). GL Assessment. Retrieved from: www.gl-assessment.co.uk/products/rivermead-perceptual-assessment-battery

Toglia, J., & Kirk, U. (2000). Understanding awareness deficits following brain injury. *Neurorehabilitation, 15*(1), 57-70.

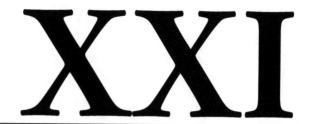

Work Rehabilitation

Bortnick, K.
*Occupational Therapy Assessments for Older Adults: 100 Instruments for
Measuring Occupational Performance* (pp. 305-312).
© 2017 Taylor & Francis Group.

Chapter 104: Work Ability Index (WAI)

Description

The Work Ability Index (WAI) is a self-administered questionnaire designed to quantify an individual's capacity for work, which is thought to occur as a result of the interaction of various determinants such as health, competence, and attitudes toward work, as well as the environment in which work takes place (Bethge, Radoschewski, & Gutenbrunner, 2012). Used as a predictive tool to identify workers at high risk for long-term sickness, absence, or disability as well as associated symptomology, the theoretical basis of the WAI is the stress/strain model, which emphasizes the important interplay of the individual and environmental factors on work ability (Bethge et al., 2012; Reeuwijk et al., 2015). The WAI has 10 items that comprise 7 dimensions and include such questions as, "Assuming that your work ability at its best has a value of 10 points how many points would you give your current work ability?" For each item a single score is obtained where the total score is a summation of all single item scores (range: 7 to 49), with higher scores indicating better work ability. Subject work ability can then be classified into 4 categories based on the total score as follows: poor (7 to 27 points), moderate (28 to 36 points), good (37 to 43 points), and excellent (44 to 49 points) (de Zwart, Frings-Dresen, & van Duivenbooden, 2002). The WAI can be completed in less than 10 minutes.

TABLE 104-1

ADAPTATION OF THE WORK ABILITY INDEX: FACTORS RELATED TO WORK SUCCESS

↑ Work ability
Work: Environment, demands, organization, leadership
Values: Attitudes and motivations
Competence: Knowledge and skills
Health: Functional capacities

Adapted from Finnish Institute of Occupational Health. (2014). Multidimensional work ability model. Retrieved from www.ttl.fi/en/health/wai/multidimensional_work_ability_model/pages/default.aspx

Psychometrics

A study of 97 construction industry workers (14% management and administrative) with a mean age of 51 years (range 40 to 60 years old) established reliability using test–retest data from a 4-week interval and found no significant differences in the mean WAI score at the group level between measurements (40.4 vs 39.9) (de Zwart et al., 2002). Exactly the same score on both measurements were reported by 25% of the subjects and 95% of the individual differences between measurements were found to be within < 7 points of each other (de Zwart et al., 2002). The study also found that the percentage of observed agreement for the classification of subjects into 1 of the 4 WAI categories on both measurements was 66% (de Zwart et al., 2002). Results also showed that a decrease in work ability was more common than an improvement (de Zwart et al., 2002). A study by da Silva Junior, Vasconcelos, Griep, and Rotenberg (2011) using results of 1436 nurse questionnaires found the Cronbach's alpha to be $\alpha = 0.80$, suggesting that all items correlated well, whereas a factorial analyses indicated a two-dimensional structure of perception of work ability/mental resources and diseases and health restrictions. A later study by Fassi et al. (2013) of 12,839 40- to 65-year-old subjects established that the convergent validity between WAI and the work ability score (the first item of the WAI) was statistically significant at $r = 0.63$. The study's multivariable analysis also found that jobs mostly characterized by physical activity increased the probability of reporting moderate or poor work ability while conversely, a work position characterized by the predominance of mental activity had a favorable impact on work ability. Finally, a study of 457 women and 579 men (mean age: 51 years) showed that poor and moderate baseline WAI scores were associated with lower health-related quality of life and more frequent use of primary health care 1 year later, and a WAI score of ≤ 37 was identified as the optimal cutoff to predict the need for rehabilitation (Bethge et al., 2012). Moreover, subjects with poor baseline work ability had 4.6 times higher odds of unemployment and 12.2 times higher odds of prolonged sick leave than the reference group with good or excellent baseline work ability (Bethge et al., 2012).

Advantages

The WAI is a fast and simple outcome measure to administer that has a significant amount of research in support of its use in clinical practice. Several studies involving large cohorts of subjects have also helped to establish norms for the WAI. For example, one study involved over > 12,000 subjects while several others involved more than > 1000. The WAI has also shown to have cross-cultural relevance evidenced by its numerous translations as well as an amount of international research studies pertaining to it.

Disadvantages

Work ability in general is a complex phenomenon and efforts to quantify it can be elusive. For example, a systematic review by van den Berg, Elders, de Zwart, and Burdorf (2009) determined that there were many important factors associated with a poor WAI score, which included lack of leisure time or vigorous physical activity, poor musculoskeletal capacity, older age, obesity, high mental work demands, lack of autonomy, a poor physical work environment, and high physical workloads. The authors went on to note that the impact of social and economic policies at the company and national level and their effect on WAI scores still remain largely unknown.

Administration

The WAI is a self-report measure where the subject is asked to consider a range of issues and their effect on work (10 questions). Scoring choices are composed of various numeric scales and are unique for each item. For example, dimension 2 contains 2 questions that are scored along a 5-point scale ranging from 1 (very poor) to 5 (very good) relative to subjective current work ability in relation to the physical and mental demands of work; dimension 4 uses a 6-point scale ranging from 1 (fully impaired) to 6 (no impairments), which is the subjective estimation of work impairment due to disease; and dimension 7 assesses a person's mental resources over a 3-month timeframe using 3 questions concerning enjoyment of regular daily activities, being active and alert, and feeling full of hope about the future and uses answering categories ranging from 0 (never) to 4 (always) (Reeuwijk et al., 2015).

TABLE 104-2
THE 7 DIMENSIONS OF THE WORK ABILITY INDEX MEASURE
1. Current work ability compared with lifetime best
2. Work ability in relation to the demands of the job
3. Number of current diseases diagnosed by a physician
4. Estimated work impairment due to diseases
5. Sick leave during the past 12 months
6. Personal prognosis of work ability 2 years from now
7. Mental resources

Adapted from de Zwart, B. C. H., Frings-Dresen, M. H. W., & van Duivenbooden, J. C. (2002). Test–retest reliability of the Work Ability Index questionnaire. *Occupational Medicine, 52*(4), 178.

Permissions

The WAI outcome measure can be obtained by contacting the Finnish Institute of Occupational Health at the information that follows for a cost of less than $15. Information regarding its use in research, publication, or other commercial purposes can also be obtained there. The instruction booklet contains information regarding background questions, the questionnaire itself, information on how to evaluate scores, suggested measures to be considered on the basis of the scores obtained as well as directions regarding data security questions that must be taken into consideration when using the questionnaire. More information can be found in the following journal article:

Bethge, M., Radoschewski, F. M., & Gutenbrunner, C. (2012). The Work Ability Index as a screening tool to identify the need for rehabilitation: longitudinal findings from the second German sociomedical panel of employees. *Journal of Rehabilitation and Medicine, 44,* 980–987.

Summary

POPULATION	General
TYPE OF MEASURE	Self-report questionnaire
WHAT IT ASSESSES	Capacity for work
TIME	< 10 minutes
COST	$15

Contact

Finnish Institute of Occupational Health

P.O. Box 40

FI-00251 Helsinki

Finland

Email: Jorma.Seitsamo@ttl.fi

Web: www.ttl.fi/en/health/wai/pages/default.aspx

CHAPTER 105: WORKER ROLE INTERVIEW 10.0 (WRI)

Description

The Worker Role Interview (WRI) by Velozo (1991) is a semi-structured interview rating scale that is designed to obtain data about a client's physical status, functional performance, and ability to return to work. It is loosely based on the Model of Human Occupation (MOHO), which conceptualizes work behavior as a function of volition that reflects the client's values, interests, and belief in his or her own work capacity and can help to identify motivational drivers and inhibitors to engage in work. Several concepts are central to the measure such as *habituation*, which explores a person's daily routines, work habits, and roles and their impact on work capacity; *performance capacity*, which is the understanding of the physical and mental basis of work ability; and lastly, the person's perception of the *physical and social environment*, which encompasses peers and family and includes the identification of physical barriers, social supports, and potential problem areas, such as social interactions with work colleagues (Forsyth et al., 2006; Lohss, Forsyth, & Kottorp, 2012). The WRI has 6 domains and comprises 17 items that assess such things as client abilities and limitations, client expectations of job success, taking responsibility, and values and commitment to work. During assessment information is gathered through a semi-structured interview where each item is then rated along a 4-point scale from (4) strongly supports to (1) strongly interferes with client returning, finding, or keeping work (Lohss et al., 2012). The assessment can be completed in less than 30 minutes with lower scores associated with poorer performance.

Psychometrics

Early research using 3 raters with 30 subjects receiving rehabilitation due to an upper extremity injury found that inter-rater reliability for the 6 domains ranged from $r = 0.46$ to 0.92 with a total value of $r = 0.81$, whereas test-retest reliability using 1 rater of 20 subjects showed intra-class correlation coefficients from $r = 0.86$ to 0.94 with a total value of $r = 0.95$ indicating high test-retest reliability (Biernacki, 1993). A subsequent study of 83 subjects found that test-retest reliability agreement varied from fair (items 5 and 12) to very good (item 7) with most showing good agreement (items 2, 4, 9, 13, and 14) or moderate agreement (items 1, 6, 8, 10, 11, and 15). No item showed poor agreement. The same study found internal consistency to be $\alpha = 0.65$ and 0.78, respectively (Ekbladh, Haglund, & Thorell, 2004). A later study by Ekbladh, Thorell, and Haglund (2010) found that at the 0- to 6-month interval 4 items showed statistically significant differences between working and non-working groups: expectations of job success, takes responsibility, adapts routine to minimize difficulties, and perception of family and peers, whereas a logistic regression analysis at 6-months found that expectations of job success together with daily routines could explain 56% of the variance of the outcome while at the 24-month interval expectations of job success and daily routines could explain 62% of the variance. In a study of 34 psychiatric patients Lohss et al. (2012) found that the distribution of scores along the 4-point rating scale had an orientation toward choice 3, supports (49%) with few observations for choice 1 strongly supports (7%), suggesting high ability level or lenient rater behavior of subjects. The same study found overall reliability to be $r = 0.83$ with an acceptable goodness of fit for most items with the exception of success in work suggesting that the WRI defines a single construct reasonably well.

Advantages

There is a significant amount of research in support of the WRI for use in clinical practice and no special training or permissions are needed. The structured interview and descriptors used in the rating scale can offer unique insights into the perceived strengths and weaknesses of the client. Finally, the MOHO Clearinghouse maintains a website devoted to the measure where supporting information can be found.

TABLE 105-1
SIX DOMAINS OF THE WORKER ROLE INTERVIEW
1. Personal causation
2. Values
3. Interests
4. Roles
5. Habits
6. Environment

Disadvantages

The WRI includes a non-standardized interview format and a standardized rating scale and because of the way information is gathered, issues with inter- and intra-rater reliability may arise, which can affect other statistical areas of the assessment as well. Also, Ekbladh et al. (2010), in their study, found a ceiling effect for the expectation of success in work question suggesting that clients might have unrealistic perceptions of their abilities and limitations.

Administration

The WRI has detailed instructions outlined in the examiner's manual, which includes three interview formats: one for workers with recent injuries or disabilities, one for clients with chronic disabilities, and a combined WRI and Occupational Circumstances Assessment Interview and Rating Scale. The guided interviews are designed to gather information as well as answer specific questions pertaining to work with the goal of developing an occupational profile of the client that can then be used to create treatment plans and interventions. The 17 items across 6 domains are then scored using the following rating scale:

TABLE 105-2

FOUR-POINT ORDINAL SCALE USED BY THE WORKER ROLE INTERVIEW

4 (SS)	Strongly supports the client returning to previous employment or finding and keeping work.
3 (S)	Supports the client returning to previous employment or finding and keeping work.
2 (I)	Interferes with a client returning to previous employment or finding and keeping work.
1 (SI)	Strongly interferes with a client returning to previous employment or finding and keeping work.
N/A	Not applicable; there is not enough information to rate the item or the item does not apply to the client's particular work situation

Adapted from Lohss, I., Forsyth, K., & Kottorp, A. (2012). Psychometric properties of the Worker Role Interview (version 10.0) in mental health. *British Journal of Occupational Therapy, 75*(4), 173.

Permissions

The WRI can be purchased from the MOHO Clearinghouse website for a price of $40. Permission to use the assessment in research or for commercial purposes can also be obtained from the MOHO Clearinghouse website. More information can be found in the following original journal article:

Velozo, C., Kielhofner, G., Gern, A., Lin, F-L., Azhar, G., & Fisher, G. (1999). Worker Role Interview: Validation of a psychosocial work-related measure. *Journal of Occupational Rehabilitation 9*, 153–168.

Summary

POPULATION	General
TYPE OF MEASURE	Semi-structured interview rating scale
WHAT IT ASSESSES	Supports and barriers to work
TIME	< 30 minutes
COST	$40

Contact

Model of Human Occupation Clearinghouse

Attn: MOHO Clearinghouse

Fax: (312) 413-0256

Web: www.cade.uic.edu/moho/productDetails.aspx?aid=11

REFERENCES

Bethge, M., Radoschewski, F. M., & Gutenbrunner, C. (2012). The Work Ability Index as a screening tool to identify the need for rehabilitation: longitudinal findings from the second German sociomedical panel of employees. *Journal of Rehabilitation and Medicine, 44,* 980–987.

Biernacki, S. D. (1993). Reliability of the worker role interview. *American Journal of Occupational Therapy, 47*(9), 797-803.

da Silva Junior, S. H. A., Vasconcelos, A. G. G., Griep, R. H., & Rotenberg, L. (2011). Validity and reliability of the Work Ability Index questionnaire in nurse's work. *Journal of Epidemiology & Community Health, 65*(Suppl 1), A457-A458.

de Zwart, B. C. H., Frings-Dresen, M. H. W., & van Duivenbooden, J. C. (2002). Test–retest reliability of the Work Ability Index questionnaire. *Occupational Medicine, 52*(4), 177–181.

Ekbladh, E., Haglund, L., & Thorell, L. (2004). The Worker Role Interview—Preliminary data on the predictive validity of return to work of clients after an insurance medicine investigation. *Journal of Occupational Rehabilitation, 14*(2), 131-141.

Ekbladh, E., Thorell, L., & Haglund, L. (2010). Return to work: The predictive value of the Worker Role Interview (WRI) over two years. *Work, 35*(2), 163-172.

Fassi, M. E., Bocquet, V., Majery, N., Lair, M. L. Couffignal, S., & Mairiaux, P. (2013). Work ability assessment in a worker population: comparison and determinants of Work Ability Index and Work Ability score. *BMC Public Health, 13*(305), 1-10.

Finnish Institute of Occupational Health. (2014). Multidimensional work ability model. Retrieved from www.ttl.fi/en/health/wai/multidimensional_work_ability_model/pages/default.aspx

Forsyth, K., Braveman, B., Kielhofner, G., Ekbladh, E., Haglund, L., Fenger, K., & Keller, J. (2006). Psychometric properties of the Worker Role Interview. *Work, 27*(3), 313-318.

Lohss, I., Forsyth, K., & Kottorp, A. (2012). Psychometric properties of the Worker Role Interview (version 10.0) in mental health. *British Journal of Occupational Therapy, 75*(4), 171-179.

Reeuwijk, K., Robroek, S., Niessen, M., Kraaijenhagen, R. A., Vergouwe, Y., & Burdorf, A. (2015). The prognostic value of the Work Ability Index for sickness absence among office workers. *PLoS ONE, 10*(5), e0126969.

van den Berg, T. I. J., Elders, L. A. M., de Zwart, B. C. H., & Burdorf, A. (2009). The effects of work-related and individual factors on the Work Ability Index: A systematic review. *Occupational and Environmental Medicine, 66,* 211–220.

Appendix: Applied Statistics

Analysis of covariance (ANCOVA): A way of statistically controlling the (linear) effects of variables one does not want to examine in a study by allowing for the removal of covariates from the list of possible explanations of variance in the dependent variable (Vogt, 2005).

Analysis of variance (ANOVA): A test of the statistical significance of the differences between the mean scores of two or more groups as they relate to one or more variables and is often used to assess the statistical significance of the relationship between independent and dependent variables (Vogt, 2005).

Baseline: The initial set of measurements with which future results are then compared.

Bias: Can be considered a lack of internal validity controls or incorrect assessment of the association between an exposure and an effect in the target population and can occur during all stages of design such as selection bias, information bias, confounding, erroneous calculation of data, or faulty analysis and interpretation of data (Delgado-Rodríguez & Llorca, 2004).

Case study: An in-depth research study of one case or a *one-patient report* discussing the patient's response to a given intervention.

Central tendency: A point in a distribution of scores that corresponds to a typical, representative, or middle score distribution such as the mode, mean, and median (Vogt, 2005).

Chi-squared test: A test applied to a two-dimensional contingency table in which one variable has two categories and the other has k ordered categories and is used to assess whether there is a difference in the trend of the proportions in the two groups (Everitt & Skrondal, 2010)

Class interval: A grouping of data on a continuous variable that makes it easier to analyze the interval between the boundaries (or limits) of the class, such as between the ages of 21 to 40 years old and 41 to 60 years old (Vogt, 2005).

Cluster sampling: A method of sampling in which the members of a population are arranged in groups. Clusters are then typically selected at random then subsampled and often consist of natural groupings, such as occupational therapy students (Everitt & Skrondal, 2010).

Coefficient of determination (R^2): A measure of the overall value of the predictor variable(s) in predicting the outcome variable in the linear regression setting. For example, an R^2 of 0.35 indicates that 35% of the variation in the outcome has been explained just by predicting the outcome using the covariates included in the model (Boslaugh, 2008).

Cohort study: A comparative study of individuals exposed to differing amounts of a suspected risk factor or intervention over a period of time.

Confidence interval (CI): A statistical method that is calculated from a given set of data that gives an estimated range of values to an unknown population parameter that is believed, with a particular probability, to contain the true parameter value (i.e., 95% CI) (Everitt & Skrondal, 2010).

Construct validity: A measure of how well an instrument measures the characteristics that in its design it has set out to do and is involved whenever a test is to be interpreted as a measure of some attribute or quality that is not operationally defined (Cronbach & Meehl, 1955).

Content validity: Degree to which the elements of an instrument are relevant to and representative of the targeted construct of what it was designed to measure where elements may be questions, response choices, or instructions (Haynes, Richard, & Kubany, 1995).

Control group: A group of subjects recruited into a study that receives no treatment, a treatment of known effect, or a placebo in order to provide a comparison for a group receiving an experimental treatment, such as a new drug (Boslaugh, 2008).

Convenience sample: A non-probability sample of subjects selected from a particular population chosen based on their accessibility to the researcher and often assembled out of expediency or when a strict probability sample cannot be constructed (Boslaugh, 2008).

Bortnick, K.
*Occupational Therapy Assessments for Older Adults: 100 Instruments for
Measuring Occupational Performance* (pp. 313-317).
© 2017 Taylor & Francis Group.

Convergent validity: Refers to the degree to which scores of one instrument correlate with score of other different instruments that are also designed to measure a similar construct.

Correlation: Considered the extent to which two or more things are related.

Correlation coefficient: Also known as *Pearson correlation coefficient.* Represents the degree of linear relationship between 2 variables being examined. It lies between –1 and +1 where –1 indicates a perfect linear negative relationship between 2 variables and +1 indicates perfect positive linear relationship. Zero (0) indicates a lack of any linear relationship.

Cronbach's alpha coefficient: Calculated as an average of all correlations among the different questions in the scale (Peacock & Peacock, 2011).

Cross-sectional study: The observation of a defined set of people at a single point in time or time period, such as a snapshot, which contrasts with a longitudinal study that follows a set of people over a period of time.

Dependent variable: Typically the variable of primary importance in an experiment because the major objective is to study the effects of treatment and/or other explanatory variables on this variable and to provide suitable models for the relationship between it and the explanatory variables (Everitt, 2006).

Discriminant validity: The numerical extent to which a test's measurements that are supposed to be unrelated are, in fact, unrelated.

Divergent validity: The extent to which a measure does not correlate strongly with another similar measure of a different construct (i.e., if it correlates too strongly than it is merely the other measure just packaged differently).

Double-blind study: Done to protect against bias, where researchers create an environment in which neither the subject nor the observer are aware of which treatment protocol is being received by the subject.

Effect size: Considered a measure of strength of a phenomenon and is the difference between the control group and experimental group mean of a response variable divided by the assumed common population standard deviation (Everitt & Skrondal, 2010).

External validity: The extent to which a study's results can be generalized to other settings and populations and is an important factor if results are to be achieved beyond merely the laboratory or population sample of the study.

Face validity: Implies an overall judgment of adequacy of a result without paying close attention to the component parts. In most studies it has a low ranking but may be important in some cases such as items intended to reflect observations and intuitions of clinical experience (de Vet, Terwee, & Bouter, 2003).

Factor analysis: A procedure that proposes that the correlations or covariance's between a set of observed variables, arise from the relationship of those variables and to a lesser extent a small number of underlying, unobservable, latent variables, usually known as common factors (Everitt & Skrondal, 2010).

Floor and ceiling effects: Represent a pooling of the lowest or highest possible scores on a test (i.e., if the construct design was too simple the representative sample will all score above the 90th percentile).

Gold standard: A method, procedure, or standardized measurement that is considered to be the best available due to the amount of evidence in support of its use.

Guttman scale: A scale based on a set of binary variables that measure a one-dimensional latent variable under the basic notion that k binary items are ordered such that a subject who answers yes to item j (< k) will probably answer yes to items j+1 (Everitt & Skrondal, 2010).

Independent variable: The variable which a researcher deliberately manipulates in an experiment in order to observe its relationship with some other quantity in the investigation.

Inter-rater reliability: The consistent measure of an instrument after several administrations by different individuals such that a highly reliable instrument should produce the same results regardless of who is administering the assessment where perfect agreement between administrations is 1.0, excellent reliability would be 0.90 or above, between 0.90 and 0.80 good, and between 0.80 and 0.70 typically considered acceptable.

Internal consistency: A measure of whether the varying items that make up the whole of a scale that proposes to measure the same general phenomenon in fact are and produce similar scores, such as questions on a questionnaire where each might address the same yet slightly different aspects of the underlying issue being measured.

Internal validity: Can be considered the extent of the accuracy of a study's results. When considered high, there is confidence to conclude that the observed change in the dependent variable was the product of the manipulation of the independent variable and not other confounding factors.

Intra-rater reliability: A measure of the consistency of an instrument after several administrations by the same individual. If the intra-rater reliability is high the instrument should produce the same results for that person upon repeated administrations, where 1.0 is perfect agreement.

Likert scale: A rating scale typically found in questionnaires in which a person is asked to use a numerical scale to judge the quality of the object being measured, such as 1 = never and 5 = always.

Mean: In a population or a sample the mean is the average of all values. It is also the measure of central tendency or location.

Median: In a population or sample the median is the value that has just as many values above it as below it.

Meta-analysis: A statistical technique where the findings of many independent studies are combined in order to present results that may be common to all.

Mode: In psychometrics mode is the value that occurs with the greatest frequency in a population or a sample.

Mokken scale: Considered a non-parametric probabilistic version of Guttman scaling and is used for the reduction of data to allow for the uni-dimensional measurement of latent variables through the analysis of pattern of responses or items that are designed to be indicators of a single latent variable (van Schuur, 2003).

Nominal scale: The placing of data into categories such as yes/no responses.

Normal distribution: Results that are typically dispersed along a classic bell-shaped curve with bilateral symmetry. Thus the mean and the median values are approximately equal and when divided into 4 equal parts the position of the cutoff values for each part is at 0.68 standard deviation above and below the mean. Also, one standard deviation on either side of the mean contains 68% of the values in the sample and the area of 1.96 standard deviations on either side of the mean contains 95% of the values (Kirch, 2008).

Ordinal scale: The sorting of data or a scoring system that uses a ranking system (i.e., first, second, third).

Outlier: An observation or result that is far away from the other results and is often termed as the number of standard deviations away from the mean score.

Psychometrics: An area of statistics concerned with the design, administration, and quantification (measurement) of psychological testing including the analysis of studies based on such measurements.

Randomized controlled trial (RCT): A comparative study in which participants are randomly allocated to intervention and control groups. Researchers then examine differences in outcomes between the groups.

Range: Can be considered the difference between the lowest and the highest numerical values of a variable or the maximum value subtracted from the minimum value. The term *range* is also used to describe the limits of the minimum and the maximum values (i.e., scores ranged from 0 to 100) (Peat, & Barton, 2005).

Receiver operating characteristics (ROC) curve: ROC curves usually plot specificity (x-axis) against sensitivity (y-axis). Using a horizontal line at 45° and a curve that joins points along the line if the diagnostic test performs well then the curve will be distinctly above the 45° line. If the curve rises steeply and is close to the y-axis and then flattens out, this is the best possible and a cutoff will give high sensitivity and specificity The area under the curve is sometimes used as a summary measure of how well a variable or set of variables predict a binary outcome (Peacock & Peacock, 2011).

Reliability: The extent to which an instrument is free of measurement error and has the ability produce consistent and reproducible results after many administrations.

Reproducibility: Comprised of two parts, reliability and agreement, where reliability represents the extent to which individuals can be clearly distinguished from each other in outcomes despite measurement errors, whereas agreement represents a lack of measurement error.

Responsiveness: An instrument's ability to detect change in the construct being measured (sensitivity).

Sensitivity: An index of performance of a diagnostic test calculated as the percentage of individuals with or without the disease (i.e., the probability of a negative test result given that the disease is absent) (Everitt, 2006).

Skewness: A measure of whether the distribution of a variable has a tail to the left- or right-hand side. Skewness values between –1 and +1 indicate slight skewness and values around –2 and +2 are a warning of a reasonable degree of skewness but possibly still acceptable. Values below –3 or above +3 indicate that there is significant skewness and that the data are not normally distributed (Peat & Barton, 2005)

Specificity: The ability of a clinical test or assessment to correctly identify subjects with or without the disease.

Standard deviation: A statistic that measures the dispersion or variation in a distribution, equal to the square root of the arithmetic mean and is a measure of spread such that it is expected that 95% of the measurements lie within 1.96 standard deviation (Peat & Barton, 2005).

Systematic review: A research document that collects and summarizes evidence according to a pre-defined protocol using systematic and explicit methods to identify, select, and appraise relevant studies.

Test-retest reliability: The consistent measure of an instrument over time. For example, taking into account confounding variables such as prior test knowledge testing at a 1-day interval should produce similar scores that significantly correlate

Type I error: Can be considered the statistically significant difference between two study groups, although the null hypothesis is still true, thus the null hypothesis is rejected in error (Peat & Barton, 2005).

Type II error: Occurs when the clinically important difference between two study groups does not reach statistical significance. Thus the null hypothesis is not rejected when it is false and often occur when the sample size is small (Peat & Barton, 2005).

Uni-dimensionality: The degree to which a test or study measures primarily a single construct considered to be the predominant factor common to all its components that may be considered along with lesser factors and subsets of components (Raykov & Pohl, 2013).

Validity: The extent to which an instrument actually measures what it is intended to measure.

Z-score: Represents the number of standard deviations the object being measured lies away from the population mean.

REFERENCES

Boslaugh, S. (Ed.). (2008). *Encyclopedia of epidemiology.* (Vols. 1-2). Thousand Oaks, CA: AGE Publications, Inc.

Cronbach, L. J., & Meehl, P. E. (1955). Construct validity in psychological tests. *Psychological Bulletin, 52,* 281-302.

Delgado-Rodríguez, M., & Llorca, J. (2004). Bias. *Journal of Epidemiology and Community Health, 58*(8), 635-641.

de Vet, H., Terwee, C., & Bouter, L. (2003). Current challenges in clinimetrics. *Journal of Clinical Epidemiology, 56,* 1137–1141.

Everitt, B. (2006). *The Cambridge dictionary of statistics.* Cambridge, United Kingdom: Cambridge University Press.

Everitt, B., & Skrondal, A. (2010). *The Cambridge dictionary of Statistics.* Cambridge, United Kingdom: Cambridge University Press.

Haynes, S. N., Richard, D., & Kubany, E. (1995). Content validity in psychological assessment: A functional approach to concepts and methods. *Psychological Assessment, 7*(3), 238-247.

Kirch, W. (2008). *Encyclopedia of Public health* (pp. 995-996). New York, New York: Springer.

Peacock, J., & Peacock, P. J. (2011). *Oxford handbook of medical statistics.* Oxford, United Kingdom: OUP Oxford.

Peat, J., & Barton, B. (2005). *Medical statistics: A guide to data analysis and critical appraisal.* Malden, MA: BMJ Books.

Raykov, T., & Pohl, S. (2013). Essential unidimensionality examination for multicomponent scales: An interrelationship decomposition approach. *Educational and Psychological Measurement, 73*(4), 581-600.

van Schuur, W. (2003). Mokken Scale analysis: Between the Guttman Scale and Parametric Item Response Theory. *Political Analysis, 11*(2), 139-163.

Vogt, W. P. (2005). *Dictionary of statistics and methodology: A nontechnical guide for the social sciences.* Thousand Oaks, CA: SAGE Publications, Inc.

Printed in the United States
by Baker & Taylor Publisher Services